T0202168

Mentalization-Based Treatment for Personality Disorders

A Practical Guide

Mentalization-Based Treatment for Personality Disorders
A Practical Guide

Anthony Bateman and Peter Fonagy

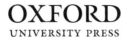

OXFORD
UNIVERSITY PRESS

OXFORD
UNIVERSITY PRESS

Great Clarendon Street, Oxford, OX2 6DP,
United Kingdom

Oxford University Press is a department of the University of Oxford.
It furthers the University's objective of excellence in research, scholarship,
and education by publishing worldwide. Oxford is a registered trade mark of
Oxford University Press in the UK and in certain other countries

Published in the United States of America by Oxford University Press
198 Madison Avenue, New York, NY 10016, United States of America

British Library Cataloguing in Publication Data
Data available

Library of Congress Control Number: 2015951912

ISBN 978-0-19-968037-5

Printed in Great Britain by
CPI Group (UK) Ltd, Croydon, CR0 4YY

Preface

The aim of our first "practical guide" to mentalization-based treatment (MBT) was to provide an understandable, accessible, and comprehensive account of MBT as used in daily clinical practice. We hoped that the book, in conjunction with only limited additional training, would make clinicians feel confident that what they were about to deliver in clinical practice was MBT, or at least resembled MBT. But over the past few years it has become apparent that we were not specific enough about some of the core components of the model, perhaps because we ourselves were unclear about some of the essential and less essential aspects of MBT; hence, the need for a completely new book. In addition, the theoretical underpinnings of MBT, the structure of treatment, and some of the interventions recommended to promote mentalizing needed clarifying. We hope that this new practical guide elucidates some of the more confusing aspects of MBT.

More importantly, there was an urgent need for a new practical guide because MBT has changed over the past decade; the model and its clinical application are continually being informed by new understanding generated from research. Indeed, MBT "looks" distinctly different now compared to a decade ago, and no doubt it will be different again in another decade. But we hope that the core components we describe here will remain as the foundation stones for further developments. In our attempt to summarize the model more accurately the book has become longer, but we hope this will not put off interested readers.

MBT has been more successful than we ever anticipated, perhaps more so than it deserves. It was initially developed for borderline personality disorder but is now used to treat patients with a range of disorders. We do not cover the adaptations for different disorders in this book, with one exception, MBT for antisocial personality disorder. This book contains an outline of the manual currently being used as the basis for a research trial of MBT for antisocial personality disorder. Other adaptations, for example, MBT for people with eating disorders, substance abuse, depression, and adolescents who self-harm, are outlined in an earlier publication (Bateman & Fonagy, 2012).

The popularity of MBT requires some explanation. First, clinicians easily understand the ideas underpinning the model and recognize that promoting mentalizing is something they are already doing in their clinical work. So it has given a clearer framework to their clinical interventions. Second, it has broad application, being rooted in developmental psychology and social cognition. Consequently, mentalizing interventions have become part of a wide range of treatments used across the lifespan, from mother–baby, to adolescence, to adulthood, through to old age. Third, MBT was developed as a psychological treatment to be delivered by skilled general mental health professionals, making it feasible for people without specialist therapeutic training to learn relatively easily. Fourth, MBT overlaps considerably with other treatments for personality disorder, and sits comfortably within the range of radical behavior therapists and psychoanalysts, all of whom have embraced it to a greater or lesser extent. Finally, MBT started out, and has continued, as a treatment that is firmly rooted in research. This has provided much-needed evidence for effectiveness, increased interest from researchers, and enabled interested practitioners to argue for its use in hard-pressed clinical services.

Introduction and summary of mentalization-based treatment

This next section of the preface introduces the reader to MBT. We recommend reading this before embarking on study of the subsequent chapters. The aim is to orient the reader to the overall treatment method and, we hope, to allow a more critical reading of the more detailed information in the chapters that follow.

MBT is a structured treatment. It has carefully managed trajectories in terms of both the time in treatment over 12–18 months, and within sessions. It is delivered in individual and group formats. The aim of treatment is to increase the resilience of individuals' mentalizing capacities.

Many techniques increase the mentalizing capacities of patients, and a wide range of psychotherapy processes facilitate mentalizing. Consequently, MBT overlaps with a number of "named" therapies, ranging from the manifestly cognitive therapies to explicitly psychoanalytic treatments. The key difference is the extent of the emphasis on mentalizing as the target of treatment.

The core of MBT is to rekindle mentalizing when it is lost, to maintain it when it is present, and to increase the resilience of the individual's capacity to keep it going when it would otherwise be lost. In the case of people with borderline personality disorder, the key area of vulnerability to losing mentalizing is the interpersonal domain, and so the clinician–patient relationship is a significant area of scrutiny.

In brief, at times the patient experiences strong affect while focusing on identified problems in individual or group sessions and his/her mentalizing appears to be limited or failing, and/or the patient's understanding of the way mental states link to behavior is inadequate. The clinician addresses this by a structured process (the sessional intervention trajectory) of (a) empathy and validation; (b) clarification, exploration, and, where necessary, challenge; and (c) following a structured process to gently expand mentalizing and encourage the patient to identify the mental states previously outside their awareness. The process is primarily in the here and now of the session but increasingly, as the patient's mentalizing improves, comes to concern core attachment relationships, including how they are activated with the clinician and key figures in the patient's life and how they influence mentalizing itself. Gradually, improvements in mentalizing serve to enable the patient to address their distorted representations of personal relationships.

First and foremost, MBT is collaborative. Nothing can occur without joint discussion, taking into account the mental experiences and ideas of both patient and clinician. The process of mentalizing necessitates an authentic desire to understand the mental processes of oneself and others. This applies as much to the clinician as to the patient. So the MBT clinician focuses on the patient's mind and attempts to understand his/her experience. Similarly, the patient is asked to do the same in relation to the clinician—for example, "Why does my clinician want me to focus on this at the moment?" may be paired with "Why does my patient *not* want to focus on this at the moment?" The therapeutic process has to become a shared endeavor. Initial goals on the road to improved mentalizing are jointly developed and focused on. The goals cannot solely be those of the patient, although his/her aims take priority unless they are antithetical to the whole process of treatment.

The assessment process and pathway to treatment prepare the patient for treatment itself. The assessment involves delineation of the patient's mentalizing vulnerabilities and a shared formulation, which includes specific detail of attachment patterns and areas of vulnerability to emotional dysregulation. This has to be understood by the patient and is for *both* patient and clinician. It is no good if it is understood only by the clinician, who may have considerable ability to make sense of the patient's problems; this would mean that the patient's nonmentalizing is being met with the clinician's mentalizing, which goes against a clear principle of MBT. Nonmentalizing in the patient cannot be met by mentalizing in the clinician; it can be met only by "switching on" mentalizing in the patient. The formulation is a work in progress and can be changed at any time. An MBT-Introductory group of 10–12 sessions assists in the development of the formulation. It covers all areas of mentalizing, attachment processes, personality disorder, emotion management, and treatment itself. This preparatory work means the patient knows what he/she is facing in trying to address his/her problems and is fully aware of the method and focus of treatment.

Following this preparatory work, the patient is offered individual and/or group MBT. Initially, this was organized around an 18-month program of weekly group and individual sessions. However, evidence that this is the optimal arrangement or the most appropriate length is not available. As a consequence, MBT is now offered for shorter lengths of time and also as individual therapy or group therapy alone. These are modifications to the research model that should be considered experimental.

At the outset of treatment, clear goals are established with the patient. The initial goal is engagement in and commitment to treatment, and this is accompanied by agreement to try to reduce harmful activities and self-destructive behavior and stabilize social circumstances where possible. Improvement of personal and social relationships, although a long-term aim, is detailed in the assessment formulation and worked on throughout treatment. In order to develop the formulation, the clinician identifies common relational fears, for example, abandonment, which stimulate the patient's attachment system and result in the use of maladaptive attachment strategies in interpersonal interactions. Identification and recognition of these strategies and patterns is done early in treatment so that they become the relational focus in treatment when appropriate. Both patient and clinician need to become sensitive to these attachment strategies when they become apparent in the treatment setting so that they can be scrutinized carefully. In short, the pattern of the patient's relationships informs an understanding of the relationship in treatment, and the relationship in treatment is used to re-appraise the relationships in life outside treatment. Finally, it is important that the patient and clinician consider establishing a goal of improving social function. This will include work, social activity, voluntary work, education, and other constructive life-affirming activity. This should be thought about at the beginning of treatment, not as an "add-on" toward the end of treatment.

Clinicians follow a number of principles when treating patients with MBT. Primarily, the clinician is alert to nonmentalizing not only in terms of the different nonmentalizing modes, namely *psychic equivalence, pretend mode,* and *teleological function,* but also in terms of the patient being fixed at one pole of any of the dimensions of mentalizing (the dimensions of mentalizing and nonmentalizing modes are discussed in Chapter 1). In general, mentalizing is optimal when the dimensions—for example, emotion and cognition, or representation of self and other—are in balance and nonmentalizing modes are inactive. The key for the clinician is to be constantly aware of imbalance and lack of flexibility in terms of the dimensions and if any dimension is operating in a nonmentalizing mode. Nonmentalizing in a dimension or mode is an indication that intervention is necessary. Second, the clinician monitors arousal levels carefully, ensuring that anxiety is neither too low nor too high, as both interfere with mentalizing. Third, the focus of a session is maintained through the clinician always noticing moments of mentalizing vulnerability, either in relation to events in the patient's life or in the session itself. Fourth, the clinician makes sure that his/her own mentalizing is maintained. It is not possible to deliver effective treatment if the clinician's mentalizing is compromised. So the MBT clinician always monitors his/her own capacities and may even have to say, for example, that his/her mind has become muddled and he/she cannot think. This type of self-disclosure of the mind state of the clinician should not be confused with sharing personal information. Sharing the effect that a patient's actions and state of mind has on the clinician is in the service of asking the patient to consider another mind as well as his/her own. In all relationships we have to be sensitive to others' states as well as our own. Without this, there can be no constructive dialogue and intimate understanding. So it is important that the effect the patient has on the clinician and what is in the clinician's mind is accessible to the patient. Finally, interventions are carefully matched to the mentalizing capacities of the patient. It is no good offering complex interventions that require considerable thought and appraisal to an individual functioning in psychic equivalence mode! This takes over their mentalizing, rather than facilitating it. As mentioned earlier, nonmentalizing in the patient cannot be met by mentalizing in the clinician, but only by reactivating mentalizing in the patient. The patient's mentalizing must be brought "on-line." This is done through a series of steps, which underpin the trajectory of every session.

The initial step in a session is listening to the patient's narrative. Sometimes, the clinician may start the narrative if there is an overriding reason to do so, for example, when the clinician is concerned about risk or the treatment breaking down, or the patient is in danger of impulsive acts, or the clinician experiences intolerable emotion, such as being frightened of the patient. Listening to the story the patient brings allows the clinician to begin working on empathic validation. Empathic validation requires the clinician to find something in the story that he/she can empathize with. This is not the same as behaving in a sympathetic manner or saying things that repeat the patient's story. Empathic validation seeks to engender in the patient a sense that the clinician has understood his/her internal state, that the clinician really "gets" the patient and the issue he/she is talking about. Often, the clinician seeks the patient's basic emotion, and it is this experience that is validated rather than subsequent social or secondary emotions. Validation is an affectively based intervention; the key component is contingency with the patient's internal emotional state. Non-contingent responsiveness on the part of the clinician at this point is likely to trigger nonmentalizing or generate avoidant attachment strategies in the patient. Once a contingent responsiveness has increased collaboration and even reduced arousal, maintaining emotions at a manageable level, the clinician can consider sensitive but non-contingent responses to try to stimulate mentalizing about the "story" the patient brings. Sessions are focused. They do not consist of free associative dialogue that seeks to illuminate unconscious process. The target area is working memory or pre-consciously held experience. It is expected that a focus for a given session will have been achieved after 10–15 minutes of the session, and this focus will then become the pivotal point around which the clinician and patient orient themselves, returning to it whenever nonmentalizing becomes to dominate the interaction.

The "story" the patient brings is then clarified. This is not clarification of events, which must also take place. It is assumed that the clinician will clarify the events and the facts as quickly as possible. For example, if the patient speaks about an act of self-harm or a suicide attempt, a drunken brawl or an emotional outburst, the clinician quickly clarifies when it occurred, who was there, what were the circumstances, and so on. This will indicate the level of risk and provide other important information. More than this, though, the MBT clinician wishes to surround the events with mentalizing. Clarification establishes the reflection the patient has on the events—what was their "pre-morbid" state of mind, what were their hopes, what was their experience when they were waiting for their boyfriend to return home, what thoughts intruded into their mind, what feelings did they identify, and can they reflect on it differently now? This process of clarification, in the service of mentalizing, links inextricably with affect identification and exploration.

Affects and interpersonal relationships reciprocally interact and are core to the personality problems characteristic of borderline personality disorder. Unmanageable emotions impinge on relationships, and relationships stimulate powerful feelings. Patients may not be able to identify their feelings accurately but experience them primarily as inchoate bodily experiences. Working with the patient to identify a range of feelings is part of the clarification and exploration component of MBT. Sometimes, emotions in specific contexts have to be normalized. Too often, patients feel that their experience is "wrong"; in effect, they invalidate their own internal perceptions and feel ashamed. It may be that their feeling is appropriate but excessive, or at other times inexplicably absent.

Clarification of current affect in the session is the next step if the patient and clinician retain capacity to mentalize around the focus. This is more than asking the patient how he/she feels at the moment, although this may be an initial component. It is identification of *current* affect *related to the session* rather than a current affect related to the *focus*. So, for example, a patient may feel sad in the session that her boyfriend was less committed to their relationship the night before and that this led her to become angry with him. This is identification of affect in relation to the focus. But, at the same time, she may have a sense of something untoward happening as she talks about it in the session, perhaps concerned that the clinician will judge her or see her as being the person at fault in the situation she describes. This is the identification of affect currently being shared between the patient and clinician in the session. This is named the *affect focus* of the session. It is an interpersonal component of affect. Commonly, this is implicit. In MBT, the clinician tries to make the implicit process more explicit; this rebalances the implicit–explicit dimension of mentalizing. All too often, relationships become stuck in the implicit pole. People reach an impasse and do not talk about something even though it influences their interactions beneath the surface. It is the task of the MBT clinician to bring important components of the interaction to the surface. For example, a patient may not feel like talking about something. As the interaction progresses, it is apparent that the clinician thinks that the patient needs to talk about the subject, but as the clinician asks questions to get the patient to expand on the subject, the patient retreats. Very soon, a reciprocal interaction is set up, characterized affectively by both patient and clinician becoming a little frustrated—but the gentle probes of the clinician and subtle retreats of the patient camouflage this. Making the affects of both patient and clinician explicit in relation to this interactional process is the affect focus. So the clinician might say, "I see that we have set up an interaction in which I keep pushing you to talk and you keep pushing me away or running off. Hazarding a guess, are you a bit frustrated that I won't leave it alone? From my part I realize that I too am a bit frustrated. I can see that we have not really agreed it is an area that we need to talk about. What do you think?"

The affect focus, that is, the identification of the interpersonal interaction in the session and the associated affect, if accurate, heightens the focus on the clinician–patient interaction in the moment of the session. Inevitably, this often indicates that a patient's attachment strategies and relational patterns, or possibly those of the clinician, are being activated. So it allows a move toward *mentalizing the relationship*. The groundwork for mentalizing the relationship will have been done through the use of *transference tracers* over time. Transference tracers are straightforward links between patterns of relationships over time, or bridging statements that establish similarities between the patient's attitudes and behaviors toward people in his/her life and the way he/she relates to the clinician—"Understandably you feel distrustful of others, and so why would you trust me? It would be a bit odd if you did." Transference tracers are not necessarily followed up with detailed exploration but are more conversational pointers to the links. The focus of the session is not disrupted by their use. In contrast, when mentalizing the relationship, the very focus is on developing an alternative perspective on an important aspect of the patient–clinician relationship. Has it arisen because of the patient's sensitivity to particular interactions?

Does it indicate an area of vulnerability for the patient in relationships which undermines his/her self-esteem and ability to enjoy relationships?

Mentalizing the relationship in a session is the training ground for managing difficult feelings in interpersonal situations in daily life through maintaining mentalizing while within an emotional interaction. We identify a number of steps for the clinician to consider. First, the clinician has to empathically validate the patient's perception of him. If the patient says that she experiences the clinician in a particular way, then the clinician needs to find part of that experience that he can validate. He actively avoids invalidating the patient's experience. Second, he needs to work out his contribution to the patient's experience of him. He does this explicitly by thinking aloud about it and asking the patient to explain how she has come to that conclusion. This questioning must be authentic and genuinely curious, and must not come from a perspective that implies that the patient's experience is distorted or inaccurate. Such an invalidating attitude will lead to disaster because invalidation, a non-contingent response, leads to excessive arousal and a consequent reduction in mentalizing. Mentalizing the relationship can meaningfully take place only in the context of mentalizing. Once the clinician has accepted his role in the relational process, the next step of more detailed exploration can occur. Here the aim is to generate a more complex understanding of the relationship, to see it from a different angle, and to see what its relevance is for the patient's life. It is not to engender insight in the sense of understanding the operation of the past in the present.

Mentalizing the *counter-relationship*, or the feeling in the clinician, is the counterweight to mentalizing the relationship. The feelings and mind state of the clinician are given considerable weight in MBT—not as representing the patient's projected feeling, but as a meaningful aspect of an interactive relationship, to be used to demonstrate how minds affect minds. This interaction becomes the subject of concern and scrutiny. For example, if the clinician is frightened of his patient with antisocial personality disorder, this is not taken, from a clinical intervention standpoint, as arising from the patient, but as an important feeling of the clinician that interferes with treatment and which may be important in the way the patient develops his relationships. The clinician finds a way of expressing his experience to the patient that makes it palatable and recognizable as something worth exploring. We recommend that this is done through a number of steps. First, the clinician works out exactly what his feeling is and what it relates to in the patient–clinician interaction. Second, he considers the patient's likely response to his explicit statement of his current state, and states this before he talks about his current feeling. Third, in the dialogue, he identifies the experience as his own, marks it, and finally he monitors the patient's reaction to his statement.

It is possible that what I am going to say may make you feel I am telling you off or being critical but I assure you that is not the case [anticipating the response of the patient].

The problem is that when you sit forward like that, stabbing the air with your finger, and raise your voice, I start to feel anxious and under threat [identifying the behavioral evidence and focus of external mentalizing, presenting his own affect and the effect it has on him].

I realize that this may be me [marking the feeling] but it makes it difficult for me to concentrate on what you are talking about [additional effect on him interfering with the relationship].

From here the patient's reaction can be taken into account and the session can continue. But if the threatening attitude and angry presentation is something that permeates all the patient's relationships, then further exploration is essential.

This concludes our brief summary of essential aspects of the basic treatment model. Adherence to the model is rated using the MBT adherence scale (Karterud et al., 2013). This scale may be used to focus discussion in clinical supervision. It is available on the Anna Freud Centre website at http://annafreud.org/training-research/mentalization-based-treatment-training/mbt-adherence-scale/.

Remember that the key is to develop a focused narrative infused with mentalizing process. Process refers simultaneously to the internal process in the patient's mind, to the interpersonal process between the minds of the patient and clinician, and to the internal process of the clinician's mind, as they relate to an agreed focus. Mentalizing with others is the basis of satisfactory social and personal relationships, which must surely be the goal of us all.

This summary would not have been possible without the work of many other people. We are grateful to all those clinicians and researchers around the world who have taken an interest in MBT and added to its evidence base. Without them, this new book would not have come about and MBT would not have traveled so far. It always seems invidious to mention individuals, and no doubt we may offend by missing out some people, so we must thank the whole teams who have made us think more, added to the clinical model, and enthusiastically questioned the whole endeavor. Groups in Australia, Denmark, the Netherlands, Norway, New Zealand, Sweden, the United States, and the United Kingdom have all been influential. But in particular, we thank Sigmund Karterud and the team at the clinic for personality psychiatry in Oslo for their research and work on adherence and mentalizing and groups; Finn Skårderud, Bente Sommerfeldt, and Paul Robinson for their work in eating disorders; Dawn Bales and her colleagues in the Netherlands for their assiduous adherence to the model and their informative research and training programs delivered from MBT Netherlands; John Gunderson, Lois Choi-Kain, and Brandon Unruh at

McLean Hospital in Boston, United States, for their integrative approach to MBT and for developing a successful MBT clinic and training program; Robin Kissell and her team for trying to bring MBT to the west coast of the United States, and Jon Allen, John Oldham, Efrain Bleiberg, and Carla Sharp for making a home for MBT at the Menninger Clinic in Texas, United States; Robert Green, Dave Carlyle, and Robin Farmar for their research on MBT in general mental health services and enthusiasm for developing the model in New Zealand; Linda Mayes, Arietta Slade, Norka Malberg, and Nancy Suchman at Yale University, United States, for their work on MBT and parenting; Morten Kjølbye, Henning Jordet, Sebastien Simonsen, and Erik Simonsen in Denmark, for their research and clinical developments; and Michael Daubney, Lynn Priddis, Clara Bookless, and Margie Stuchbery in Australia for their adaptations and clinical wisdom. There are many others too numerous to name, but thank you. Last but not least, we should thank our colleagues in London, United Kingdom, who have worked with us over the past decade to develop MBT as both a theory and a practice: Liz Allison, Eia Asen, Dickon Bevington, Martin Debbané, Pasco Fearon, Peter Fuggle, George Gergely, Alessandra Lemma, Patrick Luyten, Nick Midgley, Trudie Rossouw, and Mary Target.

Finally, whenever you think that this book "reads" well, it is a result of the assiduous work of Chloe Campbell and Clare Farrar, both of whom spent considerable time trying to make sense of our work, insisting we eliminated inconsistency and frank errors, and clarifying our many confusing statements. Any parts that do not read well are those paragraphs that we slipped past them. We also thank our publishers, who waited patiently for the final manuscript.

Above all, we want to thank the patients and their families, who have taught us all we know about these cruel conditions.

Anthony Bateman
Peter Fonagy
London, United Kingdom
December 2015

References

Bateman, A. W., & Fonagy, P. (Eds.). (2012). *Handbook of mentalizing in mental health practice*. Washington, DC: American Psychiatric Publishing.

Karterud, S., Pedersen, G., Engen, M., Johansen, M. S., Johansson, P. N., Schluter, C., ... Bateman, A. W. (2013). The MBT Adherence and Competence Scale (MBT-ACS): Development, structure and reliability. *Psychotherapy Research, 23*, 705–717.

Contents

Part 1

The mentalizing framework

Chapter 1

What is mentalizing?

Introduction

Mentalization-based treatment (MBT) was originally developed in the 1990s and initially used to treat patients with borderline personality disorder (BPD) in a partial (day) hospital setting. More recently, MBT has grown into a more comprehensive approach to the understanding and treatment of personality disorders in a range of clinical contexts, including antisocial personality disorder (ASPD), the mentalization-based treatment of which we are including in this new edition.

The mentalizing approach has changed—and, we hope, progressed considerably—over the past several years. Recent advances have in particular been influenced by new findings in developmental psychology, psychopathology, and the neurosciences, and of course the lessons we have learned from our own clinical experiences in the practice and training of MBT.

In this chapter, we will explain the concept of mentalizing and describe the theory of mentalizing in its up-to-date and clinically relevant form. We will show how these developments in thinking on mentalizing have influenced both our understanding and clinical practice in relation to BPD and ASPD.

Mentalizing is the ability to understand actions by both other people and oneself in terms of thoughts, feelings, wishes, and desires; it is a very human capability that underpins everyday interactions (see Box 1.1). Without mentalizing there can be no robust sense of self, no constructive social interaction, no mutuality in relationships, and no sense of personal security (Fonagy, Gergely, Jurist, & Target, 2002). Mentalizing is a fundamental psychological process that has a role to play in all major mental disorders. Indeed, mentalizing techniques are now being used for the treatment of post-traumatic stress disorder (PTSD), drug addiction, eating disorders, personality disorder in adolescents, particularly those who self-harm, and in work with families in crisis (much of this work is summarized in Bateman & Fonagy, 2012).

Mentalizing involves an awareness of mental states in oneself or in other people, particularly when it comes to explaining behavior. It is beyond question that mental states influence behavior. Beliefs, wishes, feelings, and thoughts, whether within or outside our awareness, always influence what we do. Mentalizing involves a whole spectrum of capacities: critically, this includes the ability

---

Box 1.1 What is mentalizing?

- ◆ Mentalizing is *perceiving and interpreting behavior as explained by intentional mental states* (e.g., a belief: *He believes that . . .*)
- ◆ Requires a careful analysis of:
  - • Circumstances of actions
  - • Prior patterns of behavior
  - • The experiences the individual has been exposed to
- ◆ Demands complex cognitive processes, but is mostly preconscious
- ◆ Is an imaginative mental activity and is based on assumptions that mental states influence human behavior.

---

to see one's *own* behavior as coherently organized by mental states, and to differentiate oneself psychologically from others. These capacities often tend to be conspicuously absent in individuals with a personality disorder, particularly at moments of interpersonal stress.

Mentalizing is a uniquely human capacity—it can be seen as what defines humanity and separates us from other higher-order primates. However, this capacity is not an entirely stable, consistent, or one-dimensional thing (see Box 1.2). We are not all able to mentalize to the same extent; many of us have strengths or weaknesses in particular aspects of mentalizing, and most of us are more likely to struggle to mentalize in moments of stress or anxiety. All of us have experienced mentalizing lapses to a greater or lesser extent. Trying to understand other people's behavior in terms of mental states is almost always more difficult and more liable to go wrong than explanations based on the impact of the physical environment—that is, the visibly contingent world of cause and effect. We can all act according to mistaken beliefs about others' mental states in particular interpersonal situations, leading to everyday misunderstandings, difficulties, and social faux pas, or in situations of heightened threat of violence, leading to more tragic consequences.

Mentalizing is a mostly preconscious, imaginative mental activity: we have to imagine what other people might be thinking or feeling. The ways in which different people mentalize can vary enormously, because each person's history and ability to imagine may lead them to different conclusions about the mental states of others. Sometimes, we may also need to make an imaginative leap to understand our *own* experiences, particularly when we are dealing with emotionally charged issues or find ourselves being overwhelmed by our own irrational, nonconsciously

Box 1.2 Characteristics of mentalizing

- Central concept is that *internal states (emotions, thoughts, etc.) are opaque*. We make inferences about them.
- Inferences are prone to error and so mentalizing easily goes awry.
- Mental states (e.g., beliefs), unlike most aspects of the physical world, are relatively readily changeable—for example, changing one's belief in the light of new evidence.
- A focus on the products of mentalizing is more prone to error than focus on physical circumstances because it concerns only a representation of reality rather than reality itself.
- Overarching principle of mentalizing is to take an "inquisitive stance." This can be defined as *interpersonal behavior characterized by an expectation that one's mind may be influenced, surprised, changed, and enlightened by learning about another's mind*.

driven reactions to situations. In essence, mentalizing is *seeing ourselves from the outside and others from the inside*. It helps us to understand misunderstandings by recapturing the mind states that led to misapprehensions. From a clinical perspective, at its core is "mind-centeredness"—a focus on acquiring a clear and coherent view of what our patient sees, having his/her mind in mind, being mind-minded, and being mindful of minds. Mentalizing is a key skill because our sense of personal continuity is dependent on envisioning the thoughts and feelings we had in the past and how these relate to our current experiences, and because how we envision ourselves in the future is rarely in terms of physical attributes (after middle age, certainly) but rather in terms of projecting ourselves as a thinking and feeling person. Mentalizing, the representation of our mental states, is the spine of our sense of self and identity (Fonagy & Target, 1997b). Seeing oneself and others as agentive and intentional beings driven by mental states that are meaningful and understandable creates the psychological coherence about self and others that is essential for navigating a complex social world.

Central ideas in the mentalizing approach to personality disorders

The mentalizing approach aims to provide a comprehensive account of the phenomenology and origins of BPD and APSD from a developmental perspective.

This fits with increasing interest, over recent years, in the emergence of BPD in childhood and adolescence, particularly as there is growing evidence to suggest that the disorder may have roots in genetic vulnerability and early development (Fonagy & Luyten, 2016).

A developmental and attachment-based approach

A developmental perspective is at the heart of the mentalizing approach to BPD and ASPD. The mentalizing model was first outlined in a large empirical study in which the security of infants' attachment to their parents proved to be strongly predicted not only by the parents' security of attachment during the pregnancy (Fonagy, Steele, & Steele, 1991) but even more by the parents' capacity to understand their childhood relationships with their *own* parents in terms of states of mind (Fonagy, Steele, Steele, Moran, & Higgitt, 1991).

This study paved the way for a systematic program of research demonstrating that the capacity to mentalize, which emerges in the context of early attachment relationships, may be a key determinant of self-organization and affect regulation. The concept of mentalizing is based around the idea that one's understanding of others depends on whether one's own mental states were adequately understood by caring, attentive, nonthreatening adults. We have particularly emphasized the central relevance of the "marked mirroring" of the child's emotional reactions by an adult with the capacity to represent the child's affect in a manner that conveys understanding at the same time as communicating a sense of coping with, rather than merely reflecting back, the child's affect (Fonagy et al., 2002; Gergely & Watson, 1996). Problems in affect regulation, attentional control, and self-control stemming from dysfunctional attachment relationships are thought to develop through a failure to acquire robust mentalizing skills. From this perspective, mental disorders in general can be seen as arising when the mind misinterprets its own experience of itself and of others, to the extent that a mental picture of others is inferred from one's experience of oneself (Bateman & Fonagy, 2010).

The capacity for automatic mentalizing seems to be an early emerging and possibly innate human characteristic, but the extent to which the potential for full mentalizing is achieved is unlikely to be genetically determined and appears to be highly responsive to environmental influences (Hughes et al., 2005). The development of mentalizing is thought to depend on the quality of the social learning environment, the child's family relationships, and, in particular, his/her early attachments, as these reflect the extent to which his/her subjective experiences were adequately mirrored by a caregiver. The attachment figure's ability to respond with contingent and marked affective displays of their own experience in response to the infant's subjective experience makes possible the child's development of coherent second-order representations of these subjective experiences. A child whose mother makes proportionally more age-appropriate references to desires and emotions than to thoughts and knowledge when the child is 5 months old will have better explicit mind-reading performance at 24 months. If, at 24 months, the mother then changes to make more references to thoughts and knowledge than to desires and emotions, the child will have better explicit mind-reading skills at 33 months (Taumoepeau & Ruffman, 2006, 2008). We suggest that these developmental differences are driven by the mother's awareness of the child's needs, and that this awareness in turn drives the child's acquisition of mentalizing.

Specifically, we believe that the quality of affect mirroring by attachment figures plays a major role in the early development of affect regulative processes and self-control (including attention mechanisms and effortful control) as well as the capacity for mentalizing. Later development follows the same pattern. More generally, parents, in the role of "expert mentalizers," have the task of communicating mental state concepts, and ways of representing these concepts, to their children. As the child acquires this competence and becomes an "expert mentalizer," the knowledge and skill of mentalizing is passed on to the next generation. Thus, we see mentalizing as a *transactional* and *intergenerational* social process (Fonagy & Target, 1997a): it develops in the context of interactions with others, and its quality in relation to understanding others is influenced by how well those around us mentalize us, as well as others around them. This experience of how other people mentalize is internalized, enhancing our own capacity for understanding ourselves and hence others and thus engaging better in interactive social processes; conversely, of course, early exposure to interactions characterized by poor mentalizing will lead the child to develop poor mentalizing too. Parents do not merely teach labels for mental states. The emotional and language environment they create conveys *concepts of mental state* (what does it mean to "think" something, how does it feel to "feel" something, what is the meaning of being "happy," how does a person behave when they are "doubtful?"). The parent, through their interactions with and in the presence of the child, generates a format with which mental state concepts can be represented. In effect, they pass on a set of processes that have evolved to represent mental states, (culturally) inherited primarily from their parents but also from others in their immediate social environment (O'Brien, Slaughter, & Peterson, 2011). We predict an association between the extent to which these mechanisms specialized for the representation of mental states are acquired and the quality of the relationship between members of the family (i.e., the individuals who undertake mental state-related discourse). The quality of adult–child relationships will influence the child's assumptions about the origin, location, and functioning of mental states. This in turn will lead individuals to attend to different aspects of observable behavior, and, in addition, different appraisals of mind states will lead to different patterns of observable behavior.

The multidimensional nature of mentalizing

Neuroscientists have identified four different components, or dimensions, to mentalizing (Lieberman, 2007), which are helpful to distinguish in clinical applications of the concept. These are:

1   Automatic versus controlled mentalizing

2   Mentalizing the self versus others

3   Mentalizing with regard to internal versus external features

4   Cognitive versus affective mentalizing.

To mentalize effectively requires the individual not only to be able to maintain a balance across these dimensions of social cognition but also to apply them appropriately according to context.

In an adult with personality disorder, imbalanced mentalizing on at least one of these four dimensions would be evident. From this perspective, different types of psychopathology can be distinguished on the basis of different combinations of impairments along the four dimensions (which we can refer to as different *mentalizing profiles*; see Figure 4.1 in Chapter 4 for an example of the mentalizing profile in BPD and ASPD).

Automatic versus controlled mentalizing

The most fundamental dimension to mentalizing is the spectrum between automatic (or implicit) and controlled (or explicit) mentalizing (see Box 1.3). *Controlled mentalizing* reflects a serial and relatively slow process, which is typically verbal and demands reflection, attention, awareness, intention, and effort. The opposite pole of this dimension, *automatic mentalizing*, involves much faster processing, tends to be reflexive, and requires little or no attention, awareness, intention, or effort.

In day-to-day life and ordinary social interaction, most of our mentalizing tends to be automatic because most straightforward exchanges do not require more attention. Particularly in a secure attachment environment, when things are running smoothly on an interpersonal level, more deliberate or controlled mentalizing is not called for; in fact, the use of such a mentalizing style might hinder such interactions, making them feel unduly weighty or uncomfortably overwrought (*hypermentalized*). Both common-sense experience and neuroscience tell us that we relax controlled mentalizing and are less watchful of social intentions in a secure attachment environment; a parent playing with

Box 1.3 The mentalizing dimensions: automatic versus controlled

- Automatic:
  - Rapid and reflexive process
  - Reduced reflective mentalizing, particularly in the context of attachment activation
  - Higher sensitivity to nonverbal cues inferring others' intentions
  - Day-to-day use
  - Associated with a secure attachment environment
- Controlled:
  - Serial and slow process
  - Verbal
  - Requires reflection, attention, and effort
  - Used when mentalizing errors and misunderstandings are apparent, interaction requires attention, if there is anxiety or uncertainty, in specific contexts.

their child or close old friends reminiscing will conduct their exchanges along automatic, intuitive processes. However, when necessary, someone with normative, strong mentalizing abilities will be able to switch to controlled mentalizing if the situation demands it. For example, when a child starts to cry during play, the parent will respond by enquiring about the child's change in affect, or the friend in conversation may detect a change in tone and mood in their friend, and wonder whether the conversation has stumbled upon a difficult memory or association. In other words, well-functioning mentalizing involves the ability to switch flexibly and responsively from automatic to controlled mentalizing.

Mentalizing difficulties arise when an individual relies exclusively on automatic assumptions about the mental states of the self or others, which tend to be oversimplistic, or when the situation makes it difficult for the individual to appropriately apply their automatic assumptions. In fact, it could be that any psychological intervention in essence involves challenging such automatic, distorted assumptions, and requires that the patient makes these assumptions conscious and attempts to reflect upon these assumptions in partnership with the clinician. In other words, any effective treatment is, at that level, about getting the patient to mentalize (we will discuss this point further, in the later section, "Reconceptualization of treatment").

Most experts agree that two systems for mentalizing arise from different neurocognitive mechanisms, both specialized for thinking about mental state interpretation (Apperly, 2011). The automatic system develops early and tracks mental states in a fast and efficient way, while the explicit system develops later, operates more slowly, and makes heavier demands on executive functions (working memory and inhibitory control). Explicit mentalizing allows us to explain and predict behavior, and has a role in social regulation (McGeer, 2007). However, it is the balance of automatic and controlled mentalizing that is critical. Explicit reflection cannot feel real unless it is contextualized by an intuitive awareness of the mental states being reflected on.

Stress and arousal, especially in an attachment context, bring automatic mentalizing to the fore and inhibit the neural systems that are associated with controlled mentalizing (Nolte et al., 2013). This has important implications for clinical work: any intervention that calls for reflection, by asking for clarification or elaboration on a thought, is by its very nature asking the patient to engage in controlled mentalizing. Many patients may perform relatively well (in terms of mentalizing) under low-stress conditions. But under higher levels of stress, when automatic mentalizing naturally kicks in, the patient may find it much more difficult to activate the processes that underpin controlled mentalizing, and so will find it harder to understand and reflect on what might be happening.

Self versus others

This mentalizing dimension involves the capacity to mentalize one's own state—the *self* (including one's own physical experiences)—or the state of *others* (see Box 1.4). The two are closely connected, and an imbalance signals vulnerability in mentalizing both others and/or the self. Individuals with mentalizing difficulties are likely to preferentially focus on one end of the spectrum, although they may be impaired at both.

It is a central tenet of our attachment-based approach that a sense of self and the capacity to mentalize both develop in the context of attachment relationships. The child observes, mirrors, and then internalizes his/her attachment figures' ability to represent and reflect mental states. Hence, the self and others—and the capacity to reflect on the self and others—are inevitably closely intertwined. In line with these assumptions, neuroimaging studies suggest that the capacity to mentalize about others is closely related to the ability to reflect on oneself because the two capacities rely on common neural substrates (Lieberman, 2007). Therefore, it is not surprising that disorders that are characterized by severe impairments in feelings of self-identity—most notably, psychosis and BPD—are also characterized by severe deficits in the ability to reflect about others' mental states.

Box 1.4 The mentalizing dimensions: self versus other

- Other focus:
  - Greater susceptibility to emotional contagion
  - Associated with accuracy in reading the mind of others without any real understanding of own inner world
  - May lead to exploitation and misuse of other, or to being exploited
- Self focus:
  - Hypermentalizing of own state
  - Limited interest in or capacity to perceive others' states
  - May lead to self-aggrandizement.

However, this should not be taken to mean that an individual whose capacity to mentalize themselves is impaired will *always* show similar impairments in their ability to mentalize others. Some individuals may have fewer universal impairments in mentalizing in relation to the self and others, and have stronger skills at one end of this spectrum of mentalizing. For example, individuals with ASPD can often be surprisingly skilled in "reading the mind" of others, but typically lack any real understanding of their own inner world.

Still, following the neuroimaging literature, we can identify two distinct neural networks used in self-knowing and knowing others (Lieberman, 2007). The first of these is a *shared representation* system, in which empathic processing relies on shared representations of others' mental states. This represents a kind of "visceral recognition" that occurs while experiencing and observing others experiencing states of mind, which operates through a mirror-neuron motor-simulation mechanism (Lombardo et al., 2010). The second is the *mental state attribution* system, which relies more on symbolic and abstract processing (Ripoll, Snyder, Steele, & Siever, 2013). In line with our expectation of the way the dimensions of mentalizing function, these two systems may be mutually inhibitory (Brass, Ruby, & Spengler, 2009), in that the neural regions most often recruited in the inhibition of imitative behavior are those involved in explicit mental state attributions.

Internal versus external mentalizing

Mentalizing can involve making inferences on the basis of the *external* indicators of a person's mental states (e.g., facial expressions) or figuring out someone's *internal* experience from what we know about them and the situation they are in (see Box 1.5). This dimension does not just refer to a process of focusing on the externally visible manifestations versus the internal mental state of others, it also applies to the self—it includes thinking about oneself and one's own internal and external states. From the perspective of clinical assessment, the internal–external distinction is particularly significant in helping us to understand why some patients appear to be seriously impaired in their capacity to "read the mind" of others, yet they may be hypersensitive to facial expressions or bodily posture, giving the impression of being astute about others' states of mind. Someone who has poor access to and great uncertainty about their subjective experience may come to a conclusion about what they are feeling from observing their own behavior as well as the reactions of others: their legs feel restless, therefore they must be feeling anxious. The external focus can make a person extremely vulnerable to the observable behavior of others. The absence of confident knowledge about the internal creates a thirst for clues from others' reactions even when these are not directed at oneself. Seeing someone else anxiously fidget can stimulate an internal state of unease and worry to a greater extent than it might normally do if mentalizing was not imbalanced in favor of the external.

Mentalizing difficulties may become apparent only when the balance of internal and external cues used to establish the mental states of others is considered. For example, BPD patients often tend to hypermentalize emotions in others, including the clinician. This is because they pay more attention to external indicators of mental states and their initial ideas are left unchecked by controlled/reflective mentalizing (which might limit the possibilities for attributing

---

Box 1.5 The mentalizing dimensions: internal versus external

- ◆ Internal:
  - Ability to make mental state judgments on the basis of internal states
  - Applies to both self and other
  - Can be associated with hypermentalizing about possible motivations and mind states of others and self
- ◆ External:
  - Higher sensitivity to nonverbal communication
  - Tendency to make judgments on the basis of external features and perceptions
  - Can lead to rapid assumptions unless checked by internal scrutiny.

thoughts and feelings). For example, if the clinician leans back and opens his/her mouth even slightly, the patient may believe that this was a yawn indicating that the clinician is bored with them. Or if the clinician frowns, perhaps pensively, the patient may interpret this as looking angry or disgusted with them. There has been considerable research on BPD patients' hypersensitivity to facial cues; their performance in the "Reading the Mind in the Eyes" test can be better than normal, creating an impression in clinicians that their patients are better than average mind-readers (sometimes called the "borderline empathy paradox"; Dinsdale & Crespi, 2013). A focus on external features, in the absence of reflective mentalizing, makes an individual highly vulnerable in social contexts, as it generates the kind of interpersonal hypersensitivity well described by Gunderson and Lyons-Ruth (2008). In MBT, mentalizing interventions often need to start by examining the patient's interpretations of a person based on external cues and then go on to consider possible plausible scenarios about what their internal states of mind may be—encouraging the patient to take into account the subtleties and complexities of people's internal worlds.

Cognitive versus affective mentalizing

Intense emotion appears to be incompatible with serious reflection on mental states. This point hardly needs to be made, but, as with much that is obvious, neuroimaging studies have provided biological confirmation. For example, emotional activation has been shown to limit people's ability to "broaden and build" in the face of stress—that is, to open up their minds to new possibilities (broaden), and to build upon their personal resources that facilitate resilience and well-being. In a functional magnetic resonance imaging study of 30 healthy females, it was found that during a provocative confrontation, high emotional reactivity to threat suppressed recruitment of the mentalizing network (Beyer, Munte, Erdmann, & Kramer, 2014).

Cognitive mentalizing involves the ability to name, recognize, and reason about mental states (in both oneself or others), whereas *affective* mentalizing involves the ability to understand the *feeling* of such states (again, in both oneself or others), which is necessary for any genuine experience of empathy or sense of self (see Box 1.6). Some individuals give undue weight to either cognitive or affective mentalizing. Studies have suggested that BPD patients have a deficit of cognitive empathy (Harari, Shamay-Tsoory, Ravid, & Levkovitz, 2010; Ritter et al., 2011), which is coupled with heightened sensitivity toward any kind of emotional cue (Lynch et al., 2006). This suggests that these patients may have an emotional processing advantage, perhaps linked to a combination of amygdala overactivation and orbitofrontal cortex and prefrontal cortex regulatory deficits (Domes, Schulze, & Herpertz, 2009).

Box 1.6 The mentalizing dimensions: cognitive versus affective

- ◆ Cognitive focus:
  - Associated with less emotional empathy
  - "Mind reading" seen as an intellectual, rational game
  - Hypermentalizing tendency, devoid of an emotional core
  - Agent-attitude propositional understanding
- ◆ Affective focus:
  - Oversensitivity to emotional cues
  - Increased susceptibility to emotional contagion
  - Tendency to be overwhelmed by affect when thinking about states of mind
  - Self-affect propositional understanding.

Context/relationship-specific nature of mentalizing

Mentalizing, then, is made up of different dimensions. All of us are likely to be more or less skilled at some of these dimensions, but individuals with personality pathology tend to have pronounced impairments along some of the dimensions, resulting in an imbalance in mentalizing and occasionally outright mentalizing failures. In this section, we will discuss the situations that are more likely to trigger mentalizing failures or difficulties. As well as not being one single "thing," mentalizing changes over time, and particular situations and stimuli are more likely to lead to mentalizing difficulties. For instance, BPD patients may be able to perform mentalizing tasks relatively well in experimental settings, but when they become emotionally aroused (e.g., in a difficult interpersonal situation), they may show considerable confusion as they become dominated by automatic assumptions about other people's internal states and find it challenging to reflect on and moderate these assumptions. In other words, when in a state of emotional arousal, they typically lose the ability for controlled mentalizing and are likely to struggle to imagine a rational scenario that might explain the states of mind of others.

Heightened psychological arousal tends to cause the capacity for controlled mentalizing to become increasingly difficult to access, and automatic and non-reflective mentalizing starts to dominate. Up to a point this is a normal "fight or flight" response to stress, which has the advantage of allowing us to respond immediately to danger. However, in situations of social interpersonal stress, more complex, cognitive, and reflective functioning may be more helpful, and an inability to use these more controlled and conscious skills can lead to real difficulties in dealing with other people. We have all noticed that, given a certain amount of emotional arousal, it becomes hard to focus on someone else's point of view. When emotional, not only does it become much harder or even impossible to concern oneself with the other person's perspective; we can also be quick to make assumptions on the basis of flimsy observations. We can become convinced that our point of view is the only valid one, and ignore everything we know about the other person except what is relevant to support our point of view. Therefore, the degree to which an individual finds themselves affected by interpersonal stress may make a critical difference to their mentalizing skills across life experiences. It seems likely that the threshold for switching to an automatic (fight or flight) style of mentalizing will be lowered in people who have been exposed to stress or trauma in early life. There may also be a genetic influence on the ease with which people are likely to switch to this automatic, uncontrolled mentalizing mode.

There is also some evidence that the activation of the attachment system is linked with the deactivation of mentalizing. Imaging studies (e.g., Nolte et al., 2013) have shown that the brain areas normally associated with maternal and romantic attachments appear to suppress activity in brain regions associated with different aspects of cognitive control, including those associated with making social judgments and mentalizing. Anything that stimulates the attachment system (beyond stress-induced arousal), therefore, seems to bring with it a general loss of mentalizing capacity. A traumatic experience will arouse the attachment system, and attachment trauma may do so chronically. The hyperactivation of the attachment system in people with a trauma history may account for the dramatic loss of mentalizing capacity experienced by some individuals in emotional situations that trigger their attachment-seeking instincts. Attachment trauma probably hyperactivates the attachment system because the person to whom the child needs to turn in a state of anxiety (their attachment figure, usually a parent) is the very person causing the fear in the first place. The quick-fire triggering of the attachment system in BPD may be a result of past trauma, and it shows itself in the tendency of BPD patients both to move to positions of intimacy with undue haste and to be vulnerable to the temporary loss of mentalizing skills when in interpersonally intense situations.

Such moments of mentalizing failure are significant because they make it difficult for someone to relate to others in the context of an attachment relationship. When mentalizing fails in this way, there tends to be a re-emergence of nonmentalizing modes of behavior, which can lead to powerful complications and profound disturbances in relationships. We will discuss these nonmentalizing modes next.

The re-emergence of nonmentalizing modes

When mentalizing fails (as typically happens in individuals with BPD, particularly in high-arousal contexts), individuals often fall back on nonmentalizing ways of thinking that have parallels with the ways in which young children behave before they have developed full mentalizing capacities (hence, they may also be termed *prementalizing* modes). These modes of experiencing the self and others tend to re-emerge whenever we lose the ability to mentalize. The modes are termed *psychic equivalence mode, teleological mode*, and *pretend mode*.

While the dimensions of mentalizing can reflect anomalies in terms of mechanisms, on the whole, that is not what the clinician sees. The whole-person perspective that clinicians are obliged to take must address the phenomenology or subjectivity of our patients. Their experience is not that of a single brain mechanism out of kilter with the rest, but of a whole system functioning suboptimally. What the patient and the mentalizing clinician see is a product of a malfunctioning mentalizing system, driven by imbalances in the dimensions of mentalizing. We have grouped the outcomes of these malfunctions under three typical modes of nonmentalizing subjectivity for the purpose of clinical experience. These nonmentalizing modes are important for the clinician to recognize and understand, as they tend to emerge in the consulting room and refer to aspects of the patient's experience. It is important to address these, because they can cause considerable interpersonal difficulties and result in destructive behaviors.

In the *psychic equivalence mode*, thoughts and feelings become "too real" to a point where it is extremely difficult for the individual to entertain possible alternative perspectives (see Box 1.7). When mentalizing gives way to psychic equivalence, what is *thought* is experienced as *being* real and true, leading to what clinicians describe as "concreteness of thought" in their patients. There is a suspension of doubt, and the individual increasingly believes that their own perspective is the only one possible. Psychic equivalence is normal in a child of around 20 months who has not yet developed full mentalizing skills. Young children, and patients with BPD who are in this mode, describe an overriding sense of certainty about their subjective experience, whether this is that "there is a tiger under the bed" or "these drugs are harming me." Such a state of mind can be extremely frightening, adding a powerful sense of drama and risk to life experiences. The sometimes exaggerated reactions of patients are justified by

> ## Box 1.7 Prementalizing modes of subjectivity: psychic equivalence
>
> - Mind–world isomorphism: mental reality equals outer reality
> - Internal has the same power as the external; thoughts are felt as real
> - Subjective experience of mind can be terrifying (e.g., flashbacks)
> - Intolerance of alternative perspectives links to concrete understanding
> - Self-related negative cognitions may be felt to be "too real"—absence of "as if" quality
> - Reflects domination of self-affect state thinking with limited internal focus
> - Managed in therapy by clinician avoiding being drawn into nonmentalizing discourse.

the seriousness and "realness" with which they can experience their own and others' thoughts and feelings. The vividness and bizarreness of subjective experience can appear as quasipsychotic symptoms and are also manifest in the physically compelling memories associated with PTSD.

In the *teleological mode*, states of mind are recognized and believed only if their outcomes are physically observable (see Box 1.8). Hence, the individual can recognize the existence and potential importance of states of mind, but this recognition is limited to very concrete situations. For example, affection is perceived to be true only if it is accompanied by physical contact such as a touch or caress. A patient who experiences mentalizing failure and falls into the teleological mode may express this by "acting out," by carrying out dramatic or inappropriate actions or behaviors in order to generate outcomes from others whose claims of subjective states (e.g., of being concerned about the patient) are not credible to them. The teleological mode shows itself in patients who are imbalanced toward the external pole of the internal–external mentalizing dimension—they are heavily biased toward understanding how people (and they themselves) behave and what their intentions may be in terms of what they physically do.

In the *pretend mode*, thoughts and feelings become severed from reality (see Box 1.9). Taken to an extreme, this may lead to feelings of derealization and dissociation. A prementalizing young child creates mental models and pretend worlds, which the child can maintain only as long as these are

Box 1.8 Prementalizing modes of subjectivity: teleological mode

- A focus on understanding actions in terms of their physical as opposed to mental constraints
- Overreliance on what is physically observable
- Understanding of self and others in terms of physical behaviors
- Only a modification in the physical world is taken to be a true indicator of the intentions of the other
- Manifests itself in behaviors that generate observable outcomes
- Extreme external focus; momentary loss of controlled mentalizing
- Misuse of mentalizing for teleological ends (e.g., harming others) becomes possible because of lack of implicit as well as explicit mentalizing.

Box 1.9 Prementalizing modes of subjectivity: pretend mode

- Ideas do not form a bridge between inner and outer reality; the mental world is severed from outer reality
- To the listener, the patient's discourse feels empty, meaningless, inconsequential, and circular
- Marked by simultaneously held contradictory beliefs
- Frequently, affects do not match the content of thoughts
- "Dissociation" of thought, hypermentalizing, or pseudomentalizing is apparent
- Reflects explicit mentalizing being dominated by an implicit, inadequate internal focus
- Poor belief–desire reasoning and vulnerability to fusion with others
- Managed in therapy by interrupting nonmentalizing process when it occurs.

completely separate from the real world (e.g., as long as an adult does not interrupt or spoil the game by "getting it wrong"). Similarly, patients in pretend mode can discuss experiences without contextualizing these in any kind of physical or material reality, as if they were creating a pretend world. The patient may *hypermentalize* or *pseudomentalize*, a state in which they may say much about states of mind but with little true meaning or connection to reality. Attempting psychotherapy with patients who are in this mode can lead to lengthy but inconsequential discussions of internal experience that have no link to genuine experience. A patient who shows considerable cognitive understanding of mentalizing states but little affective understanding may often hypermentalize. This state can often be difficult to distinguish from genuine mentalizing, but it tends to involve excessively lengthy narratives, devoid of a real affective core or of any connection to reality. On first impressions, hypermentalizing can lead the clinician to believe that they are working with an individual with extraordinary mentalizing capacities, but after a little while they discover that they are unable to resonate with the feelings underlying their patient's mentalizing efforts (Allen, Fonagy, & Bateman, 2008). In addition, because in pretend mode there are no real feelings or emotional experiences providing the individual with constraints, he/she may misuse his/her cognitive capacity in self-serving ways (e.g., to get others to care for or feel compassion toward him/her, or to control or coerce others).

As the astute reader will have noticed, imbalances within the dimensions of mentalizing predictably generate the nonmentalizing modes earlier described. Psychic equivalence is inevitable if emotion (affect) dominates cognition. Teleological mode follows from an exclusive focus on external features to the neglect of the internal. Pretend mode thinking and hypermentalizing are unavoidable if reflective, explicit, controlled mentalizing is not well established. Although we cannot go into detail here, the normal predominance of nonmentalizing in the early years can be predicted from what we know about the developmental unfolding of mentalizing capacities. For example, as affect-focused mental state thinking antedates more cognitive mentalizing (Harris, de Rosnay, & Pons, 2005), psychic equivalence (and the anxieties that accompany it) will almost inevitably be part of the life of a child 3 to 5 years of age.

These three prementalizing modes are particularly important to recognize in patients as they are often accompanied by a pressure to externalize unmentalized aspects of the self (so-called *alien self* parts). This may be expressed in attempts to dominate the mind of others, self-harm, or other types of behavior that in the teleological mode are expected to relieve tension and arousal, a feature typical of BPD (Fonagy & Target, 2000).

The concept of the "alien self"

At moments of mentalizing failure, as well as falling back on prementalizing modes, we also experience a pressure for what psychodynamic clinicians would recognize as "projective identification." This term has many meanings, and this has led us to talk about one aspect of this—the *externalization of the alien part of the self.*

Because mentalizing generates self-coherence, the faltering of mentalizing can signal a sense of fragmentation, a painful state from which we often seek shelter by extreme and even violent acts. Emotional interactions are painful in part because intense emotions undermine mentalizing and the natural and understandable reaction is to try to restore a sense of cohesion by dramatic action. When I find myself in an intense quarrel with a friend and I get "emotional," only a small part of this is the emotion I feel in relation to the argument; the lion's share is likely to be me trying to maintain my sense of self and identity. I may achieve this by:

1　Being excessively assertive (raising my voice)

2　Blinding myself to the potentially "confusing" perspective of my friend

3　Creating an image of him that is highly self-serving and confirms me in my position as coherent, accurate, and, above all, beyond reproach

4　Forcing a reaction from him to affirm me still further or make me feel "even more real."

From a dispassionate, external perspective, the impression is as much of me trying to escape from a painful situation as trying to engage effectively in discussion or debate.

What am I so busy trying to protect myself from? To understand this we have to introduce the concept of the *alien self* (see Box 1.10). We assume, as suggested by Winnicott (1956), that when a child cannot develop a representation of his/her own experience via parental mirroring (of the psychological self), he/she internalizes the image of the caregiver for affirmation as part of his/her self-representation. While this is used to bolster the infantile self, it is not contingent with the self-state: it does not match it in quality, intensity, timing, or tone. This discontinuity within the self is the "alien self." We understand the excessively controlling behavior shown by children with a history of disorganized attachment as the persistence of a pattern analogous to projective identification, where the experience of incoherence within the self is reduced through externalization: that is, placing an aspect of the self on to another person by nudging them to behave according to the representation that requires externalization. As a young person, one of us (PF) used to phone home in states of distress and

Box 1.10 The alien self: practice points (1)

- Clinician must be alert to subjective experiences indicating discontinuities in self-structure (e.g., a sense of having a wish/belief/feeling that does not "feel like their own")
- Discontinuity in the self will have an aversive aspect to most patients—leads to a sense of discontinuity in identity (*identity diffusion*)
- Patients deal with discontinuous aspects of their experience by externalization (generating the feeling within the clinician)—so the clinician must actively monitor his/her feelings for this
- Tendency to externalization is usually established early in childhood and deeply entrenched
- Externalization is not reversed simply by bringing conscious attention to the process; it is futile to see these states of mind as if they were manifestations of a dynamic unconscious
- Technically, there is no interpretation of unconscious process.

talk about his situation in catastrophic terms until his parents were palpably panicked, and then he would end the conversation feeling relieved. It was not until he received similar communications from his own children that he realized fully just what power this process had on parental well-being. If the alien self is an experience of vulnerability, the person creates this experience in his communication partner by generating chronic uncertainty; if it is aggression, he simply has to irritate him; if it is depression or lack of interest and hopelessness, then he might force him to experience the potential of helping, only to dash his hopes again and again. In all these cases, the person resolves an internal incoherence, normally covered over by a capacity to create an illusion of coherence through mentalizing, by ridding oneself of its source—the alien self—on to someone in the external world.

In people with personality disorder, the need for this externalizing can feel like a matter of life and death, not just a momentary relief from discomfort. This is because the alien self can frequently become the vehicle for the experience of maltreatment, the host to a genuinely malevolent intentionality that has taken residence inside the self and expresses its malevolent intent from within through unmoderated self-destructiveness (see Box 1.11). This aspect of the alien self, too, is brought into relief by the disappearance of the "self-generating" mentalizing narrative, which normally bridges cracks in the self-structure and prevents

Box 1.11 The alien self: practice points (2)

- In patients who have experienced maltreatment, abuse, or severe neglect, disowned mental states may include the internalization of a malevolent state of mind
- The patient's experience is of a hostile/persecutory state that must be "got rid of" to stop the experience of attack by the self from within
- This process is a matter of self-survival—"life or death"
- Patient is given limited opportunity to create relationships where they involve the other in enactments
- The degree to which patients engage in externalization of the alien self must be carefully controlled; too many regressive enactments will undermine any opportunity for using that relationship to enhance mentalizing.

them from undermining self-coherence. Loss of mentalizing destabilizes the self, provoking an uncertainty—"Who am I?"; "Who are they?"; "What do they want?"; "Who am I in relation to them?" No answers are available to the individual and panic ensues. As it does so, the individual attempts to recapture a sense of self by schematic representation—"I understand this if he does not like me—he is victimizing me and I am a victim." To manage this state of mind, individuals project aspects of themselves that are destabilizing, and see them in the other. The alien aspects of the self are most dangerous to the individual's integrity and narrative structure.

Failures of mentalizing reveal discontinuities in the structure of the self. This happens simply because the narrative of intentionality that all of us continuously create for ourselves depends on mentalizing being available. When there is a break in mentalizing, discontinuities in our self-representation also become more prominent and threatening. At these points, coherence can be restored by attributing ownership of undesired aspects of oneself (those that are experienced as alien) to another person. In a personal quarrel, someone might accuse a friend of being controlling, inflexible, of caring nothing about other people's point of view, of being unable to listen to an argument, and so on. Nonmentalizing begets nonmentalizing. Relationships become rigid and fixed, and the other has to be controlled, almost forced, to keep and not give up playing the roles of alien parts of the self. In fact, unfair accusations will only anger the friend and rile him exactly to the level of angry unreasonableness that the person finds hard to tolerate in himself. It is at odds with the person's normal self-representation, because it is a part of the self that a frequently tired and short-tempered mother, responding to the person (when a young child's) pleas for comforting, might have created there. The alternative to this successful externalization would be destructive nonmentalized self-criticism, experienced as truly persecutory in psychic equivalence mode. In a teleological mode, this state can represent a genuine risk—that is, a physical risk, through self-harm or even suicide. The need for the other as a vehicle for the alien self can be overwhelming, as the patient experiences it as a matter for survival, and an adhesive, addictive pseudo-attachment to this individual can develop.

Ostensive cues and epistemic trust

The most recent theoretical developments in our thinking about mentalizing and therapeutic change have important implications for how we approach our clinical practice. This new thinking involves the theory of *epistemic trust*. In short, this theory emphasizes the social and emotional significance of the trust we place in the information about the social world that we receive from another person—that is, the extent and ways in which we are able to consider social knowledge as genuine and personally relevant to us (see Box 1.12). The theory builds on the ground-breaking work of the Hungarian psychologists Gergely and Csibra about the evolutionary importance of human infants' capacity to learn from their primary caregivers. According to the theory, human beings have evolved to both teach and learn new and relevant cultural information, and to do this we have evolved particular sensitivity to forms of communication that indicate opportunities for this kind of learning. As part of this process of communication, a caregiver signals to the child that what they are conveying is relevant and can be considered useful and valid cultural knowledge (see Box 1.13). To do this, the caregiver uses what we term *ostensive cues*. Human infants are attuned to respond with particular attention to these signals (Csibra & Gergely, 2011). Ostensive cues include eye contact, turn-taking contingent reactivity, and the use of a special vocal tone (*motherese*), all of which appear to trigger a special mode of learning in the infant (see Box 1.14). We believe that this happens because the ostensive cues indicate to the infant that the caregiver recognizes the child as an individual, and as a mentalizing (thinking and feeling) "agent." In brief, sensitive responding to the child's need fosters not just a general confidence that he/she matters as a person, but also serves to open his/her mind more generally to receive new information as relevant and alter his/her beliefs and modify his/her future behavior accordingly.

Box 1.12 Epistemic trust (1)

- ◆ A human-specific, cue-driven social cognitive adaptation of mutual design dedicated to ensure efficient transfer of relevant cultural knowledge
- ◆ Humans are predisposed to "teach" and "learn" new and relevant cultural information from each other
- ◆ Human communication is specifically adapted to allow the transmission of:
  - Cognitively opaque cultural knowledge
  - Kind-generalizable generic knowledge
  - Shared cultural knowledge.

Ostensive cues trigger *epistemic trust*: they signal that what the caregiver is trying to convey is relevant and significant, and should be remembered. A securely attached child is more likely to treat the caregiver as a reliable source of knowledge, and this trust is likely to generalize to other people in a position to teach and learn from. But what of individuals whose social experiences have led them to a state of chronic *epistemic mistrust*, in which (perhaps because of hypermentalizing) they imagine the motives of the communicator to be malign?

Box 1.13 Epistemic trust (2)

- ◆ Attachment to a person who responded sensitively in early development provides a special condition for generating epistemic trust—provides cognitive advantage of security
- ◆ Communication that is "marked" by recognition of the listener as an intentional agent will increase epistemic trust and the likelihood of the communication being coded as:
  - Relevant to the listener
  - Generalizable to situations beyond the immediate one
  - To be retained in memory as relevant
- ◆ Ostensive cues trigger epistemic trust, which triggers a special kind of attention to knowledge that is understood as relevant to "me."

Box 1.14 Receptivity to learning triggered by ostensive communicative cues

- Examples of ostensive communicative cues from caregiver to infant/child:
  - Eye contact
  - Turn-taking contingent reactivity
  - Special tone of voice ("motherese") to address the child
- Ostensive cues function:
  - To signal that the caregiver has a communicative intention addressed to the infant/child
  - To get across new and relevant information.

Such individuals will appear to be resistant to new information, and might come across as rigid, stubborn, or even bloody-minded, because they treat new knowledge from the communicator with deep suspicion and will not internalize it (i.e., they will not modify their internal mental structures to accommodate it). Their epistemic trust has been undermined by their previous experiences, and as a consequence an evolutionarily prepared channel for the acquisition of personally relevant information is partially blocked. We suspect that it is less likely to be the frank brutality of abuse that undermines epistemic trust (although of course it can do), and that genetic predisposition, in combination with neglect and emotional abuse, will play a larger role in making an individual excessively vulnerable to distrusting information from others (see Box 1.15). Paradoxically, some people whose attachment system is disorganized (as is characteristic of those with BPD) often initially react to people in an excessively trusting way. This is because the hyperactivation of the attachment system disrupts the capacity for epistemic vigilance, making the individual unusually vulnerable.

Everybody seeks social knowledge to help navigate the interpersonal world. We are all often insecure in relation to our own beliefs and intuitions, and seek input and reassurance from others. This, of course, is more likely to be the case for someone whose consistent insecurity has left them at the edge of the interpersonal lattice of social understanding. Yet, even though this individual's need for confirmation may be more intense than normal, and anxiously sought, the content of such reassuring communications may be rejected, their meanings confused, or they may even be misinterpreted as

Box 1.15 Epistemic mistrust

- *Not believing what one is told*
- High levels of *epistemic vigilance* (the overinterpretation of motives, and a possible consequence of hypermentalizing)
- Recipient of a communication assumes that the communicator's intentions are other than those declared; this means that the communication is not treated as coming from a deferential source
- Misattribution of intention and seeing the reasons for someone's actions as malevolent; communication is treated with *epistemic hypervigilance.*
- Process of modifying stable beliefs about the world (oneself in relation to others) remains closed.

having hostile intent, leaving the person in a state of chronic uncertainty yet without means of meaningful redress. A person whose channels for learning about the social world have been disrupted—for example, one whose social experiences with caregivers during childhood have caused a breakdown in epistemic trust—is stuck in a general state of uncertainty and permanent epistemic vigilance. An individual with a history of trauma has little reason to trust, and will reject information that is inconsistent with their existing beliefs. Precluding themselves from social information in this way will create an apparent rigidity, or reluctance to change. This rigidity is underpinned by epistemic mistrust and a state that may be characterized by "hearing but not listening" (see Box 1.16).

As clinicians, we may end up calling these individuals "hard to reach," yet they are simply showing what may be a reasonable adaptation to a social environment where information from most attachment figures is "tagged" as likely to be misleading (see Box 1.17). Notwithstanding the behavior of a parent or a partner as faultlessly supportive and invariably acting in the patient's interest, or a clinician who consistently offers valuable and accurate advice, the patient apparently takes no notice, ignores the evidence of cooperativeness and support, and continues (from the point of view of others, "persists") to feel abandoned, betrayed, and unsupported. It is as if the patient is blind to the evidence, as it runs contrary to their belief. According to this perspective, we can see the destruction of trust in social knowledge as a key mechanism in pathological personality development. This has significant implications for how we understand how and why psychological therapies for BPD and ASPD work.

Box 1.16 Epistemic mistrust and personality disorder

- Social adversity (most profoundly, trauma following neglect) causes destruction of trust in social knowledge of all kinds—manifests as rigidity, individual is "hard to reach"
- The individual cannot change because he/she is unable to accept new information as relevant to other social contexts (i.e., to generalize)
- Personality disorder is not a "disorder of personality" but an *inaccessibility to cultural communication relevant to the self from the social context*:
  - Partner
  - Clinician } epistemic mistrust
  - Teacher

Box 1.17 Epistemic trust and nature of psychopathology

- Epistemic mistrust is epistemic "hunger" combined with mistrust
- Clinicians ignore this knowledge at their peril!
- Personality disorder is a failure of communication:
  - It is *not* a failure of the individual, but a failure of learning relationships (patient is "hard to reach")
  - It is associated with an unbearable sense of isolation in the patient, generated by epistemic mistrust
  - Clinician's inability to communicate with the patient causes frustration in clinician and a tendency to blame the patient
  - Clinician feels that the patient is not listening, but the reality is that the patient finds it hard to trust and consider the truth or otherwise of what he/she hears.

Reconceptualization of treatment: three systems

In the case of BPD, a considerable number of different therapies have now been found to be effective (Stoffers et al., 2012). What these treatments have in common is a clear theoretical framework and a reliable model for the delivery of treatment. Beyond this, though, it is not yet known whether there is a single factor, common to all these therapies, that makes them effective. Clearly,

Box 1.18 Three therapeutic communication systems

- ◆ All three systems address the epistemic mistrust of patients with BPD
- ◆ Communication system 1: communication of therapeutic model-based content:
  - • This varies according to the treatment model (e.g., MBT versus DBT)
  - • Serves as an ostensive cue that increases the patient's epistemic trust and thus acts as a catalyst for therapeutic success ("therapeutic alliance by any other name")
- ◆ Communication system 2: mentalizing as a common factor:
  - • The therapeutic setting serves to increase the patient's mentalizing
- ◆ Communication system 3: social learning in the context of epistemic trust:
  - • The patient applies his/her restored mentalizing in the wider (social) environment, which reinforces and builds upon what he/she has learned in therapy.

understanding what makes interventions effective (or what renders them ineffective) would be of great value in the formulation of future interventions and the refinement of existing practice.

In the light of our earlier argument about epistemic trust, we suggest that successful treatments all involve three essential systems of communication relating to epistemic trust and social learning (see Box 1.18). MBT has been informed by these three principles of change. Over the past few years, specific components have been increasingly emphasized to take into account our understanding of the processes underpinning effective treatment. In the following sections we identify how MBT interventions relate to each component of the change system. Different techniques are emphasized at different stages of treatment and change; for example, communication change system 1 is of greatest importance at the beginning of treatment, although it maintains a place for the clinician and patient throughout treatment.

Communication change system 1: the teaching and learning of content and the increase of epistemic openness

All evidence-based psychotherapies provide a coherent framework that enables the patient to examine the issues that are deemed to be central to him/her, according to a particular theoretical approach, in a safe and low-arousal context.

These psychotherapies provide the patient with helpful skills or knowledge, such as strategies to handle emotional dysregulation or restructure thinking about interpersonal relationships. Perhaps more importantly, however, all *evidence-based* psychotherapies implicitly provide for the patient a model of mind and an understanding of their disorder, as well as a hypothetical appreciation of the process of change, that are accurate enough for the patient to feel recognized and understood as an agent, empowered to make decisions and to alter the course of their path through life. The conceptual model of each treatment contains considerable personally relevant information so the patient experiences feeling markedly mirrored or "understood." Helpful, directive approaches may be more likely to communicate a clear recognition of the patient's position than a generic exploratory style (McAleavey & Castonguay, 2014).

MBT initially takes a more directive and informative approach, and we summarize some examples of how MBT addresses communication system 1 here (see also Box 1.19). MBT requires the clinician and patient to:

1 Collaboratively develop a formulation early in the assessment process. This is written by the clinician and shared with the patient, and is constantly revised when new understanding develops.

2 Identify mentalizing vulnerabilities using examples personal to the patient. Pathways to the loss of mentalizing are identified and established as "vulnerability points" to be monitored carefully.

Box 1.19 Communication system 1 and MBT

MBT requires the clinician and patient to:

- Collaboratively develop a formulation early in the assessment process
- Identify mentalizing vulnerabilities using examples that are personal to the patient
- Discuss the patient's diagnosis in terms of the patient's symptoms and history
- Map attachment patterns and how they play out in current relationships
- Engage the patient in an introductory phase, which combines psycho-education with some interpersonal process
- Establish a developmental narrative of the patient's problems
- Jointly agree goals that are relevant to the patient.

3 Discuss the diagnosis in terms of the patient's symptoms and history. The diagnosis is less important than agreeing a lens through which the variability of symptoms can be understood.

4 Map attachment patterns and how they play out in current relationships. The identification of attachment strategies is essential if the patient and clinician are to recognize their deployment during treatment.

5 Engage the patient in an introductory phase, which combines psychoeducation with some interpersonal process. The MBT-Introductory (MBT-I) group (see Chapter 11) offers the patient and clinician a shared framework for understanding BPD and the whole process of therapy.

6 Establish a developmental narrative of problems. The patient's background and context support a compassionate view of the problems.

7 Jointly agree goals relevant to the patient so that therapy is about what is important to the patient.

In essence, we suggest that such explanations and suggestions may be seen as ostensive cues that signal to the patient the relevance to them of information that is being conveyed. These cues serve to trigger in the patient a feeling of being personally recognized by the clinician or the therapeutic situation. This process is important because it allows the patient to reduce his/her epistemic hypervigilance as he/she increasingly sees the model's relevance to his/her own state of mind. Thus, acquiring new skills and learning new and useful information about oneself, as well as doubtless being useful in its own right, has the nonspecific effect of creating openness. This openness makes it easier for the patient to learn the specific suggestions conveyed within the model. A virtuous cycle is created: *the patient "feels" the personal truth of the content conveyed within the therapeutic model, which, because it is accurate and helpful, generates epistemic openness.* The growth of epistemic trust, in turn, allows the patient to take in further information that also serves to reassure and validate him/her. The learning process is facilitated by the patient's experience of feeling mentalized by the "felt truth" of the content being communicated, either through its correspondence with phenomenology or through practical experience.

However, the fact that so many different therapies using widely differing theoretical models have been found to have considerable beneficial effects indicates that the significance of system 1 lies not so much in the essential truth of the wisdom conveyed by the clinician and the therapeutic model, but more importantly in the fact that it allows the patient to apply this new *received learning* in a more or less concrete way, changing the nature of the communication between patient and clinician in the direction of increased epistemic trust. This brings us to system 2.

Communication change system 2: the re-emergence of robust mentalizing

As noted earlier, through passing on knowledge and skills that feel appropriate and helpful to the patient, the clinician implicitly recognizes the patient's agency. The clinician's presentation of information that is personally relevant to the patient serves as a form of ostensive cueing that conveys the impression that the clinician seeks to understand the patient's perspective; this in turn enables the patient to listen to and hear the clinician's intended meaning. In effect, the clinician is demonstrating how he/she engages in mentalizing in relation to the patient. It is important that in this process both patient and clinician come to see each other more clearly as intentional agents (i.e., individuals seeking to mentalize). For example, when the clinician shows that his/her mind has been changed by the patient, the clinician gives agency to the patient and increases his/her faith in the value of social understanding. The context of an open and trustworthy social situation facilitates achievement of a better understanding of the beliefs, wishes, and desires underpinning the actions of others and of the self. This allows a more trusting relationship to develop between clinician and patient. Ideally, the patient's feeling of having been sensitively responded to by the clinician opens a second virtuous cycle in interpersonal communication in which *the patient's own capacity to mentalize is regenerated* (see Box 1.20). This is the core of MBT.

MBT recommends an authentic "not-knowing" stance that forms the bedrock for exploration of the patient's perspective. Empathic validation and establishing a shared affective platform held between patient and clinician increases the patient's experience that he/she is not alone and indicates that another mind can be useful to clarify mental states and increase a sense of agency. Increasing focus on affect and interpersonal interaction during a session and over time provides the context in which to explore ever more complex states of mind within an attachment context that would normally trigger loss of mentalizing. The mind of the clinician is open to the patient to the extent that the clinician actively demonstrates mentalizing about the patient, stating what is in his/her mind and giving his/her perspective. Subjectivity is held to be of importance and not subjugated. The patient has to consider the clinician's viewpoint just as the clinician has to consider the patient's. Perspectives are expected to change when new information becomes available; minds change minds in a transactional manner.

However, the mentalizing of patients—that is, acting in accordance with the patient's perspective—may be a common factor across psychotherapies not because patients need to learn about the contents of their minds or those of others, but because mentalizing may be a generic way of increasing epistemic trust

Box 1.20 Communication system 2 and MBT

- Authentic "not-knowing" stance that forms the bedrock for exploration of the patient's perspective
- Empathic validation
- Establishing a shared affective platform held between patient and clinician
- Focus on the principle that another mind can be useful to clarify mental states and increase a sense of agency
- Increasing focus on affect and interpersonal interaction—both during a session and over time
- Attachment context in which to explore ever more complex states of mind that would normally trigger loss of mentalizing
- Mind of the clinician is "open" to the patient
- Subjectivity is held to be of importance and not subjugated
- Patient has to consider the clinician's viewpoint, just as the clinician has to consider the patient's
- Perspectives are expected to change when new information becomes available; minds change minds in a transactional manner.

and therefore achieving change in mental function. We would maintain that the patient's capacity to mentalize improves in all effective therapies. This is likely to have generic benefits in that it increases the patient's self-control and sense of self-coherence; it increases the accuracy of their social understanding, reduces their experience of mental pain, and improves their ability to think coherently in the context of attachment relationships. This has been a key part of our understanding of the mechanisms of change since we advanced the MBT model (Fonagy & Bateman, 2006). Understanding the patient's subjectivity is vital to this process, as the patient's self-discovery as an active agent occurs through the social interchange where they experience themselves as an agent in the way their clinician thinks of them—it could be said that they "find themselves in the mind of the clinician." It is also vital to a further function of therapy: the rekindling of the patient's wish to learn about the world, including the social world. We believe that this is a complex and nonlinear process, but it can be summarized briefly as follows: the insight obtained in therapy, whatever its content, creates or recreates the potential for the patient to have a learning experience, which in turn makes other similar learning experiences more productive because it *enables the patient to adopt a stance of learning from experience by increasing their capacity to mentalize.*

Here we would like to emphasize a point that may seem initially puzzling, given our own declared commitment to mentalization-based psychotherapy: *mentalizing in itself is only an intermediate step, not the ultimate therapeutic objective.* Simply instructing the clinician to focus the patient on his/her own thoughts and feelings, or the thoughts and feelings of those around them, will not achieve change by itself. It may, along with other techniques, initiate change by changing the mindset of the person undergoing treatment. However, the process of creating a more robust mentalizing function in therapy (system 2), although a likely necessary step, can no more assure enduring change in the patient than system 1. True and lasting improvement, we believe, rests on a third communication system: learning from experience beyond therapy.

Communication change system 3: the re-emergence of social learning with improved mentalizing

We hypothesize that rekindling epistemic trust through improved mentalizing, which permits the person to understand better and opens them up to feeling understood, in turn reopens the key evolutionarily determined route to information transmission and the possibility of taking in knowledge that is felt to be personally relevant and generalizable. Overcoming epistemic mistrust, so that positive social information that has previously been disavowed is now registered, enables the patient to alter his/her beliefs. This is the vital component of change; it is what brings about genuine alteration in previously rigidly held beliefs. In essence, the experience of feeling thought about enhances mentalizing, which in turn enables us to learn new things about our social world (see Box 1.21).

Box 1.21 Communication system 3 and MBT

- Stabilization of patient's wider social context
- Exploration of patient's current relationships outside the therapeutic relationship
- Focus on sensitive responses from others
- Recognition that negative responses are no more than that
- Emphasis on self-agency and self-determination
- Openness to others' states of mind, including those of the clinician.

The therapeutic situation teaches about sources of knowledge. It provides a clear social illustration of trust, making the clinician a "deferential source" of knowledge (Wilson & Sperber, 2012) with the capacity to undo previously rigidly held beliefs about the self and about others, and to reduce the patient's experience of epistemic isolation, which is embodied in the rigidity of their subjective experience. This initiates a third virtuous cycle. Improved understanding of social situations through improved mentalizing leads to better understanding of significant others in the patient's life, which in turn creates potential for the person to notice a sensitive response and feel understood. Reopening the potential to experience feeling sensitively responded to, both within and outside the therapeutic setting, may in itself initiate more trusting interpersonal relationships, and thus open the patient up to new understandings of specific social situations as they encounter these in day-to-day life.

MBT recommends that early in therapy the patient's social context is stabilized. Change will be impossible if housing, financial, employment, probation, and other stressors are dominant. The MBT clinician is an active advocate for the patient's link to the wider social system. Once treatment is stable and when mentalizing is established with greater constancy and less vulnerable to daily assaults, the clinician and patient consistently work on interpersonal process both within and outside the patient–clinician relationship. Exploration about attachment process in the therapy relationship is seen as not the end point but merely a stage to focus meaningfully on current relationships in the patient's life. How does the patient understand a negative response from an important person in his/her life; how does he/she respond to sensitive reactions from others? Too often, epistemic hypervigilance interferes with getting what is good in an interaction and finding what might propel a joint relational endeavor forward.

We hypothesize that, as the patient's state of epistemic hypervigilance relaxes, his/her capacity for trust increases and he/she can discover new ways of learning about others. This facilitates an increase in the patient's willingness to modify his/her cognitive structures for interpreting others' behavior. Social experiences that may have been positive but were in the past discounted as a result of the patient's epistemic hypervigilance and rigidity now have the potential to have a positive impact and be learned from. This is the third system of communication, which becomes available once the second system, tied to the therapeutic situation, has improved the patient's capacity to mentalize. As patients begin to experience social interactions as more benign and interpret social situations more accurately (e.g., being able to see an experience of temporary social disappointment as simply this, rather than a total rejection of themselves), they update their knowledge of both themselves and others.

It is the recovery of the capacity for social information exchange that, we feel, may be at the heart of effective psychotherapies for BPD, of which MBT is one. They impart an ability to benefit from benign social intentions, and to update and build on knowledge about the self and others in social situations. The improved sense of epistemic trust derived from mentalizing enables learning from social experience; in this way the third virtuous cycle is maintained beyond therapy.

As clinicians we often assume that the process in the consulting room is the primary driver of change, but experience shows us that change is also brought about by what happens beyond therapy, in the person's social environment. Studies in which change was monitored session by session have suggested that the patient–clinician alliance in a given session predicts change in the next (Falkenstrom, Granstrom, & Holmqvist, 2013). This indicates that the change that occurs between sessions is a consequence of changed attitudes to learning engendered by therapy, influencing the patient's behavior between sessions. The implication is that the extent to which a patient benefits from therapy depends partly on what he/she encounters in his/her social world during and after treatment. Because of this, we predict that psychotherapy for BPD is much more likely to succeed if the individual's social environment at the time of treatment is largely benign. Clinical experience suggests that there is likely to be some validity to this assertion, although there is not yet evidence from research to support it.

This admittedly speculative model offers a way to integrate the specific and nonspecific factors in effective psychotherapy. Specific factors associated with "therapies that work" create experiences of truth, which in turn encourage the patient to learn more. In this process, via a nonspecific pathway, the patient's capacity to mentalize is fostered. Both of these systems would be expected to lead to symptomatic improvement. Improved mentalizing and reduced symptomatology both improve the patient's experiences of social relationships. However, it is likely that these new and improved social experiences, rather than just what happens within therapy, serve to erode the epistemic hypervigilance that has previously prevented benign social interactions from changing the patient's experience of themselves and of the social world. *Meaningful change is thus possible only if the person can use their social environment in a positive way (and if the social environment is sufficiently supportive to allow this to happen).* For this to happen, recognition of self-agency is key, and this recognition is best achieved through the ostensive cues that are provided by feeling appropriately mentalized by another person. For the social environment to be accurately interpreted so that it can provide opportunities for new learning, mental state understanding of others' actions and reactions is critical—and only improved mentalizing will achieve this. For the benefit of social experience to be preserved through the maintenance of improved relationships, emotion regulation and good behavioral control are key—and, once again, only improved mentalizing will deliver these. This is essentially why MBT focuses on this capacity, and why its realization is the focus of this practical guide.

References

Allen, J. G., Fonagy, P., & Bateman, A. W. (2008). *Mentalizing in clinical practice.* Washington, DC: American Psychiatric Press.

Apperly, I. A. (2011). *Mindreaders: The cognitive basis of "Theory of Mind."* Hove, UK: Psychology Press.

Bateman, A., & Fonagy, P. (2010). Mentalization based treatment for borderline personality disorder. *World Psychiatry, 9*, 11–15.

Bateman, A. W., & Fonagy, P. (Eds.). (2012). *Handbook of mentalizing in mental health practice.* Washington, DC: American Psychiatric Publishing.

Beyer, F., Munte, T. F., Erdmann, C., & Kramer, U. M. (2014). Emotional reactivity to threat modulates activity in mentalizing network during aggression. *Social Cognitive and Affective Neuroscience, 9*, 1552–1560.

Brass, M., Ruby, P., & Spengler, S. (2009). Inhibition of imitative behaviour and social cognition. *Philosophical Transactions of the Royal Society of London. Series B, Biological Sciences, 364*, 2359–2367.

Csibra, G., & Gergely, G. (2011). Natural pedagogy as evolutionary adaptation. *Philosophical Transactions of the Royal Society of London. Series B, Biological Sciences, 366*, 1149–1157.

Dinsdale, N., & Crespi, B. J. (2013). The borderline empathy paradox: Evidence and conceptual models for empathic enhancements in borderline personality disorder. *Journal of Personality Disorders, 27*, 172–195.

Domes, G., Schulze, L., & Herpertz, S. C. (2009). Emotion recognition in borderline personality disorder—A review of the literature. *Journal of Personality Disorders, 23*, 6–19.

Falkenstrom, F., Granstrom, F., & Holmqvist, R. (2013). Therapeutic alliance predicts symptomatic improvement session by session. *Journal of Counseling Psychology, 60*, 317–328.

Fonagy, P., & Bateman, A. W. (2006). Mechanisms of change in mentalization-based treatment of BPD. *Journal of Clinical Psychology, 62*, 411–430.

Fonagy, P., Gergely, G., Jurist, E., & Target, M. (2002). *Affect regulation, mentalization, and the development of the self.* New York, NY: Other Press.

Fonagy, P., & Luyten, P. (2016). A multilevel perspective on the development of borderline personality disorder. In D. Cicchetti (Ed.), *Developmental psychopathology* (3rd ed.). New York, NY: John Wiley & Sons.

Fonagy, P., Steele, H., & Steele, M. (1991). Maternal representations of attachment during pregnancy predict the organization of infant-mother attachment at one year of age. *Child Development, 62*, 891–905.

Fonagy, P., Steele, M., Steele, H., Moran, G. S., & Higgitt, A. C. (1991). The capacity for understanding mental states: The reflective self in parent and child and its significance for security of attachment. *Infant Mental Health Journal, 12*, 201–218.

Fonagy, P., & Target, M. (1997a). Attachment and reflective function: Their role in self-organization. *Development and Psychopathology*, **9**, 679–700.

Fonagy, P., & Target, M. (1997b). Research on intensive psychotherapy with children and adolescents. *Child and Adolescent Psychiatric Clinics of North America*, **6**, 39–51.

Fonagy, P., & Target, M. (2000). Playing with reality: III. The persistence of dual psychic reality in borderline patients. *International Journal of Psychoanalysis*, **81**, 853–874.

Gergely, G., & Watson, J. S. (1996). The social biofeedback theory of parental affect-mirroring: The development of emotional self-awareness and self-control in infancy. *International Journal of Psychoanalysis*, **77**, 1181–1212.

Gunderson, J. G., & Lyons-Ruth, K. (2008). BPD's interpersonal hypersensitivity phenotype: A gene-environment-developmental model. *Journal of Personality Disorders*, **22**, 22–41.

Harari, H., Shamay-Tsoory, S. G., Ravid, M., & Levkovitz, Y. (2010). Double dissociation between cognitive and affective empathy in borderline personality disorder. *Psychiatry Research*, **175**, 277–279.

Harris, P. L., de Rosnay, M., & Pons, F. (2005). Language and children's understanding of mental states. *Current Directions in Psychological Science*, **14**, 69–73.

Hughes, C., Jaffee, S. R., Happe, F., Taylor, A., Caspi, A., & Moffitt, T. E. (2005). Origins of individual differences in theory of mind: From nature to nurture? *Child Development*, **76**, 356–370.

Lieberman, M. D. (2007). Social cognitive neuroscience: A review of core processes. *Annual Review of Psychology*, **58**, 259–289.

Lombardo, M. V., Chakrabarti, B., Bullmore, E. T., Wheelwright, S. J., Sadek, S. A., Suckling, J.,. . . Baron-Cohen, S. (2010). Shared neural circuits for mentalizing about the self and others. *Journal of Cognitive Neuroscience*, **22**, 1623–1635.

Lynch, T. R., Rosenthal, M. Z., Kosson, D. S., Cheavens, J. S., Lejuez, C. W., & Blair, R. J. (2006). Heightened sensitivity to facial expressions of emotion in borderline personality disorder. *Emotion*, **6**, 647–655.

McAleavey, A. A., & Castonguay, L. G. (2014). Insight as a common and specific impact of psychotherapy: Therapist-reported exploratory, directive, and common factor interventions. *Psychotherapy*, **51**, 283–294.

McGeer, V. (2007). The regulative dimension of folk psychology. In D. Hutto & M. M. Ratcliffe (Eds.), *Folk psychology re-assessed* (pp. 137–156). Dordrecht, The Netherlands: Springer.

Nolte, T., Bolling, D. Z., Hudac, C. M., Fonagy, P., Mayes, L., & Pelphrey, K. A. (2013). Brain mechanisms underlying the impact of attachment-related stress on social cognition. *Frontiers in Human Neuroscience*, **7**, 816.

O'Brien, K., Slaughter, V., & Peterson, C. C. (2011). Sibling influences on theory of mind development for children with ASD. *Journal of Child Psychology and Psychiatry*, **52**, 713–719.

Ripoll, L. H., Snyder, R., Steele, H., & Siever, L. J. (2013). The neurobiology of empathy in borderline personality disorder. *Current Psychiatry Reports*, **15**, 344.

Ritter, K., Dziobek, I., Preissler, S., Ruter, A., Vater, A., Fydrich, T.,. . . Roepke, S. (2011). Lack of empathy in patients with narcissistic personality disorder. *Psychiatry Research*, **187**, 241–247.

Stoffers, J. M., Vollm, B. A., Rucker, G., Timmer, A., Huband, N., & Lieb, K. (2012). Psychological therapies for people with borderline personality disorder. *Cochrane Database of Systematic Reviews*, **8**, CD005652.

Taumoepeau, M., & Ruffman, T. (2006). Mother and infant talk about mental states relates to desire language and emotion understanding. *Child Development*, **77**, 465–481.

Taumoepeau, M., & Ruffman, T. (2008). Stepping stones to others' minds: Maternal talk relates to child mental state language and emotion understanding at 15, 24, and 33 months. *Child Development*, **79**, 284–302.

Wilson, D., & Sperber, D. (2012). *Meaning and relevance*. Cambridge, UK: Cambridge University Press.

Winnicott, D. W. (1956). Mirror role of mother and family in child development. In D. W. Winnicott (Ed.), *Playing and reality* (pp. 111–118). London, UK: Tavistock.

Chapter 2

Using the mentalizing model to understand personality disorder

Introduction

At the heart of the mentalizing approach to borderline personality disorder (BPD) is our belief that problems in social cognition, and particularly a compromised capacity to understand oneself and others in terms of mental states, play an important role in various psychiatric disorders involving pathology of the self. In this chapter, we will describe the mentalizing difficulties encountered by people with BPD and antisocial personality disorder (ASPD), and how mentalizing might relate to the lived experiences of an individual who has either of these disorders (see Box 2.1). We will begin by discussing the main symptoms of the two disorders and provide an understanding of these from a mentalizing perspective.

Borderline personality disorder

BPD is a severe condition with a lifetime prevalence estimated at up to 6% (Grant et al., 2008). BPD is often diagnosed alongside mood disorders, anxiety disorders, bipolar disorder, and schizotypal and narcissistic personality disorders (see also Chapter 3 for discussion of some of the common comorbidities). It may be particularly common in outpatient and forensic psychiatric populations, where between one-quarter and one-third of individuals may be expected to meet criteria for the diagnosis.

The DSM-5 (American Psychiatric Association, 2013) lists nine criteria, of which at least five must be present for a diagnosis of BPD to be made. These are:

1 A pattern of unstable intense relationships

2 Inappropriate, intense anger

3 Frantic efforts to avoid abandonment

4 Affective instability

5 Impulsive actions

6 Recurrent self-harm and suicidality

Box 2.1 Mentalizing and personality disorder

- Personality disorder is defined in DSM according to functional impairment and pathological personality traits
- Personality disorder is a disorder in the dimensions of mentalizing
- BPD and ASPD show an imbalance of the mentalizing dimensions
- Core features of emotional dysregulation, impulsivity, and social/interpersonal dysfunction.

---

7 Chronic feelings of emptiness or boredom (dysphoria)

8 Transient, stress-related paranoid thoughts

9 Identity disturbance and severe dissociative symptoms.

A proposal included in Section III of the DSM-5 indicates that further research is warranted on the model for personality disorder, and sets out a new model based on impairments in personality *functioning* and pathological personality *traits*. The proposed alternative model reflects an increasing interest in understanding each personality disorder as a dimensional rather than a monolithic disorder, with individuals showing different traits to different degrees. The impairments in functioning described in the alternative model are also of relevance in the context of this book because they are strikingly consistent with a mentalizing perspective. The alternative model sets out four possible elements of impairment in functioning. The first two elements relate to the self; the second two elements are interpersonal.

1 *Identity* is the first area of functional impairment, involving potentially extreme difficulties in experiencing the self as a unique entity with boundaries and a coherent sense of personal history. In Chapter 1 we described in some detail the self–other dimension of mentalizing: patients with BPD characteristically experience difficulties in retaining a judicious balance between the self and other polarities.

2 The second interpersonal element is that of *self-direction*. This involves impairments in the pursuit of both short-term and long-term life goals; operating within constructive and prosocial ways of behavior; and self-reflection.

3 *Empathy* is one of the interpersonal elements of functioning described in the DSM-5 alternative model. It is conceptualized as the ability to comprehend and appreciate others' experiences; the capacity for tolerating differing

perspectives; and understanding the social effects of one's behavior. These are all underpinned by mentalizing—the accurate understanding of the thoughts and feelings that direct behavior.

4 Problems with *intimacy*—a lack of depth or the short duration of connection with others and a limited desire or capacity for closeness—constitutes the fourth element of functional impairment. To relate this to our thinking, this characteristic points to failures in forming attachment relationships resulting from disruptions of the attachment system.

The alternative model further describes five pathological personality traits related to personality disorder: negative affectivity, detachment, antagonism, disinhibition, and psychoticism. Finally, the model proposes consideration of the pervasiveness and stability of these traits, impairments in functioning, and pathological personality traits.

The group of patients captured by the DSM-5 BPD criteria for diagnosis is wide. This creates problems for clinicians and academics alike. For example, it is unlikely that the various available evidence-based treatments are equally applicable to all subtypes of BPD. There is, however, increasing consensus that BPD consists of three related core features: emotion dysregulation, impulsivity, and social dysfunction. We will discuss these features in turn, giving a mentalizing perspective on the processes at work when these features are prominent.

Before describing the core features of BPD, however, we would like to briefly emphasize that the reality of living with BPD is that these characteristics—while helpful from a clinical and theoretical perspective—are often blurred, and one may end up triggering another. An example of this is the way in which emotion dysregulation can easily be the cause as well as the consequence of dysfunctional social relationships. Intense emotion almost invariably causes social dysfunction. When an individual with BPD behaves in an emotionally dysregulated way, it is likely to severely disrupt social relationships, particularly intimate ones. Whoever the person is with is quite likely to act in a way that causes further emotional reaction, and a spiral of dysregulation might follow. Or the attempt to control the emotion dysregulation may entail initiating impulsive behaviors such as self-harm.

Core related features of BPD

Emotion dysregulation

Emotion dysregulation often shows itself as intense, inappropriate anger. Affective instability and intensity of affect may underlie the frantic efforts to avoid abandonment that are a key characteristic of the disorder, but may also drive many other BPD symptoms (e.g., impulsive actions). Experimental studies have indeed confirmed that patients with a diagnosis of BPD are less willing to experience distress in order to pursue goal-directed behavior (Gratz, Rosenthal, Tull, Lejuez, & Gunderson, 2006; Salsman & Linehan, 2012), have significantly prolonged anger reactions (Jacob et al., 2008), are less able to inhibit their response to negative emotional stimuli (Gratz, Breetz, & Tull, 2010), show abnormalities in processing unpleasant emotional stimuli (Baer, Peters, Eisenlohr-Moul, Geiger, & Sauer, 2012; Hazlett et al., 2007) and are more likely to behave impulsively when in a negative mood (Chapman, Leung, & Lynch, 2008). Over any specific time period they are likely to experience dramatic shifts in mood states (Reich, Zanarini, & Fitzmaurice, 2012; Santangelo, Bohus, & Ebner-Priemer, 2014) and increases in heart rate not associated with metabolic activity (Reisch, Ebner-Priemer, Tschacher, Bohus, & Linehan, 2008; Trull et al., 2008). BPD patients also report more complex emotions, and experience greater problems in identifying specific emotions associated with higher levels of distress (Bornovalova, Matusiewicz, & Rojas, 2011; Ebner-Priemer et al., 2008; Preissler, Dziobek, Ritter, Heekeren, & Roepke, 2010), although this may be the effect rather than the cause of emotional hyperreactivity (Domes, Schulze, & Herpertz, 2009).

Emotion dysregulation is a well-recognized core feature of BPD. But from a clinical point of view, we need to explain emotion dysregulation from a mentalizing perspective (see Box 2.2). Overwhelming emotional arousal, we argue, causes significant mentalizing imbalances. In terms of the mentalizing dimensions, this involves being temporarily restricted to the affective polarity of the cognitive–affective dimension, with thinking also characterized by an automatic, non-reflective form of mentalizing (on the automatic–controlled dimension). When someone is in a state of stress, it is natural for automatic mentalizing

---

Box 2.2 Emotional dysregulation and mentalizing

- Emotional arousal causes significant mentalizing imbalance
- Cognitive–affective dimension fixed at affective pole
- Automatic–controlled dimension fixed at automatic (non-reflective) pole
- Inability to access representation of states of mind of the other and to be constrained by them
- Psychic equivalence is the nonmentalizing mode most often associated with high emotion.

to come to the fore. Up to a point this is a normal "fight or flight" response to stress, which has the evolutionary advantage of allowing a person to respond to physical danger immediately and without reflection. However, in situations of social interpersonal stress, being able to function in a more cognitive and reflective way is clearly important, and an inability to use the more controlled and conscious mentalizing skills can lead to real difficulties. For example, before we act on the desire to scream we think about how it might frighten a child we are with, and evoking the child's mental state has a calming, regulating effect. If it is difficult for the individual to access the sense of perspective that can help to regulate his/her heightened affect by appraising the context, it may also make him/her behave in a way that generates responses that escalate interpersonal stress and worsen social difficulties and dysfunctions. Going back to the example, shouting or screaming would dysregulate the child, which may in turn further dysregulate us.

The nonmentalizing mode that may be most closely linked to emotion dysregulation is *psychic equivalence*. As described in Chapter 1, in this mode emotion is felt as overly "real," and when sufficiently intense, it leaves no room for any doubt. It makes the experience of internal events (thoughts and feelings) seem concrete rather than subjective, as being of the same weight and significance as a physical incident; this may be what makes the impact of emotional arousal so overwhelming. It is one thing to *feel* tired and unattractive first thing in the morning, but quite another to regard that feeling as proof positive that one *is* ugly and undesirable. When this emotional way of experiencing the world is extended to cognitions—when both thoughts and feelings become "too real"—it leads to a state of mind that allows no alternative perspective. It makes the emotions themselves feel highly immediate and completely unquestionable; this experience can be powerful and overwhelming. When such points arise in therapy, the best strategy for the clinician is to avoid being drawn into a nonmentalizing discourse. We see dysregulated emotional thinking as triggering the concreteness of the psychic equivalence mode, which in turn makes it hard for the individual to accept alternative perspectives that could help to contextualize and down-regulate the intensity of the experience.

Impulsivity

Impulsivity is the second core feature of BPD, the most disquieting aspect of which is suicidality (see Box 2.3). Three-quarters of BPD patients attempt suicide at least once (Black, Blum, Pfohl, & Hale, 2004). Affective instability, particularly negative mood amplitude and the intensity of negative mood (Links, Eynan, Heisel, & Nisenbaum, 2008), has been associated with an increased likelihood of impulsivity (Gratz et al., 2010). A diagnosis of major depressive

---

Box 2.3 Impulsivity and BPD

- *Not attending*: decreased attention—easily getting bored, inability to concentrate on a task, difficulty keeping to topic when something else comes into the mind
- *Not planning*: lack of premeditation; limited consideration about or concern for consequences; excitement about risky activities that precludes considering negative consequences
- *Action*: action without reflection—going into an action rapidly, acting rashly; sometimes related to pleasing as well as displeasing emotions.

---

disorder, substance use disorder, or post-traumatic stress disorder, the presence of self-harm, being sexually assaulted in adulthood, having had a caretaker who completed suicide, affective instability, and more severe dissociation have each been shown to increase suicidal behavior (Wedig, Frankenburg, Bradford Reich, Fitzmaurice, & Zanarini, 2013; Wedig et al., 2012). Suicide risk has been associated with poor social adjustment and the absence of supportive family, work, and social relationships (Soloff & Fabio, 2008; Soloff, Feske, & Fabio, 2008; Wedig et al., 2013).

We understand impulsivity in terms of imbalance among the dimensions of mentalizing: it involves a heavy emphasis on the automatic pole of the automatic–controlled dimension (see Box 2.4). Impulsive behavior will result if there is insufficient reflection concerning the impact of one's actions on others or on oneself. What reflection there is will most likely be disconnected from reality: that is, it is likely to be *hypermentalizing* or *pseudomentalizing*. If I have done something for which I can find no explanation, I will develop a reason retrospectively, usually in terms of my "intentions" and "beliefs" and/or those of others around me. For example, if the context for my actions was an imagined slight because my partner did not respond immediately to a text message I sent them, my explanation will be marked by extravagant assumptions about what might have been going on. If I discuss this event in therapy, I will entangle myself and my clinician in extended analyses, but offer little compelling evidence for any of my assertions. I urgently seek validation for my view, but even when this is forthcoming, it is meaningless because I am simultaneously aware that I made up my explanation; thus, confirming or elaborating it only increases my sense of emptiness and meaninglessness. My clinician would help me most by interrupting this nonmentalizing process— and the sooner the better. This style of functioning, when mentalizing becomes highly impaired, develops into the *pretend mode* of prementalizing, where there is an inadequate link between inner and outer reality: this can often result in impulsive behavior as it is not tempered by a measured hold on external reality.

Impulsivity can also result from the *teleological stance*. The teleological mode of prementalizing involves a heavy emphasis on observable, physical outcomes. In teleological mode, the individual cannot accept anything other than a physical action as a true expression of someone's intentions. In the case of such a patient, a partner or parent might constantly assure him/her of their love and support, and yet none of that feels real: it does not address the "hole" that the patient "falls into" at certain, especially lonely, times when he/she feels terrible emptiness. For such a patient, what does seem to help are physical actions that make him/her feel real, for example, scratching himself/herself a little too violently. Intentions can be accepted only if they are proven by actions and are meaningless unless they produce physically observable outcomes—this can explain acts of self-harm, demonstrating to oneself that one still has the power of self-agency, or acts of aggression toward others for similar reasons. Imagine feeling that interpersonal affection can only be real if it is accompanied by physical behavior—this certainly explains some risky sexual behavior, but also the need to create physical distraction that helps with the feeling that all verbal expressions of interpersonal affection are without real meaning. The teleological stance is a state of nonmentalizing that is highly fixed on the exterior pole of the internal–external dimension of mentalizing and reflects the momentary loss of controlled mentalizing.

Box 2.4 Impulsivity and mentalizing in BPD

- Suicide and self-harm are common behaviors in BPD linked to impulsivity
- Impulsivity indicates "short circuiting" of the reflective mentalizing system
- Over-reliance on the automatic pole of the automatic–controlled dimension
- Hypermentalizing explanations of action when discussed retrospectively, which can fix as pretend mode
- Teleological nonmentalizing mode fuels impulsivity.

Social dysfunction

Social dysfunction is typically seen as the third factor in the core triad of BPD symptom clusters. For example, patients with BPD experience heightened social problem-solving difficulties compared to other clinical groups and report high levels of disturbances in romantic relationships. Difficulties in social problem-solving are likely to be directly connected to *dysfunctional attachment processes* (see Box 2.5). In one study of a sample of patients with BPD (Fonagy et al., 1996), which controlled for conditions that commonly co-occur with BPD, a particular association between BPD and preoccupied attachment was reported (75% of patients who met criteria for BPD fell into the rarely used adult attachment subgroup of "fearfully preoccupied with respect to trauma"). Numerous studies have reported that individuals with BPD appear to anxiously expect, readily perceive, and intensely react to social rejection. We, along with many others working in this area of clinical practice and research, have highlighted a characteristic pattern in BPD patients of *fearful attachment* (attachment anxiety and relational avoidance), painful *intolerance of aloneness*, a marked *hypersensitivity* to social situations, *alertness to a hostile response* from others, and greatly *reduced positive memories* of dyadic interactions (e.g., Gunderson & Lyons-Ruth, 2008).

As mentalizing is at the heart of social cognition, it is clear that these social difficulties are more likely to arise in poorly mentalizing individuals who find it difficult to moderate their automatic assumptions about others by using reflective thought. Furthermore, social dysfunction will inevitably arise if undue emphasis is placed on mentalizing based on exterior cues as indicators of mental states. Difficulties in understanding and connecting with one's own thoughts and feelings can drive a constant and intense need for reassurance to protect against feelings of

---

Box 2.5 Social dysfunction and mentalizing in BPD

- Social and interpersonal problems indicate dysfunctional attachment processes
- Patients with BPD show fearful attachment patterns
- Attachment patterns are related to mentalizing processes
- Difficulties moderating automatic mentalizing using controlled mentalizing → hypersensitivity to negative experience
- Excessive focus on external mentalizing of self and other → hypervigilance and need for reassurance
- Requirement of other to establish own internal mental state.

emptiness and meaninglessness. This can lead to the neediness and dependence on others that is a common aspect of the social dysfunction associated with BPD. The focus on exterior cues can create an attitude of hypervigilance, which, combined with what might seem to others unreasonable demands for reassurance, can actually increase the likelihood of being rejected. The dependence on others is driven by hypersensitivity to others' moods and what they say, the chameleon effect (the unconscious tendency to mimic others' behavior), and the attendant fear of the self disappearing. A rejection triggers panic that others' affirmations and reassurance will cease. The threat that others represent to the sense of self is hard to overestimate: an impingement can feel existential. One way to meet this vulnerability may be through brittle and assertive actions that seek to force recognition of one's identity in interactions with others. However understandable this may be, this kind of aggressive or dominating behavior will cause others to respond defensively, often leading to conflict and intense affect, which serves to further undermine the individual's mentalizing capacity.

Attachment, mentalizing, and BPD

Our approach to BPD is based on three key ideas (see also Box 2.6):

1 We assume that a history of early (in particular emotional) neglect, and a disrupted early social environment in general, is common in people with BPD, and we assume that it can undermine the ability of some individuals to develop full mentalizing capacities.

2 We assume that, particularly in these individuals, subsequent adversity or trauma could further disrupt mentalizing, in part as an adaptive maneuver on the part of the individual to limit exposure to a brutalizing psychosocial environment, and in part because the high level of arousal generated by attachment hyperactivation and disorganized attachment strategies serve to disrupt less well-practiced and less robustly established higher cognitive capacities.

3 Mentalizing is a multidimensional capacity, and thus different BPD patients will be characterized by specific impairments in these capacities.

Several predictions follow from these views. In BPD patients we expect to see:

◆ Higher levels of insecure attachment strategies, and attachment disorganization in particular

◆ An association with high levels of early (emotional) neglect and later trauma

◆ A complex pattern of mentalizing deficits, which vary according to the nature of the task, the emotional and (in particular) attachment demands the task places on the individual, and the nature of the individual's attachment history.

> ## Box 2.6 Attachment and mentalizing in BPD
>
> We assume:
>
> - Early (especially emotional) neglect and disrupted social environment undermine development of full mentalizing capacities
> - Later adversity or trauma can further disrupt mentalizing
> - Attachment hyperactivation and disorganized attachment strategies disrupt higher cognitive capacities
> - Mentalizing is multidimensional. Different subtypes of BPD patients are characterized by specific impairments in mentalizing dimensions.
>
> This predicts:
>
> - Higher levels of insecure attachment strategies, and attachment disorganization in particular
> - An association with high levels of early (emotional) neglect and later trauma
> - A complex pattern of mentalizing deficits, which vary according to:
>   - The nature of the task
>   - The emotional and attachment demands the task places on the individual
>   - The nature of the attachment history of the individual.

As this book is primarily a guide to treatment rather than a comprehensive review of research evidence, we would like to refer the reader to Fonagy and Luyten (2016) for a detailed review of each of these assumptions.

The mentalizing profile of BPD across the four dimensions

To return to the four dimensions of mentalizing discussed in Chapter 1— automatic versus controlled, self versus other, internal versus external, and cognitive versus affective—we will briefly reconsider how the mentalizing strengths and weaknesses of a typical individual with BPD may be apparent across these dimensions (see Figure 2.1).

Automatic versus controlled: the overvaluing of intuition in the absence of adequate capacity for reflection

Individuals with BPD often tend toward a form of mentalizing that is unhelpfully automatic or implicit (see Box 2.7). This can appear simplistic; it is

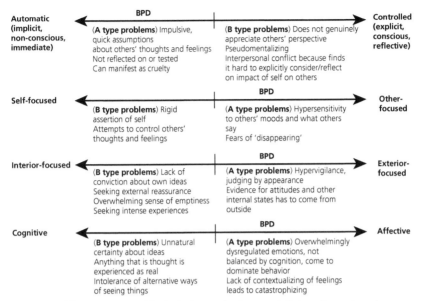

Fig. 2.1 Problems generated by imbalances in the mentalizing dimensions in people with BPD. The unbalanced emphasis on one pole in each dimension has mentalizing outcomes across the whole dimension. (*A type problems* arise from the undue focus on the favored pole and *B type problems* are consequent dysfunctions in tasks normally underpinned by the opposite, underused pole).

Box 2.7 Automatic versus controlled mentalizing in BPD

- Excessive or inappropriate use of automatic mentalizing unmoderated by controlled mentalizing
- Vigilant when arousal is high
- Overly sensitive and either distrustful or too trusting
- Quick decision-making, non-reflective of the other's response
- Logic is intuitive, unreasoned, and nonverbal.

normally automatic, non-questioning, and nonconscious; it is impossible to genuinely verbally explicate because the logic is intuitive, unreasoned, and non-verbal; it is marked by an unwarranted certainty, which betrays its unreflective origin. Particularly when arousal increases, as is typical in the context of intense attachment relationships, individuals with BPD may easily find themselves switching to automatic mentalizing. As a consequence, they often show severe impairments in social cognition; for example, they may be overly distrustful (paranoid) or, conversely, overly trustful (naive). Their thinking is impulsive: they make quick assumptions about others' thoughts and feelings, which are not reflected upon or tested. Because these individuals are likely to find it challenging to consider and reflect on the impact they are having on others around them, interpersonal conflicts can arise. Furthermore, because of their lack of perspective-taking, a degree of (unintended) cruelty can enter into the person's thinking and actions. In place of genuine reflectiveness, pseudomentalizing can occur. In addition, as it is not circumscribed by being tested against reality, their mentalizing is frequently excessive; this has been described as *hypermentalizing*, and it may be particularly characteristic of adolescents with personality disorder (Sharp, 2014).

Self versus other: asserting the self because of the excessive influence of the other

Patients with some borderline traits may show excessive concern about their own internal state (i.e., they hypermentalize in relation to the self) (see Box 2.8). At the same time, these views of the self develop without reference to social reality (an awareness of how others perceive oneself). Failure to balance self-perception with sincere curiosity about how one is perceived by others can lead to exaggerations of the self-image, in both positive and negative directions. A balanced, adaptive form of self-mentalizing is lost, and the reality of the individual's identity becomes dissolved in hypermentalized fantasy.

Box 2.8 Self versus other mentalizing in BPD

- Concern about self internal state and self-coherence—fears "disappearing"
- Mind states of others can be overly influential
- Sensitive to others' moods
- Rigid control of others' thoughts and feelings to protect the self
- Hypermentalizing of self with little constraint from external reality.

Internal versus external: hypersensitivity to the external at the expense of the internal

BPD patients tend to perform poorly on tasks that require them to understand the intentions of other people. However, they can be hypersensitive to facial expressions (in fact, in some studies of individuals' sensitivity to visual cues about emotional states, subjects with BPD outperform those without BPD). The heightened sensitivity to emotional experiences in BPD seems to be intrinsically related to an increased sensitivity to external features of self and others as a source of knowledge about mental states, and perhaps links to BPD patients' tendency to be excessively affected by the emotional states of those around them. Excessive focus on the external may make an individual hypervigilant about what others feel or think, yet unable to make accurate assessments based on anything other than surface judgments (see Box 2.9).

This type of mentalizing impairment may become apparent only when the balance of internal and external cues used to establish the mental states of others is assessed. For example, an accurate depiction of how committed one's clinician is can come only from considering the level of motivation normally required to attend regularly, receiving relatively low compensation, and receiving little by way of explicitly expressed gratitude. However, if such evaluations of *internal* states are inaccessible to a person, then *external* indicators of attitudes feel crucial. Tiny indicators of a lack of commitment, such as the clinician arriving late for a session, can be considered to be devastating evidence of betrayal. In mentalization-based treatment (MBT), mentalizing interventions often need to start by accepting the patient's subjective experience, which can often be overwhelming, rather than yielding to the temptation to review the evidence, which, in more balanced circumstances, would be accepted as evidence that the other person's internal state is different from what the patient, in his/her state of high emotional arousal, holds to be true.

Box 2.9 Internal versus external mentalizing in BPD

- Hypersensitive to external cues at the expense of internal understanding
- Make judgments on the basis of appearance, facial expression, eye movement, and tone of voice
- Evidence for attitudes and other internal states has to come from outside
- Increased evidence of own thoughts and feelings about the other person.

Cognitive versus affective: a failure of cognitive mentalizing

Patients with borderline traits are often overwhelmed by automatic, feeling-driven mentalizing and lack the ability to balance this with more reflective, cognitive modes of function (see Box 2.10). What we see clinically are overwhelmingly dysregulated emotions that are inadequately balanced (or not balanced at all) by cognition, and these emotions come to dominate behavior. This leads to catastrophizing. Cognitions serve to help us differentiate between what we feel and what is reality. If I am aware that I am thinking of something, it means that I know that the thought is just a thought and that my expectation might not be true. Reality comes in a "combined package" with emotions. If I feel pain, it will be hard to convince me that this is a product of my imagination; try to tell me that I am just imagining that my back hurts. But with cognition there is always doubt. Cognition is firmly located in the self—I know that beliefs are in my mind. But emotions reverberate and are distorted by social context. If I sense ("feel") that someone sees me as "second-rate," and if I simply experience this thought without reflecting on it, the thought will carry with it some of the inner conviction of the back pain—it will become something I cannot argue with.

To compound this problem, intense emotion can disrupt the process that normally helps to regulate it: that is, cognitive appraisal. If my sense of being thought of as "second-rate" by a friend creates an intense emotional response in me, I am no longer capable of testing my assumptions against everything else I know about that person and our past experiences with each other. The absence of cognition can also lead to an oversensitivity to emotional cues and, in a social context, overwhelming experiences of "emotion contagion" when one person's intense emotional experience triggers an emotional reaction in another, which, in turn, can become challenging to regulate. I may respond to my friend's

---

Box 2.10 Cognitive versus affective mentalizing in BPD

+ Overwhelming dysregulated emotions with self-affect propositions
+ Absence of doubt about experience
+ Emotions not balanced by cognition; cognitive appraisal decreased
+ Lack of contextualizing of feelings leads to catastrophizing
+ Pretend mode.

imagined slight by slighting (or even overtly insulting) him, something to which he understandably does not take kindly. In this situation, a person may lose the capacity for boundaries around the self and may more readily attribute their own mental states to others. I see my friend's response as a clear indication of his vulnerable sense of self, and his modest attempt to protect himself as an equally clear indication of his untrustworthiness and unreliability. I end up feeling let down by him and quite abandoned and isolated. Thus, despite an apparent emotionality shown by people with BPD in relation to others, emotional storms can lead to serious limitations in their capacity for genuine empathy, and they may show self-oriented distress when confronted with sadness or pain in others, in place of genuine other-oriented empathy.

Antisocial personality disorder

The DSM-5 lists four diagnostic criteria for ASPD. These are:

1 A pervasive disregard for and violation of the rights of others, occurring since the age of 15, as indicated by three of the following:

  a Failure to conform to social norms with respect to lawful behaviors, as indicated by repeatedly performing acts that are grounds for arrest

  b Deceitfulness, as indicated by repeated lying, use of aliases, or conning others for personal profit or pleasure

  c Impulsivity or a failure to plan ahead

  d Irritability and aggressiveness, as indicated by repeated physical fights or assaults

  e Reckless disregard for safety of self or others

  f Consistent irresponsibility, as indicated by repeated failure to sustain work behavior or honor financial obligations

  g Lack of remorse, as indicated by being indifferent to or rationalizing having hurt, mistreated, or stolen from another

2 The individual is at least 18 years old

3 There is evidence of conduct disorder with onset before the age of 15

4 The occurrence of antisocial behavior is not exclusively during the course of schizophrenia or bipolar disorder.

The descriptive clinical features of ASPD—a failure to conform to social norms in relation to lawful behavior, impulsivity, irritability, aggressiveness, recklessness, irresponsibility, and remorselessness—understandably make others wary of individuals with the disorder (see Box 2.11).

Box 2.11 Clinical features of ASPD

- Failure to conform to social norms with respect to lawful behaviors
- Deceitfulness
- Impulsivity or failure to plan ahead
- Irritability and aggressiveness
- Reckless disregard for safety of self or other
- Consistent irresponsibility
- Lack of remorse.

   None of these features is endearing to others. The self-serving attitude of people with ASPD and their unpredictability makes people wary of them.

The prevalence of ASPD has been reported to be 0.6% in the general population of the United Kingdom (National Institute for Health and Clinical Excellence, 2010), although the disorder may be underdiagnosed in the community. Nonetheless, there is a wide disparity between the prevalence of ASPD among the general population and among offenders: in the prison population in the United Kingdom, 63% of male remand prisoners, 49% of male sentenced prisoners, and 31% of female prisoners have been reported to have ASPD (Singleton, Neltzer, Gatward, Coid, & Deasy, 1998). The contribution of ASPD to violent criminal behavior is clear: it is associated with a significantly increased likelihood of violent behaviors and is highly predictive of future violence, future reconviction, or re-incarceration upon release from prison. The treatment of ASPD is a well-recognized priority, but at the time of writing no intervention has been established as the treatment of choice for addressing its symptoms (National Institute for Health and Clinical Excellence, 2010). Treatment of ASPD is considered difficult, and individuals with the disorder receive poor mental health care from psychiatric and psychological services.

   Here we will show how many of the descriptive characteristics of ASPD relate to abnormalities in mentalizing, and that understanding these may offer a route to effective treatment. First we review evidence suggesting an association between ASPD and a limited capacity for mentalizing.

   An early study using the Reflective Functioning Scale to assess Adult Attachment Interview transcripts from offenders showed reduced reflective functioning in comparison to individuals with personality disorders and no history of offending, and normal controls (Levinson & Fonagy, 2004). The psychological functioning of people with ASPD appears less rigid than that of individuals with other personality disorders, for example, paranoid personality disorder. Their mentalizing shows flexibility at times, but when uncertainty arises, they use prementalizing modes of thinking to organize their mental processes and interpret the world and their relationships. The balance of components of mentalizing can also be distorted. Patients with narcissistic personality disorder have a well-developed self-focus but a very limited mentalized understanding of others (Dimaggio, Lysaker, Carcione, Nicolo, & Semerari, 2008). In contrast, individuals with ASPD are experts at reading the inner states of others, even to the point that they can misuse this capacity to coerce or manipulate them, while being unable to develop any real understanding of their own inner world. In addition, they lack the ability to read certain emotions accurately (an external component of mentalizing) and fail to recognize fearful emotions from facial expressions: a robust link has been shown between antisocial behavior and specific deficits in recognizing fearful expressions (Marsh & Blair, 2008). Laboratory findings also indicate that violent offenders fail to mentalize a victim's desperation (Blair, Jones, Clark, & Smith, 1997).

Limited capacity to mentalize is part of the picture presented by individuals with histories of antisocial offending behavior, and this is marked in those who meet criteria for a diagnosis of ASPD. A recent study tested the hypothesis that individuals with antisocial (particularly violent) histories have specific problems in relation to accurately envisioning mental states (Newbury-Helps, Feigenbaum, & Fonagy, in press). Eighty-two male offenders (65% of whom met the threshold for ASPD) on community license, recruited from probation services in London, United Kingdom, completed a battery of computerized mentalizing tests requiring perspective-taking, mental state recognition from facial expression, and identification of mental states in the context of social interaction. They were compared with a matched sample of 43 controls with no history of offending. The offender group showed mentalizing impairments in all the tasks when compared with the control group, and also in comparisons with samples drawn from published studies. Three of the mentalizing subscales had modest ability to predict the severity of ASPD: the Sensitivity to Others' Perspectives task, the Movie for the Assessment of Social Cognition absence of mentalizing subscale, and the Reading the Mind in the Eyes Test accuracy score.

Another study confirmed the mediating role of mentalizing in the association between experience of childhood abuse and aggression in 97 adolescents with conduct problems (Taubner & Curth, 2013). Results showed that reflective functioning was a complete mediator of the relationship between early abuse and aggressive behavior. Conversely, mentalizing capacity is a protective factor in the relationship between early abusive experience and the development of aggressive behavior. A further study of 104 adolescents (both sexes) with a mean age of 16.4 years assessed mentalizing capacities using the Reflective Functioning Scale on the Adult Attachment Interview (Taubner, White, Zimmermann, Fonagy, & Nolte, 2013). Psychopathic traits and aggressive behavior were measured via self-report. Deficits in mentalizing were significantly associated with psychopathic traits and proactive aggression. Mentalizing played a moderating role, such that individuals with more profound psychopathic tendencies did not display greater proactive aggression when they had higher mentalizing capacities. The effects of mentalizing on reactive aggression were fully accounted for by its shared variance with proactive aggression. Psychopathic traits only partially explain aggression in adolescence. Mentalizing may serve as a protective factor preventing the emergence of proactive aggression in spite of psychopathic traits, and may represent a target for intervention to reduce aggression in such individuals (Taubner & Curth, 2013).

The mentalizing profile of ASPD across the four dimensions

In a sense it is self-evident that ASPD entails mentalizing difficulties and that a common path to violence is via momentary inhibition of the capacity to mentalize. However, it would be too simplistic to assert that individuals with ASPD have an outright mentalizing deficit. For example, there is evidence to suggest that, however paradoxically, better mentalizing ability in some areas (as alluded to earlier) may be linked with violence in mental disorders (see Box 2.12). Violent patients with schizophrenia, for example, tend to outperform their nonviolent counterparts on complex Theory of Mind tasks. As with BPD, we need to think in terms of mentalizing profiles and the subjective states they engender, rather than of "mentalizing" as a single entity. Individuals with ASPD can be better at external rather than internal, cognitive rather than affective, and impulsive-intuitive (automatic) rather than reflective (controlled) forms of mentalizing.

Since clinically normal people's mentalizing fluctuates according to context and mood, it follows that personality pathology does not arise simply because of a loss of mentalizing. First, it matters how easily individuals lose the capacity to mentalize. Some people are sensitive and reactive, and rapidly move to nonmentalizing modes in a wide range of contexts. Second, also it matters how quickly they regain mentalizing once it has been lost. We have suggested that a combination of frequent, rapid, and easily provoked losses of mentalizing within interpersonal relationships, with associated difficulties in regaining mentalizing and a consequent lengthy exposure to nonmentalizing modes of experience, is characteristic of BPD (Bateman & Fonagy, 2004). Third, mentalizing can become rigid, lacking flexibility. People with paranoid personality

---

Box 2.12 Mentalizing and ASPD

- Violent offenders show lower reflective functioning than nonviolent offenders
- Mentalizing in ASPD is more flexible than in paranoid, and possibly narcissistic, personality disorders
- People with ASPD may be expert at reading the minds of others, leading to misuse of mentalizing
- However, they show:
  - General reduction in ability to read emotions accurately
  - Failure to recognize fearful emotions from facial expressions
  - Lack of concern about victim distress
- Mentalizing may mediate between abuse and aggression in conduct disordered adolescents; mentalizing is a protective factor.

---

disorder, for example, often show rigid hypermentalizing with regard to their own internal mental states and lack any real understanding of others (Dimaggio et al., 2008; Nicolo & Nobile, 2007). At best they are suspicious of others' motives, and at worst they see people as having malign motives and cannot be persuaded otherwise.

From the point of view of implementing an MBT program for people with ASPD, we have to try to identify more explicitly the nature of their mentalizing deficits in terms of the dimensions of mentalizing. This is the aim of the second part of this chapter. To summarize our view: we believe that antisocial characteristics stabilize mentalizing by "rigidifying" otherwise unpredictable interpersonal relationships with the use of prementalistic modes of thinking.

Automatic versus controlled: a regular failure of automatic mentalizing

Controlled or explicit mentalizing, particularly when it is of a higher order, can be the apparent substance of psychological therapy. For example, a patient might be asked to reflect upon his/her awareness of what someone else might think about the same situation, or be asked to evaluate his/her own thoughts and appraise them more carefully against some agreed criteria. It is important to note that explicit mentalizing can be considered genuine and productive only when the link between these cognitions and direct experience of physical reality is comprehensive and strong. Cognitions, because of their "disembodied" character, can readily be distorted in largely self-serving ways, so that they end up extensively distorting, rather than representing, reality. If it suits me to ignore critical aspects of reality, such as the safety of the person I am with, I can drive at a dangerously high speed and report that my companion enjoyed the trip as much as I did. In this process, I ignored external cues from my companion as well as the intuitive products of implicit mentalizing, which I might have become aware of in relation to his experience as he was gripping, white-knuckled, the dashboard of the car. My elaboration of his mental state was thoroughly self-serving as, for whatever reason, I wanted to have company. If confronted, I might have partially acknowledged his distress, but this would not affect my behavior because the acknowledgement is merely intellectual.

This is a problem for people with ASPD, who may be asked in the course of treatment to undertake explicit mentalizing but who do not attach any emotional salience to the understanding (see Box 2.13). The link between cognition and emotional experience in both the self and others is tenuous. So asking a person with ASPD to consider others' mental states and to be compassionate about them can be done meaningfully only when their mentalizing is sufficiently robust for them to establish this link. However, beyond the weak contribution that automatic mentalizing makes—albeit greater relative to that made by controlled mentalizing—there may be a direct link between antisocial behavior and the imbalance between automatic and controlled mentalizing. As we have stressed earlier, to feel "real" and "meaningful," controlled/reflective mentalizing requires an appreciation of the wider context, based on intuitive awareness of the mental states of others. In a sense, the imbalance of automatic and controlled mentalizing permanently places individuals with ASPD in a position where they believe they do not experience explicit mentalizing as meaningful because it is not grounded in an intuitive, implicitly acquired experience of the other's intentional state. People with ASPD, who are limited in their capacity to resonate with others, feel that their explicit ideas about the

---

Box 2.13 Automatic versus controlled mentalizing in ASPD

- Persistent imbalance between implicit and explicit mentalizing
- Weak contribution and meaning is given to automatic mentalizing
- Controlled mentalizing processes are not experienced as meaningful
- Clinician should exercise caution about demanding explicit mentalizing in treatment until mentalizing is better established.

other—however accurate these might be—lack meaning, and therefore do not serve to regulate their own behavior. Even if I am aware that I am causing harm and distress because I turn up to work according to my convenience rather than my boss's need and I am aware that he sees me as someone who cannot be relied upon, this recognition has no power to alter my future behavior. Experience of the other's reaction and feeling does not constrain me.

Self versus other: a failure to see the self in the other

As we have said, individuals with ASPD are often adept at reading cognitive aspects of the inner states of others—even to the point that they misuse this capacity in self-serving ways or to coerce or manipulate others—while often being reluctant and probably unable to develop any real understanding of their own inner worlds (see Box 2.14). People with ASPD may be expert at reading other people's minds and misuse this, for example, in skillful lying. When I dissemble, I have to be ultra-aware of what the person I am lying to knows and does not know. This requires perspective-taking, which, as we have seen, individuals with ASPD are generally poor at. In fact, some individuals with ASPD are very poor liars precisely for this reason. However, others are excellent at distorting the truth. For example, some can maintain several identities, and to maintain each one are able to hold in mind what aspect of their past experience is shared by whoever it is they are talking to. So how can we account for this mixture of exceptional mentalizing and evidently quite limited capacity for social collaboration? We assume that the sacrifice of certain types of mentalizing frees up capacity for other domains to develop, along the same principles that Treffert (2010, 2014) described for the so-called savant syndrome. Just as

---

Box 2.14 Self versus other mentalizing in ASPD

- Ability to read others and to use this ability in self-serving ways—misuse of mentalizing
- Read minds from cognitive perspective but lack compassion for affective experience of other
- Paradox of skillful liars and poor liars
- Aim is not to facilitate social and personal collaboration but to exploit
- Reluctance to explore and understand their own inner world
- Overall, focus on own internal states by becoming selective experts in what others can do for them to meet *their* requirements.

only one in ten people with autism has savant skills (Treffert, 2014), so only a minority (perhaps, again, one in ten) of those with ASPD who show a pervasive disregard for the rights of others will also have unusual reflective, cognitive mentalizing abilities in relation to others. But, just as with the savant syndrome, it is the result of the unlocking of a genetically predefined capacity that these individuals have, rather than something they acquire in the same way as normally developing individuals do (via attachment relationships).

Leaving aside the paradox of the exceptional mentalizing capacity of some individuals, in general, the purpose of mentalizing the other for people with ASPD—regardless of ability—is primarily not to facilitate social collaboration but to exploit it for their own gain. Individuals with ASPD are relative experts at reading the inner states of others from a cognitive perspective but are unable to identify empathically with their states and be compassionate toward them. This asymmetry facilitates pervasive disregard for the rights of others (see later). In addition, they misuse their cognitive/other-focused mentalizing abilities to coerce or manipulate others. It is this sense of *partial* recognition of the mind of the other that is critical in permitting antisocial behavior. Recognition of the other person as having a separate mind will inhibit violence; the loss of mentalizing makes it possible to use the other to fulfill one's own needs, or to carry out a physical attack on them, as the other person becomes no more than a body or threatening presence. Individuals with ASPD may focus on themselves and their own internal states and become selective experts in getting others to do things for them to meet *their* requirements.

Thus, excessive concentration on either the self or the other leads to one-sided relationships and distortions in social interaction. Inevitably, this will be reflected in how individuals present for treatment and interact with their clinicians. People with ASPD tend to "fix" at one pole or other of the self–other dimension, sometimes depending on context.

Internal versus external: a failure to see the inside from outside

Internal mentalizing is a focus on one's own or others' internal states—that is, thoughts, feelings, and desires. External mentalizing implies a reliance on external features, such as facial expressions and behavior. As we described earlier, people with ASPD have been shown to have a limited response to expressed facial or otherwise externally depicted emotion; this suggests that mechanisms for acquiring information about mental states quickly and easily are profoundly compromised in these individuals (see Box 2.15).

Individuals with ASPD show a particular inability to read facial expressions that convey affect. If we mentalize someone so that we "feel" what they feel, it obviously makes it harder to hurt them, as we are constrained by their feelings.

> **Box 2.15 Internal versus external mentalizing in ASPD**
>
> ♦ Limited response to externally expressed emotions
> ♦ Less concern about external evidence of danger to self
> ♦ Most violent individuals have few concerns about the internal states of self and others
> ♦ Fewer references to internal states, related to low reporting of psychiatric symptoms and interpersonal problems
> ♦ More interest in understanding others from within increases engagement with treatment.

Aggressive acts are possible only if mentalizing is temporarily inhibited or decoupled. This makes good evolutionary sense. In a prospective study of 66 violent patients with personality disorder who were detained in a high-security hospital, who were interviewed in relation to their index offense, McGauley, Ferris, Marin-Avellan, and Fonagy (2013) found that the degree to which patients held internal (as opposed to external) representations of interpersonal violence and malevolence predicted subsequent violent behavior. Interestingly, those who were most likely to be violent—who were the least able to refer to internal states when describing their index offense—were also the patients who rated themselves as having fewer psychiatric symptoms and fewer problems in interpersonal relationships. This underscores our belief that prioritizing the external, as opposed to the internal, applies equally to the self and the other. It is also of note that in this sample patients who expressed a richer representation of the victim of their index offense from within also engaged better with treatment.

Mentalizing enables social collaboration by improving interpersonal understanding (Tomasello, 2014). Violence obviously reduces the chance of productive collaboration. So a capacity that has the potential simultaneously to advance a culture of collaboration *and* to inhibit violence will carry with it massive selective advantage from an evolutionary perspective. However, in certain circumstances, such as in a life-and-death struggle, being unable to be violent is a self-evident handicap. In such a situation, there is an advantage to being an individual with impaired sensitivity to the internal states of others. To be successful in such a situation, a social group has to contain both kinds of people. There is an obvious selective advantage in the group containing a certain proportion of individuals who are able to seriously harm others because they are unbothered by the external cues of distress they observe as they carry out a violent act. However, equally obviously, too many individuals like this would be dangerous and would threaten the capacity of the social group to work collaboratively. It is more desirable to vary the proportion of such individuals according to context: in some environments, having a larger pool of individuals who are capable of violence is an advantage; in other situations it will be disastrous. In the human species, such individuals may develop in two ways: genetics and early development. Later in this chapter (see section "ASPD, attachment, violence, and psychopathy"), we will return to the question of how natural selection may have solved the problem of environmental variability by using the attachment system as an "early warning system" to indicate to an infant the degree to which violent conduct may be required later in life.

Cognitive versus affective: a failure of affective mentalizing

Individuals with ASPD show considerable cognitive understanding of mental states, but are not in touch with the affective core of human experience (see Box 2.16). This makes the possibility of genuine empathy elusive for them. Youths with conduct problems have been shown to have a low reaction of their amygdala (the region of the brain that has a key role in processing emotions) in response to pictures that are normally considered emotionally arousing—for example, an image depicting a potentially painful aggressive act (Jones, Laurens, Herba, Barker, & Viding, 2009). In contrast, amygdala *hyperresponsiveness* has been observed in some youths with aggressive conduct disorder who were shown footage of, say, a hand being shut in a door (Decety, Michalska, Akitsuki, & Lahey, 2009). These amygdala responses correlated with parents' ratings of the youths' daring behavior and sadism. Such an increased amygdala response may indicate excitement in response to, or enjoyment of, others' pain. Both under- and over-responsiveness of the amygdala as found in these studies appears to be linked with antisocial behavior and dysfunction in terms of empathy.

Box 2.16 Cognitive versus affective mentalizing in BPD

- Understanding of cognitive mental states but relegation of the affective core of human experience (self and other)
- Cognitive understanding is used to control the mind states of others
- Avoidance of self-affect states—particularly of humiliation
- Reduced identification of a range of own emotions.

ASPD and the prementalizing modes

The significant characteristics of ASPD all reflect a shift to nonmentalizing (or prementalizing) ways of operating. We assume that in some individuals, perhaps those who have experienced attachment-related trauma such as severe parental maltreatment or exposure to domestic violence, activation of the attachment system inhibits aspects of mentalizing.

As described in Chapter 1, prementalizing mental function is characterized by psychic equivalence, pretend mode, and teleological mode (see Box 2.17). In *psychic equivalence*, the suspension of the sense of "as if" and the experience that everything is "for real" makes individuals' apparently exaggerated reactions understandable in view of the seriousness with which they experience their own and others' thoughts and feelings. Particularly relevant to ASPD is the impact of shame: when experienced in psychic equivalence, shame can be truly devastating; it is simply impossible to tolerate.

This state of affairs is a reflection of chronic imbalances in the dimensions of mentalizing. In individuals with antisocial behavior, the failure to detect underlying intentions of others and the tendency to assume motives based merely on external appearance can cause real social problems. What is often described as concrete thinking—another aspect of psychic equivalence—is a consequence of mentalizing that is excessively based on external cues and is implicit and non-reflective. The extreme reactions of individuals with ASPD are understandable

---

Box 2.17 Prementalizing modes in ASPD

- Psychic equivalence:
  - Due to imbalance in mentalizing dimensions
  - Shame and other emotions become potentially devastating
- Pretend mode:
  - Victim's mind detached from perpetrator's mind
  - Violence is possible, as not constrained
  - Lack of reflection on action, as there is no representation of the other's mind and no affective identification with the experience of the other
- Teleological mode:
  - Experience is valid only when consequences are apparent
  - Retribution needs to be physical (acceptance that others, e.g., justice system, prison, act according to same rules).

given their overemphasis on external indicators of internal states, which is unchecked by reflection; this can generate deeply disturbing expectations of other people's intentions.

Pretend mode allows the individual to undertake violence in a disconnected way, as if there is no psychological victim involved in a crime or the victim's mind is so alien and different from the perpetrator's that no continuity between the two could be established. In the absence of an appropriate balance between mentalizing the self and the other, thoughts and feelings can become dissociated almost to the point of meaninglessness. Emotional capacities such as guilt, love of others, and fear of consequences normally help to restrain violent behavior, but the loss of mentalizing and the stunted ability of some violent individuals to fully experience and resonate with such feelings prevent these inhibitory mechanisms from being mobilized. This is particularly the case if fear for one's self is absent and the dangers associated with violence become secondary. The onset of pretend mode makes the risk of being caught committing an offense seem unreal and creates an illusory sense of safety. The internal state no longer links with external reality: "It happened like in the movies"; "It didn't seem real."

Individuals with ASPD can sometimes reflect on their own antisocial actions in this mode and find nothing compelling to reflect on. A person with ASPD does not experience mental pain when thinking about someone else's state of mind; thus, attempting to generate behavior change in people with ASPD by "thinking about thinking" will typically be ineffective. Importantly, ordinary psychological therapy can be fruitless because the discussion of internal states carries little genuine connection with reality and is not experienced as having meaning.

The *teleological mode* tends to dominate motivation for actions in individuals with ASPD. In this mode, experience is felt to be valid when only its consequences are visibly and palpably apparent. Retribution has to be physical and observable. Intriguingly, the justice system has, by and large, adopted the same teleological stance. The logic of "justice being seen to be done" is acceptable to prisoners and guards in equal measure. Deviating from these simple principles and attempting to introduce psychological mindedness into the system is disconcerting to all and can create confusion (Gilligan, 2000). The stereotypical depiction of a successful antisocial individual as wearing ostentatious jewelry or an expensive watch, driving a luxury car, and demonstrating loyalty through violent attacks on enemies (and, similarly, requiring others to demonstrate loyalty to him in a similar way) may be a fantasy of scriptwriters, but it is based on an appreciation of the massive value placed by antisocial individuals on appearance and "face" (Gilligan, 2000).

ASPD and the alien self

Individuals with ASPD need relationships, whether within a gang-like group or in a more personal context. These relationships tend to be hierarchical and rigidly organized. However, the controlled and often limited nature of inter-actions within such relationships should not lead us to underestimate their intensity and significance; they are often characterized by a strong sense of loy-alty to and identification with the other. Such relationships can be of great importance to people with ASPD because they stabilize their sense of self, for two reasons: first, they can affirm and validate the individual's state (and this sense of affirmation and validation is often a rare experience for individuals with ASPD, given that their behavior often serves to alienate others). Second, social relationships often function as a place where the alien self can be exter-nalized. The other is made to host the unbearable feelings that might otherwise destabilize the person with ASPD's sense of self (see Figure 2.2; see Chapter 1 for further discussion of the alien self). In ASPD, the alien self has to be exter-nalized. This may occur in relation to a partner, who is made mindless and sub-servient ("Women needed to be treated like dogs. They need training and can only gradually be let off the lead"), or it may be in relation to a system ("The police pick on me, they follow me around and want to break me down"). These characterizations of relationships tend to be rigidly held, and anything that seems to threaten them can trigger arousal: for example, a partner wanting more independence. This arousal generates a fear of the loss of agency and sense of self, further impairing mentalizing. In a downward spiral, this further loss of mentalizing strengthens the sense of loss of agency and self, heightening the

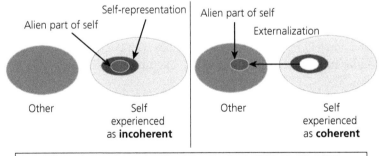

Fig. 2.2 The alien self and recovering self-coherence in ASPD.

perception of threat. The resolution of this spiral lies in externalizing the unbearable feelings of vulnerability, shame, or weakness on to someone else. The imperative to externalize the alien self creates challenges for treatment: the rigidity with which relationships are conceptualized needs to be challenged by the clinician, but with great care, as such a challenge may arouse feelings of violence and aggression because any perceived changes in relationships unleash a need for the violent assertion of control as an automatic response.

ASPD, attachment, violence, and psychopathy

Human infants are born with the potential to be aggressive and violent. As we discussed earlier, interpersonal aggression is a crucial evolutionary adaptation. In certain human environments, violence is likely to contribute materially to the survival of the individual's genes. However, in other contexts, violence is seriously maladaptive. Thus, violence is something that we should be potentially capable of, but able to desist from if our environment does not require us to be physically aggressive in order to survive. Given these moving goalposts, it not surprising that there is variation between individuals in the development of aggression and violence. Most preschool children make extensive use of physical aggression (Tremblay et al., 2004). Longitudinal studies such as the National Institute of Child Health and Human Development (NICHD) study (NICHD Early Child Care Research Network, 2004) have demonstrated that the earlier the onset of problem behaviors, the higher the risk for continued aggression and violence. Only a small proportion of individuals (perhaps 5–10%) are persistently physically aggressive; the remainder increasingly desist from aggression over the course of the first 10 years. Those who persist on a trajectory of violence have family environments that markedly differ from those who gradually desist. In a longitudinal study of over 10,000 individuals followed between 2 and 11 years, parenting-related factors differentiated children with persistently aggressive trajectories (Cote et al., 2007): children with high levels of stable aggression had far less positive interactions with their parent and experienced more hostile, ineffective parenting and substantially greater family dysfunction.

The quality of early attachment probably plays a critical role in guiding a young child's development toward or away from a more violent trajectory (see Box 2.18). Following John Bowlby's (1982) biological model of attachment, we have suggested that the early attachment relationship serves as a signaling system to the newborn, identifying the kind of environment they might expect to experience. An early choice of developmental trajectory is necessary because, as we have discussed, there is an evolutionary (reproductive) cost to following a trajectory of physical aggression. Secure attachment ensures that social

---

Box 2.18 ASPD and attachment

◆ Preschool children make extensive use of violence in their interactions

◆ Attachment has a critical role in the developmental trajectory toward low levels of violence

◆ Individuals with ASPD and a history of violence:

  • Have insecure-dismissing patterns of adult attachment

  • Tend to disavow the importance of attachment relationships

  • May deactivate attachment processes when possible.

---

cognitive capacities, such as emotional understanding, are adequately learned. But an environment where the caregivers do not have the time, resources, or inclination to devote attention to the infant is far more likely to call for the later use of violence than an environment where the infant's needs are attended to.

People with ASPD have typically never had the opportunity to learn about mental states in the context of appropriate attachment relationships. Alternatively, their attachment experiences may have been cruelly or consistently disrupted; for others, a nascent capacity for mentalizing may have been destroyed by an attachment figure who created sufficient anxiety in the child about their thoughts and feelings toward him/her for the child to wish to avoid thinking about the subjective experience of others. In a longitudinal analysis of a substantial high-risk sample, maternal withdrawal in infancy predicted the extent of ASPD features 20 years later, and did so independently of later childhood abuse (Shi, Bureau, Easterbrooks, Zhao, & Lyons-Ruth, 2012). In a follow-up of this sample in middle childhood, disorganized attachment behavior and maladaptive behavior at school added to the prediction of ASPD features in later life. These findings confirm how attachment can undermine social adaptation, which, in turn, increases the risk of violence. There is reasonable evidence from several cross-sectional studies that individuals with ASPD, especially those who have a history of violence, have insecure-dismissing patterns of adult attachment representations; that is, they cut themselves off from, and disavow the importance of, attachment relationships (Frodi, Dernevik, Sepa, Philipson, & Bragesjo, 2001; Levinson & Fonagy, 2004; van IJzendoorn et al., 1997). The early years of individuals who later develop ASPD are characterized by threats to the developing attachment system in the form of losses, separations, neglect, and physical and sexual abuse (Luntz & Widom, 1994; Pert, Ferriter, & Saul, 2004). Numerous studies have reported that psychosocial deprivation, including abuse, in childhood is associated with features of ASPD in adulthood (e.g., Kumari et al., 2013; Liu et al., 2012). Genetic factors may also be involved. Parents who demonstrate lower-quality caregiving may also pass on genes that confer risk for antisocial behavior. Twin and adoption studies will be necessary to determine whether environmental factors themselves confer risk for antisocial behavior, or whether there may be confounding genetic factors. There is also accumulating evidence indicating that the association between childhood maltreatment and externalizing problems is probably mediated by inadequate interpersonal understanding (social competences) and limited behavioral flexibility in response to environmental demands (e.g., Mayberry & Espelage, 2007).

Taking these observations together, we suggest that for individuals with ASPD the attachment system is kept deactivated by a process of denigration whereby the "other" is seen as less than human and is frequently left unmentalized, treated as a "thing" rather than a person. In failing to see the other as an intentional agent, he/she is relatively readily dehumanized; this removes (or temporarily reduces) a critical inhibitory barrier to violence against the other. In the presence of an enfeebled capacity to mentalize, nonmentalizing thinking predominates. Nonmentalized thinking in ASPD is characterized by poor intuition about mental state drivers of behavior, failure to envision the experience of the other linked to self-experience, failure to depict the internal experience of the other based on external cues, and failure to mentalize emotion fully. There is a shift from the mental to the physical, such that individuals with ASPD experience their own mental states and those of others in physical and bodily modes; again, this opens the way to violent behavior. Violent acts are likely to occur either as a response to misperceiving the world, including the actions or intentions of others (e.g., experiencing a dismissing comment in psychic equivalence as destructively shaming), or to evacuate intolerable mental affects or bodily sensations, linked to the alien self, that cannot be thought about.

In relation to early childhood experience we will also address the issue of *psychopathy* here. Psychopaths share many of the features of ASPD, but manifest additional interpersonal and affective features (shallow affect, low anxiety/fear, impulsivity, dominance, callousness, superficial charm, and manipulativeness). Some individuals diagnosed with ASPD have psychopathic traits, but most do not. It has been suggested by some clinicians that although psychopathy and ASPD share many features, the underlying psychobiological processes may be distinct and, furthermore, that these features place them beyond what would be accessible to modification by a psychosocial treatment. Studies looking at populations of offenders can reliably delineate and validate meaningful subgroups with different types of ASPD based on personality traits identified with psychopathy. These are: non-psychopathic ASPD; a small group of primary psychopaths; a group in which psychopathy appears secondary to antisocial behavior; and a group characterized by fearful psychopathy, probably reflecting a dual diagnosis (Cox et al., 2013; Poythress et al., 2010). It is the proclivity for instrumental aggression (planned aggression to obtain a goal) that best distinguishes psychopaths from their non-psychopathic antisocial and conduct disordered counterparts. In contrast to reactive (affective) aggression, which typically is impulsive and stems from frustration and anger, instrumental aggression is deliberate, calculated, and goal-directed. The lack of responsiveness to socialization—nothing deters it—plays a major role in the etiology of such behavior.

Numerous findings highlight the importance of affective–interpersonal traits in distinguishing psychopathy from ASPD. In one study, psychopathic participants (nearly all of whom also met criteria for comorbid ASPD) manifested a diminished defensive response to threat compared to non-psychopathic ASPD participants (Drislane, Vaidyanathan, & Patrick, 2013). Non-psychopathic ASPD participants responded in the same way as typical adults, and the deficit in defensively responding to threat was associated with the affective–interpersonal features of the disorder. Magnetic resonance imaging studies also suggest that violent individuals diagnosed with comorbid psychopathy and ASPD have structural brain anomalies (significantly reduced gray matter volume), but the brain structure of those with only an ASPD diagnosis appears similar to that of non-offenders (Gregory et al., 2012). In contrast to the history reported by individuals with psychopathy, trauma plays a greater role in *reactive aggression*, inasmuch as trauma sensitizes individuals to stress, lowering the threshold for emotional reactivity (Allen, 2004). Blair (2008) proposes that psychopaths are *less* vulnerable to potentially traumatic stressors by virtue of their emotional under-reactivity.

We have considered psychopathy at some length here in order to advise clinicians against including individuals with personality features usually identified with psychopathy in MBT treatment programs. We are convinced that the model outlined in this book poorly fits the group described as primary psychopaths (Poythress et al., 2010), whether for biological or other etiological reasons. However, we should be cautious about expanding this group too widely. A child or young person may show an apparent callousness that is rooted in anxiety about attachment relationships: they may not actually be callous and unemotional (Frick & Viding, 2009), but terrified and perhaps striving for a more reliable attachment (Fonagy, 2004). It is such cases that we would be primarily concerned with here. As described earlier, a harsh early childhood environment could have signaled a greater future need for interpersonal violence, as well as undermining the normal development of cognitive and affective means of expressing underlying mental states. In summary, in the treatment of ASPD, we suggest that the clinician has to understand the pathway that leads to loss of control and has to accept the individual's need to structure their interactions with others in a way that maintains externalization of the alien self. The individual with ASPD has experienced developmental disturbance in their attachment relationship(s), with experiences of shame and humiliation at the fore. Robust development of mentalizing is lost, leaving a lifelong sensitivity to internal emotional states. Within psychic equivalence, any experience of shame, however small, is experienced as a collapse of the self in a mental context in which there is no buffer of secondary representational levels to cope with the experience. The threat to the self, which is in effect a return of the shameful alien self, has to be controlled to survive. Rather than managing the underlying mental state of terror through representation and emotional processing, the inner alarm is relieved by controlling the physical environment (e.g., via coercion and violence). The essence of treatment is to stimulate affiliative bonds *without* simultaneously provoking the threat of shame and humiliation. At the same time, feelings of trust, honesty, and openness within the context of the attachment process have to be nurtured.

Summary of outcome studies of MBT

Borderline personality disorder

There have been several recent reviews of psychosocial interventions for BPD. These recognize the evidence base for MBT for BPD as generally inferior only to the evidence base for dialectical behavior therapy (e.g., Budge et al., 2013; Nelson et al., 2014; Stoffers et al., 2012), although not from a health economic perspective (Brettschneider, Riedel-Heller, & Konig, 2014). Encouragingly, a large qualitative study of patients' treatment goals established that the goals of MBT were closely allied with what patients hoped to gain from their therapies (Katsakou et al., 2012).

A small number of randomized controlled trials (RCTs) and a number of naturalistic studies have tested the effectiveness of the MBT approach for BPD patients. In an RCT of MBT for BPD in a partial hospital setting (Bateman & Fonagy, 1999, 2001), an 18-month program achieved significant and enduring changes in mood states and interpersonal functioning. Outcome measures included frequency of suicide attempts and acts of self-harm, number and duration of inpatient admissions, service utilization, and self-report measures of depression, anxiety, general symptom distress, interpersonal function, and social adjustment. The benefits, relative to treatment as usual (TAU), were large, with a number needed to treat of approximately two; in addition, the benefits were observed to increase during the follow-up period of 18 months. Analysis of participants' healthcare use suggested that day hospital treatment for BPD was no more expensive than general psychiatric care and showed considerable cost savings after treatment. A follow-up study of BPD patients 5 years after all treatment was completed and 8 years after initial entry into treatment, comparing patients treated with MBT and those receiving TAU, found that those who received MBT remained better than the TAU group. Superior levels of improvement were shown on levels of suicidality (23% in the MBT group vs. 74% in TAU group), diagnostic status (13% vs. 87%), service use (2 years vs. 3.5 years), and other measurements such as use of medication, global functioning, and vocational status (Bateman & Fonagy, 2008).

Two well-controlled single-blind trials of outpatient MBT have been conducted, one with adults with BPD (Bateman & Fonagy, 2009) and the second with adolescents presenting to clinical services with self-harm, the vast majority of whom met BPD criteria (Rossouw & Fonagy, 2012). In both trials, MBT was found to be superior to TAU in reducing self-harm (including suicidality) and depression. Importantly, in the adult trial, the control group received a manualized, highly efficacious treatment, structured clinical management (Bateman & Fonagy, 2009); MBT was superior to this intervention, particularly in the long term (Bateman & Fonagy, 2013). A post hoc analysis of moderators found that the number of personality disorder diagnoses in addition to BPD was the key indicator of severity that predicted the need for the MBT approach, as structured clinical management appeared to have little benefit on most outcome measures among these patients (Bateman & Fonagy, 2013). Furthermore, in the trial with an adolescent sample, improvements generated by MBT appear to have been mediated by improved levels of mentalizing, reduced attachment avoidance, and amelioration of participants' emergent BPD features; participants treated with MBT showed a recovery rate of 44%, compared to 17% of those who received TAU (Rossouw & Fonagy, 2012). It should be noted that the evidence for mentalizing mediating therapeutic change in MBT is currently limited, and more evidence is available in relation to mentalizing mediating change in other treatment modalities (Forster, Berthollier, & Rawlinson, 2014; Goodman, 2013). Ongoing follow-ups of both these trials indicate that improvements in the MBT groups have been at least maintained, and in most cases improvements continued after treatment termination and differences relative to the comparison group remain significant.

Three recent studies provide further support for the efficacy of MBT in BPD. An RCT from Denmark investigated the efficacy of MBT versus a less intensive, manualized supportive group therapy in patients diagnosed with BPD

(Jørgensen et al., 2013). Patients were randomly allocated to MBT (n = 58) or the manualized supportive therapy (n = 27). Each intervention was delivered in combination with psychoeducation and medication. Both the combined MBT and the less intensive supportive therapy brought about significant improvements on a range of psychological and interpersonal measures (e.g., general functioning, depression, and social functioning) and decreased the number of diagnostic criteria met for BPD; effect sizes were large (d = 0.5–2.1). The combined MBT was superior to the less intensive supportive group therapy on clinician-rated Global Assessment of Functioning. An 18-month naturalistic follow-up found that treatment effects at termination were sustained at 18 months (Jørgensen et al., 2014). Half of the patients in the MBT group met criteria for functional remission at follow-up, compared with less than one-fifth in the supportive therapy group, but three-quarters of both groups achieved diagnostic remission, and almost half of the patients had attained symptomatic remission. A limitation of this study is that the same clinicians delivered both interventions (and thus there was a high risk of spillover effects between the two treatments); incomplete data was a further significant limitation. In another study from Denmark (Petersen et al., 2010), a cohort of patients treated with partial hospitalization followed by group MBT showed significant improvements after treatment (average length 2 years) on a range of measures including Global Assessment of Functioning, hospitalizations, and vocational status, with further improvement at 2-year follow-up.

A quality improvement study examined the outcomes for BPD patients treated in an MBT program in a Norwegian specialist treatment unit compared with a former psychodynamic treatment program (Kvarstein et al., 2015). This longitudinal comparison had a sample of 345 BPD patients, including 281 patients treated on the psychodynamic program and 64 who received MBT, who had comparable baseline severity and impairments of functioning on all measures. Outcome measures included Symptom Checklist-90 symptom distress, interpersonal problems, and global functioning assessed routinely throughout treatment, and suicidal/self-harming acts, hospital admissions, medication, and occupational status assessed at baseline and discharge. The change in program from traditional psychodynamic therapy to MBT led to a reduction in unplanned discharges (MBT had a low dropout rate of 2%). Measured benefits from the change of program included greater improvements in symptom distress and interpersonal, global, and occupational functioning. Although the change was associated with the introduction of MBT, specific causal attributions are hard to establish in such a design.

A naturalistic study by Bales et al. (2012) in the Netherlands investigated the effectiveness of an 18-month manualized program of MBT in 45 patients diagnosed with severe BPD. There was a high prevalence of comorbidity of DSM-IV Axis I and Axis II disorders. Results showed significant positive change in symptom distress, social and interpersonal functioning, and personality pathology and functioning; effect sizes were moderate to large ($d = 0.7$–1.7). The study also showed that the use of additional treatments and psychiatric inpatient admissions decreased significantly during and after treatment. The lack of a control group in this study limits the ability to draw conclusions about the efficacy of MBT. Another study (Bales et al., 2015) applied propensity score matching to determine the best matches for 29 MBT patients from within a larger (n = 175) group who received other specialized psychotherapeutic treatments. These other specialized treatments yielded improvement across domains, which was generally only moderate; in contrast, pre–post effect sizes were consistently large for MBT, with Cohen's d for reduction in psychiatric symptoms of -1.06 and -1.42 at 18 and 36 months, respectively, and ds ranging from 0.81 to 2.08 for improvement in domains of personality functioning. Given the nonrandomized study design and the variation in treatment dose received by participants, the between-condition difference in effects should be interpreted cautiously. A multisite randomized trial by the same group comparing intensive outpatient and partial hospitalization-based MBT for patients with BPD is currently underway (Laurenssen, Westra, et al., 2014).

A recent naturalistic pilot trial studied the feasibility and effectiveness of an inpatient adaptation of MBT in 11 female adolescents (aged 14–18 years) with borderline symptoms (Laurenssen, Hutsebaut, et al., 2014). One year after the start of treatment, significant decreases in symptoms and improvements in personality functioning and quality of life were observed; effect sizes were between $d = 0.58$ and 1.46, representing medium to large effects. Further, 91% (n = 10) of the adolescents showed reliable change on the Brief Symptom Inventory and 18% (n = 2) moved to the functional range on this measure. A report of the application of MBT principles to a therapeutic community also yielded positive results (Jones, Juett, & Hill, 2013). Patients who completed 18 months of treatment showed significant self- and clinician-rated symptomatic improvement and significant change on clinician-administered measures of social and occupational functioning.

Antisocial personality disorder

Research into treatment for ASPD up to the year 2009 is summarized in the UK NICE clinical guideline for ASPD (National Institute for Health and Clinical Excellence 2010), which confirmed that interventions for ASPD are poorly researched and that evidence on its treatment is scarce. The authors of the NICE guideline concluded that the evidence for treatments for ASPD was extremely

limited, and did not support the development of any treatment recommendations (National Institute for Health and Clinical Excellence 2010). We have rep-
licated the NICE search but focusing on papers published from 2009 on, using
a search strategy consisting of RCT and systematic review filters combined with
subject heading and free-text phrases for ASPD. The search yielded only five
results meeting the selection criteria: three trials and two Cochrane reviews.
Only one paper mentioned research conducted in a community setting (Davidson et al., 2009); this study of cognitive behavioral therapy was an exploratory
trial rather than a full RCT. The two Cochrane reviews concluded that there was
no consistent evidence for any intervention for ASPD, and recommended that
research to test interventions for the disorder is urgently needed (Gibbon et al.,
2010; Khalifa et al., 2010).

A feasibility study of MBT for ASPD by McGauley, Yakeley, Williams, and
Bateman (2011) reports findings from a small sample (n = 9) receiving group
and individual MBT at the Tavistock and Portman Foundation Trust in London, United Kingdom. Preliminary results on the Overt Aggression Scale suggested that the participants rated the severity of their aggression toward others
and themselves as decreasing over the first 6.5 months of treatment; in contrast,
their rating of irritability did not change. Psychiatric symptom severity on the
Brief Symptom Inventory showed a reduction in the distress participants experienced in relation to their symptoms at 6-month follow-up, with participants
reporting greatest decreases in distress resulting from symptoms of depression,
anxiety, and hostility.

Finally, we note that a significant subsample of the participants in the outpatient treatment trial of MBT for BPD described earlier (Bateman & Fonagy,
2009) also met criteria for ASPD. A separate analysis of these individuals with
comorbid ASPD revealed that they benefited significantly from MBT.

References

Allen, J. G. (2004). *Coping with trauma: A guide to self-understanding* (2nd ed.).
Washington, DC: American Psychiatric Press.

American Psychiatric Association. (2013). *Diagnostic and statistical manual of mental
disorders* (5th ed.). Washington, DC: American Psychiatric Association.

Baer, R. A., Peters, J. R., Eisenlohr-Moul, T. A., Geiger, P. J., & Sauer, S. E. (2012).
Emotion-related cognitive processes in borderline personality disorder: A review of the
empirical literature. *Clinical Psychology Review*, **32**, 359–369.

Bales, D., van Beek, N., Smits, M., Willemsen, S., Busschbach, J. J., Verheul, R., & Andrea,
H. (2012). Treatment outcome of 18-month, day hospital mentalization-based
treatment (MBT) in patients with severe borderline personality disorder in the
Netherlands. *Journal of Personality Disorders*, **26**, 568–582.

Bales, D. L., Timman, R., Andrea, H., Busschbach, J. J., Verheul, R., & Kamphuis, J. H. (2015). Effectiveness of day hospital mentalization-based treatment for patients with severe borderline personality disorder: A matched control study. *Clinical Psychology and Psychotherapy*, **22**, 409–417.

Bateman, A., & Fonagy, P. (1999). Effectiveness of partial hospitalization in the treatment of borderline personality disorder: A randomized controlled trial. *American Journal of Psychiatry*, **156**, 1563–1569.

Bateman, A., & Fonagy, P. (2001). Treatment of borderline personality disorder with psychoanalytically oriented partial hospitalization: An 18-month follow-up. *American Journal of Psychiatry*, **158**, 36–42.

Bateman, A., & Fonagy, P. (2004). *Psychotherapy for borderline personality disorder: Mentalization-based treatment*. Oxford, UK: Oxford University Press.

Bateman, A., & Fonagy, P. (2008). 8-year follow-up of patients treated for borderline personality disorder: Mentalization-based treatment versus treatment as usual. *American Journal of Psychiatry*, **165**, 631–638.

Bateman, A., & Fonagy, P. (2009). Randomized controlled trial of outpatient mentalization-based treatment versus structured clinical management for borderline personality disorder. *American Journal of Psychiatry*, **166**, 1355–1364.

Bateman, A., & Fonagy, P. (2013). Impact of clinical severity on outcomes of mentalisation-based treatment for borderline personality disorder. *British Journal of Psychiatry*, **203**, 221–227.

Black, D. W., Blum, N., Pfohl, B., & Hale, N. (2004). Suicidal behavior in borderline personality disorder: Prevalence, risk factors, prediction, and prevention. *Journal of Personality Disorders*, **18**, 226–239.

Blair, J. (2008). Empathic dysfunction in psychopathy. In C. Sharp, P. Fonagy & I. Goodyer (Eds.), *Social cognition and developmental psychopathology* (pp. 175–197). Oxford, UK: Oxford University Press.

Blair, R. J., Jones, L., Clark, F., & Smith, M. (1997). The psychopathic individual: A lack of responsiveness to distress cues? *Psychophysiology*, **34**, 192–198.

Bornovalova, M. A., Matusiewicz, A., & Rojas, E. (2011). Distress tolerance moderates the relationship between negative affect intensity with borderline personality disorder levels. *Comprehensive Psychiatry*, **52**, 744–753.

Bowlby, J. (1982). *Attachment and loss. Volume I: Attachment* (2nd ed.). New York, NY: Basic Books.

Brettschneider, C., Riedel-Heller, S., & Konig, H. H. (2014). A systematic review of economic evaluations of treatments for borderline personality disorder. *PLOS ONE*, **9**, e107748.

Budge, S. L., Moore, J. T., Del Re, A. C., Wampold, B. E., Baardseth, T. P., & Nienhuis, J. B. (2013). The effectiveness of evidence-based treatments for personality disorders when comparing treatment-as-usual and bona fide treatments. *Clinical Psychology Review*, **33**, 1057–1066.

Chapman, A. L., Leung, D. W., & Lynch, T. R. (2008). Impulsivity and emotion dysregulation in borderline personality disorder. *Journal of Personality Disorders*, **22**, 148–164.

Cote, S. M., Boivin, M., Nagin, D. S., Japel, C., Xu, Q., Zoccolillo, M., . . . Tremblay, R. E. (2007). The role of maternal education and nonmaternal care services in the prevention of children's physical aggression problems. *Archives of General Psychiatry*, **64**, 1305–1312.

Cox, J., Edens, J. F., Magyar, M. S., Lilienfeld, S. O., Douglas, K. S., & Poythress, N. G. (2013). Using the Psychopathic Personality Inventory to identify subtypes of antisocial personality disorder. *Journal of Criminal Justice*, **41**, 125–134.

Davidson, K. M., Tyrer, P., Tata, P., Cooke, D., Gumley, A., Ford, I., . . . Crawford, M. J. (2009). Cognitive behaviour therapy for violent men with antisocial personality disorder in the community: An exploratory randomized controlled trial. *Psychological Medicine*, **39**, 569–577.

Decety, J., Michalska, K. J., Akitsuki, Y., & Lahey, B. B. (2009). Atypical empathic responses in adolescents with aggressive conduct disorder: A functional MRI investigation. *Biological Psychology*, **80**, 203–211.

Dimaggio, G., Lysaker, P. H., Carcione, A., Nicolo, G., & Semerari, A. (2008). Know yourself and you shall know the other . . . to a certain extent: Multiple paths of influence of self-reflection on mindreading. *Consciousness and Cognition*, **17**, 778–789.

Domes, G., Schulze, L., & Herpertz, S. C. (2009). Emotion recognition in borderline personality disorder—A review of the literature. *Journal of Personality Disorders*, **23**, 6–19.

Drislane, L. E., Vaidyanathan, U., & Patrick, C. J. (2013). Reduced cortical call to arms differentiates psychopathy from antisocial personality disorder. *Psychological Medicine*, **43**, 825–835.

Ebner-Priemer, U. W., Kuo, J., Schlotz, W., Kleindienst, N., Rosenthal, M. Z., Detterer, L., . . . Bohus, M. (2008). Distress and affective dysregulation in patients with borderline personality disorder: A psychophysiological ambulatory monitoring study. *Journal of Nervous and Mental Disease*, **196**, 314–320.

Fonagy, P. (2004). Early life trauma and the psychogenesis and prevention of violence. *Annals of the New York Academy of Sciences*, **1036**, 1–20.

Fonagy, P., Leigh, T., Steele, M., Steele, H., Kennedy, R., Mattoon, G., . . . Gerber, A. (1996). The relation of attachment status, psychiatric classification, and response to psychotherapy. *Journal of Consulting and Clinical Psychology*, **64**, 22–31.

Fonagy, P., & Luyten, P. (2016). A multilevel perspective on the development of borderline personality disorder. In D. Cicchetti (Ed.), *Developmental psychopathology* (3rd ed.). New York, NY: John Wiley & Sons.

Forster, C., Berthollier, N., & Rawlinson, D. (2014). A systematic review of potential mechanisms of change in psychotherapeutic interventions for personality disorder. *Journal of Psychology and Psychotherapy*, **4**, 133.

Frick, P. J., & Viding, E. (2009). Antisocial behavior from a developmental psychopathology perspective. *Development and Psychopathology*, **21**, 1111–1131.

Frodi, A., Dernevik, M., Sepa, A., Philipson, J., & Bragesjo, M. (2001). Current attachment representations of incarcerated offenders varying in degree of psychopathy. *Attachment and Human Development*, **3**, 269–283.

Gibbon, S., Duggan, C., Stoffers, J., Huband, N., Vollm, B. A., Ferriter, M., & Lieb, K. (2010). Psychological interventions for antisocial personality disorder. *Cochrane Database of Systematic Reviews*, **6**, CD007668.

Gilligan, J. (2000). *Violence: Reflections on our deadliest epidemic*. London, UK: Jessica Kingsley.

Goodman, G. (2013). Is mentalization a common process factor in transference-focused psychotherapy and dialectical behavior therapy sessions? *Journal of Psychotherapy Integration*, **23**, 179–192.

Grant, B. F., Chou, S. P., Goldstein, R. B., Huang, B., Stinson, F. S., Saha, T. D., . . . Ruan, W. J. (2008). Prevalence, correlates, disability, and comorbidity of DSM-IV borderline personality disorder: Results from the Wave 2 National Epidemiologic Survey on Alcohol and Related Conditions. *Journal of Clinical Psychiatry*, **69**, 533–545.

Gratz, K. L., Breetz, A., & Tull, M. T. (2010). The moderating role of borderline personality in the relationships between deliberate self-harm and emotion-related factors. *Personality and Mental Health*, **4**, 96–107.

Gratz, K. L., Rosenthal, M. Z., Tull, M. T., Lejuez, C. W., & Gunderson, J. G. (2006). An experimental investigation of emotion dysregulation in borderline personality disorder. *Journal of Abnormal Psychology*, **115**, 850–855.

Gregory, S., Ffytche, D., Simmons, A., Kumari, V., Howard, M., Hodgins, S., & Blackwood, N. (2012). The antisocial brain: Psychopathy matters. *Archives of General Psychiatry*, **69**, 962–972.

Gunderson, J. G., & Lyons-Ruth, K. (2008). BPD's interpersonal hypersensitivity phenotype: A gene-environment-developmental model. *Journal of Personality Disorders*, **22**, 22–41.

Hazlett, E. A., Speiser, L. J., Goodman, M., Roy, M., Carrizal, M., Wynn, J. K., . . . New, A. S. (2007). Exaggerated affect-modulated startle during unpleasant stimuli in borderline personality disorder. *Biological Psychiatry*, **62**, 250–255.

Jacob, G. A., Guenzler, C., Zimmermann, S., Scheel, C. N., Rusch, N., Leonhart, R., . . . Lieb, K. (2008). Time course of anger and other emotions in women with borderline personality disorder: A preliminary study. *Journal of Behavior Therapy and Experimental Psychiatry*, **39**, 391–402.

Jones, A. P., Laurens, K. R., Herba, C. M., Barker, G. J., & Viding, E. (2009). Amygdala hypoactivity to fearful faces in boys with conduct problems and callous-unemotional traits. *American Journal of Psychiatry*, **166**, 95–102.

Jones, B., Juett, G., & Hill, N. (2013). Initial outcomes of a therapeutic community-based outpatient programme in the management of personality disorder. *Therapeutic Communities: The International Journal of Therapeutic Communities*, **34**, 41–52.

Jørgensen, C. R., Bøye, R., Andersen, D., Døssing Blaabjerg, A. H., Freund, C., Jordet, H., & Kjølbye, M. (2014). Eighteen months post-treatment naturalistic follow-up study of mentalization-based therapy and supportive group treatment of borderline personality disorder: Clinical outcomes and functioning. *Nordic Psychology*, **66**, 254–273.

Jørgensen, C. R., Freund, C., Bøye, R., Jordet, H., Andersen, D., & Kjølbye, M. (2013). Outcome of mentalization-based and supportive psychotherapy in patients with borderline personality disorder: A randomized trial. *Acta Psychiatrica Scandinavica*, **127**, 305–317.

Katsakou, C., Marougka, S., Barnicot, K., Savill, M., White, H., Lockwood, K., & Priebe, S. (2012). Recovery in borderline personality disorder (BPD): A qualitative study of service users' perspectives. *PLOS ONE*, **7**, e36517.

Khalifa, N., Duggan, C., Stoffers, J., Huband, N., Vollm, B. A., Ferriter, M., & Lieb, K. (2010). Pharmacological interventions for antisocial personality disorder. *Cochrane Database of Systematic Reviews*, **8**, CD007667.

Kumari, V., Gudjonsson, G. H., Raghuvanshi, S., Barkataki, I., Taylor, P., Sumich, A., . . . Das, M. (2013). Reduced thalamic volume in men with antisocial personality disorder or schizophrenia and a history of serious violence and childhood abuse. *European Psychiatry*, **28**, 225–234.

Kvarstein, E. H., Pedersen, G., Urnes, O., Hummelen, B., Wilberg, T., & Karterud, S. (2015). Changing from a traditional psychodynamic treatment programme to mentalization-based treatment for patients with borderline personality disorder—does it make a difference? *Psychology and Psychotherapy*, **88**, 71–86.

Laurenssen, E. M., Hutsebaut, J., Feenstra, D. J., Bales, D. L., Noom, M. J., Busschbach, J. J., . . . Luyten, P. (2014). Feasibility of mentalization-based treatment for adolescents with borderline symptoms: A pilot study. *Psychotherapy*, **51**, 159–166.

Laurenssen, E. M., Westra, D., Kikkert, M. J., Noom, M. J., Eeren, H. V., van Broekhuyzen, A. J., . . . Dekker, J. J. (2014). Day hospital mentalization-based treatment (MBT-DH) versus treatment as usual in the treatment of severe borderline personality disorder: Protocol of a randomized controlled trial. *BMC Psychiatry*, **14**, 149.

Levinson, A., & Fonagy, P. (2004). Offending and attachment: The relationship between interpersonal awareness and offending in a prison population with psychiatric disorder. *Canadian Journal of Psychoanalysis*, **12**, 225–251.

Links, P. S., Eynan, R., Heisel, M. J., & Nisenbaum, R. (2008). Elements of affective instability associated with suicidal behaviour in patients with borderline personality disorder. *Canadian Journal of Psychiatry*, **53**, 112–116.

Liu, N., Zhang, Y., Brady, H. J., Cao, Y., He, Y., & Zhang, Y. (2012). Relation between childhood maltreatment and severe intrafamilial male-perpetrated physical violence in Chinese community: The mediating role of borderline and antisocial personality disorder features. *Aggressive Behavior*, **38**, 64–76.

Luntz, B. K., & Widom, C. S. (1994). Antisocial personality disorder in abused and neglected children grown up. *American Journal of Psychiatry*, **151**, 670–674.

Marsh, A. A., & Blair, R. J. (2008). Deficits in facial affect recognition among antisocial populations: A meta-analysis. *Neuroscience and Biobehavioral Reviews*, **32**, 454–465.

Mayberry, M. L., & Espelage, D. L. (2007). Associations among empathy, social competence, & reactive/proactive aggression subtypes. *Journal of Youth and Adolescence*, **36**, 787–798.

McGauley, G., Ferris, S., Marin-Avellan, L., & Fonagy, P. (2013). The Index Offence Representation Scales; a predictive clinical tool in the management of dangerous, violent patients with personality disorder? *Criminal Behaviour and Mental Health*, **23**, 274–289.

McGauley, G., Yakeley, J., Williams, A., & Bateman, A. (2011). Attachment, mentalization and antisocial personality disorder: The possible contribution of mentalization-based treatment. *European Journal of Psychotherapy and Counselling*, **13**, 371–393.

National Institute for Health and Clinical Excellence. (2010). *Antisocial personality disorder: Treatment, management and prevention*. London, UK: The British Psychological Society and the Royal College of Psychiatrists. Retrieved from http://www.nccmh.org.uk/downloads/ASPD/ASPD%20published%20full%20guideline%20-%20amended%20June%202013.pdf

Nelson, K. J., Zagoloff, A., Quinn, S., Swanson, H. E., Garber, C., & Schulz, S. C. (2014). Borderline personality disorder: Treatment approaches and perspectives. *Clinical Practice*, **11**, 341–349.

Newbury-Helps, J., Feigenbaum, J., & Fonagy, P. (in press). Offenders with antisocial personality disorder display more impairments in mentalizing. *Journal of Personality Disorders*.

NICHD Early Child Care Research Network. (2004). Trajectories of physical aggression from toddlerhood to middle childhood: Predictors, correlates, and outcomes. *Monographs of the Society for Research in Child Development*, **69**, 1–129.

Nicolo, G., & Nobile, M. (2007). Paranoid personality disorder: model and treatment. In G. Dimaggio & A. Semerari (Eds.), *Psychotherapy of personality disorders: Metacognition, states of mind and interpersonal cycles* (pp. 188–220). Hove, UK: Routledge.

Pert, L., Ferriter, M., & Saul, C. (2004). Parental loss before the age of 16 years: A comparative study of patients with personality disorder and patients with schizophrenia in a high secure hospital's population. *Psychology and Psychotherapy*, **77**, 403–407.

Petersen, B., Toft, J., Christensen, N. B., Foldager, L., Munk-Jorgensen, P., Windfeld, M., . . . Valbak, K. (2010). A 2-year follow-up of mentalization-oriented group therapy following day hospital treatment for patients with personality disorders. *Personality and Mental Health*, **4**, 294–301.

Poythress, N. G., Edens, J. F., Skeem, J. L., Lilienfeld, S. O., Douglas, K. S., Frick, P. J., . . . Wang, T. (2010). Identifying subtypes among offenders with antisocial personality disorder: A cluster-analytic study. *Journal of Abnormal Psychology*, **119**, 389–400.

Preissler, S., Dziobek, I., Ritter, K., Heekeren, H. R., & Roepke, S. (2010). Social cognition in borderline personality disorder: Evidence for disturbed recognition of the emotions, thoughts, and intentions of others. *Frontiers in Behavioral Neuroscience*, **4**, 182.

Reich, D. B., Zanarini, M. C., & Fitzmaurice, G. (2012). Affective lability in bipolar disorder and borderline personality disorder. *Comprehensive Psychiatry*, **53**, 230–237.

Reisch, T., Ebner-Priemer, U. W., Tschacher, W., Bohus, M., & Linehan, M. M. (2008). Sequences of emotions in patients with borderline personality disorder. *Acta Psychiatrica Scandinavica*, **118**, 42–48.

Rossouw, T. I., & Fonagy, P. (2012). Mentalization-based treatment for self-harm in adolescents: A randomized controlled trial. *Journal of the American Academy of Child and Adolescent Psychiatry*, **51**, 1304–1313.e3.

Salsman, N. L., & Linehan, M. M. (2012). An investigation of the relationships among negative affect, difficulties in emotion regulation, and features of borderline personality disorder. *Journal of Psychopathology and Behavioral Assessment*, **34**, 260–267.

Santangelo, P., Bohus, M., & Ebner-Priemer, U. W. (2014). Ecological momentary assessment in borderline personality disorder: A review of recent findings and methodological challenges. *Journal of Personality Disorders*, **28**, 555–576.

Sharp, C. (2014). The social-cognitive basis of BPD: A theory of hypermentalizing. In C. Sharp & J. L. Tackett (Eds.), *Handbook of borderline personality disorder in children and adolescents* (pp. 211–226). New York, NY: Springer.

Shi, Z., Bureau, J. F., Easterbrooks, M. A., Zhao, X., & Lyons-Ruth, K. (2012). Childhood maltreatment and prospectively observed quality of early care as predictors of antisocial personality disorder features. *Infant Mental Health Journal*, **33**, 55–96.

Singleton, N., Neltzer, H., Gatward, R., Coid, J., & Deasy, D. (1998). *Psychiatric morbidity among prisoners in England and Wales*. London, UK: Office of National Statistics, HM Government.

Soloff, P. H., & Fabio, A. (2008). Prospective predictors of suicide attempts in borderline personality disorder at one, two, and two-to-five year follow-up. *Journal of Personality Disorders*, **22**, 123–134.

Soloff, P. H., Feske, U., & Fabio, A. (2008). Mediators of the relationship between childhood sexual abuse and suicidal behavior in borderline personality disorder. *Journal of Personality Disorders*, **22**, 221–232.

Stoffers, J. M., Vollm, B. A., Rucker, G., Timmer, A., Huband, N., & Lieb, K. (2012). Psychological therapies for people with borderline personality disorder. *Cochrane Database of Systematic Reviews*, **8**, CD005652.

Taubner, S., & Curth, C. (2013). Mentalization mediates the relation between early traumatic experiences and aggressive behavior in adolescence. *Psihologija*, **46**, 177–192.

Taubner, S., White, L. O., Zimmermann, J., Fonagy, P., & Nolte, T. (2013). Attachment-related mentalization moderates the relationship between psychopathic traits and proactive aggression in adolescence. *Journal of Abnormal Child Psychology*, **41**, 929–938.

Tomasello, M. (2014). *A natural history of human thinking*. Cambridge, MA: Harvard University Press.

Treffert, D. A. (2010). *Islands of genius: The bountiful mind of the autistic acquired and sudden savant*. London, UK: Jessica Kingsley.

Treffert, D. A. (2014). Savant syndrome: Realities, myths and misconceptions. *Journal of Autism and Developmental Disorders*, **44**, 564–571.

Tremblay, R. E., Nagin, D. S., Seguin, J. R., Zoccolillo, M., Zelazo, P. D., Boivin, M., . . . Japel, C. (2004). Physical aggression during early childhood: Trajectories and predictors. *Pediatrics*, **114**, e43–50.

Trull, T. J., Solhan, M. B., Tragesser, S. L., Jahng, S., Wood, P. K., Piasecki, T. M., & Watson, D. (2008). Affective instability: Measuring a core feature of borderline personality disorder with ecological momentary assessment. *Journal of Abnormal Psychology*, **117**, 647–661.

van IJzendoorn, M. H., Feldbrugge, J. T., Derks, F. C., de Ruiter, C., Verhagen, M. F., Philipse, M. W., . . . Riksen-Walraven, J. M. (1997). Attachment representations of personality-disordered criminal offenders. *American Journal of Orthopsychiatry*, **67**, 449–459.

Wedig, M. M., Frankenburg, F. R., Bradford Reich, D., Fitzmaurice, G., & Zanarini, M. C. (2013). Predictors of suicide threats in patients with borderline personality disorder over 16 years of prospective follow-up. *Psychiatry Research*, **208**, 252–256.

Wedig, M. M., Silverman, M. H., Frankenburg, F. R., Reich, D. B., Fitzmaurice, G., & Zanarini, M. C. (2012). Predictors of suicide attempts in patients with borderline personality disorder over 16 years of prospective follow-up. *Psychological Medicine*, **42**, 1–10.

Chapter 3

Comorbidity

Depression

Depression and borderline personality disorder (BPD) are highly comorbid: depressive mood is a key feature of BPD. Research also suggests that comorbidity of depression with features of BPD can negatively influence both the course and response to treatment for depression (Levenson, Wallace, Fournier, Rucci, & Frank, 2012; Stringer et al., 2013). In terms of clinical work, we suggest that the extent to which a patient with depression has features of BPD should determine how best to manage their treatment (see Box 3.1).

Although from a research perspective the precise nature of the relationship between depression and BPD requires further elucidation (there is uncertainty about the extent to which depression and BPD should be considered as part of the same spectrum of affective disorder), from a clinical perspective, the relationship is too important to neglect. Depressed patients with comorbid BPD have greater affective instability; this makes the relationship between stressful experiences and the onset of depression less obvious than that typically seen in depressed patients without borderline features (Kopala-Sibley, Zuroff, Russell, Moskowitz, & Paris, 2012). Research has also indicated that patients with BPD features experience more intensely painful depressive feelings; this is evidenced by higher scores on self-report measures of depression, although not on observation-based measures (Levy, Edell, & McGlashan, 2007; Silk, 2010; Zanarini et al., 1998). They also experience stronger feelings of emptiness and diffuse negative affectivity, higher levels of self-criticism, and a greater focus on fears of abandonment (Levy et al., 2007; Wixom, Ludolph, & Westen, 1993) and shame.

From the perspective of MBT theory, the symptoms of depression are massively amplified by the limitations of balanced mentalizing in individuals with BPD. The greater intensity of the depressive feelings is the result of the nonmentalizing way in which BPD patients respond to their subjective experience (see Box 3.2). With the loss of mentalizing, failure, rejection, and abandonment are experienced in *psychic equivalence mode* (see Chapter 1), giving them an unshakeable force and intensity; on the other hand, when mentalizing is recovered, these feelings can improve far more rapidly than would be expected in major depression.

Box 3.1 BPD and comorbidity

- BPD is associated with many other mental health conditions
- BPD interferes with effective treatment for other conditions
- Treatment of BPD is required if comorbid disorder is to be treated
- However, treating the comorbid disorder does not improve BPD.

We understand the common association of depression with self-harm in terms of the disorganized self-structure characteristic of BPD. Greater self-harm and destructiveness result as the patient seeks to mitigate, distract from, and perhaps "externalize" (perceive as coming from outside) these highly critical experiences, which nevertheless continue to feel internal yet not part of the experiencing self (the "alien self"; see Chapter 1). Depressed patients without comorbid BPD also experience mentalizing difficulties, and they may too sometimes function in the psychic equivalence mode; for such patients, this will show itself in a marked absence of "pretend" or "play" ways of seeing the world, a heavy sense of depressive reality, and a static view of inner mental states (see Box 3.3). In patients with marked comorbid BPD features, the psychic equivalence spirals into more extreme accounts of inner pain and devastation—this may also make sense of the higher levels of physical pain and fatigue associated with depression in BPD patients (Hudson, Arnold, Keck, Auchenbach, & Pope, 2004; Van Houdenhove & Luyten, 2009). Similarly, in the psychic equivalence mode, perceived criticisms are felt as highly threatening attacks on the self: rejection can be felt as literally painful (Eisenberger, Lieberman, & Williams, 2003).

Box 3.2 BPD and depression

- Depressive symptoms are amplified by BPD—for example, greater affective instability
- BPD nonmentalizing modes make depressive symptoms subjectively more severe
- Self-harm and suicide attempts are increased
- Depression improves more rapidly than BPD
- Standard techniques for the treatment of depression are ineffective unless BPD is taken into account.

Box 3.3 BPD, depression, and nonmentalizing modes

- Psychic equivalence:
  - Self-harm arises in the context of the disorganized self-structure of BPD
  - Self-critical thoughts feel real
  - Fear of abandonment and loss are experienced as a fact
- Pretend mode:
  - Hypomentalizing followed by rebound hypermentalizing
  - Self-fulfilling logic of failure and futility
  - Suicide as part of a hypermentalizing process
- Teleological mode:
  - Insistent demand for attachment figures
  - Requirement for extra sessions
  - Potential boundary violations.

If the *teleological mode* is dominant, it will cause BPD patients who feel depressed to attempt to deal in a concrete fashion with the sense of loss and consequent feelings of being unloved, rejected, or excluded. This might be apparent as desperate attempts to gain closeness to attachment figures, including the clinician, for example, by demanding more sessions or wishing to be hugged or touched; this has obvious potential risks for boundary violation. While such impulses may be similarly experienced in depressed patients without BPD, the feelings will be easier to resist and more likely to be felt as inappropriate.

The same amplification of a shared characteristic is true with the third nonmentalizing mode, *pretend mode*. Hypomentalizing is often cyclically followed by hypermentalizing. In depressed patients without comorbid BPD, this hypermentalizing may strike the clinician as reasonably accurate or connected to reality, even if these patients tend to produce repetitive, overly analytical, and self-critical accounts. In contrast, in BPD patients this pretend mode will commonly be disassociated from reality; it may often be quite self-serving or coercive and be emotionally overwhelming.

In other words, we can identify nonmentalizing in depressed patients both with and without BPD features, and these modes of functioning can come to dominate as the individual experiences breakdowns in his/her mentalizing abilities. However, patients without BPD have a stronger capacity for explicit, controlled, conscious, reflective thinking, and they can self-correct and restore the balance of their mentalizing more easily. Additionally, they experience a far less intense pressure to externalize their alien self. Finally, patients without BPD tend to have lower levels of epistemic hypervigilance (as discussed in Chapter 1), meaning that they may be more open to respond to their social context and social cues (including therapy), which can in turn support a speedier return to more balanced mentalizing.

The mentalizing impairments associated with depressed patients with BPD features are apparent in a heightened cycle of hypomentalizing and hypermentalizing, and an intense pressure to externalize a painful alien self. Suicidal ideation reflects these problems: studies have found increased levels of suicidal behavior in depressed patients with comorbid BPD features (Bolton, Pagura, Enns, Grant, & Sareen, 2010). Similarly, Stringer and colleagues (2013) found, in a study of 1838 patients, that the rate of suicide attempts increased by the astonishingly high value of 33% for every unit increase in BPD features. The high rates of suicide and suicidal ideation in BPD patients are probably linked to higher levels of impulsivity and aggression, both of which reflect the stronger grip that the teleological mode has over subjectivity. Suicidal thoughts and behavior in depressed patients without comorbid BPD are more "object related," often directly connected to their interpersonal circumstances, to harsh feelings of self-criticism, feelings about "killing off" hated parts of the self, or reuniting with lost loved ones. In BPD patients, suicidal impulses are more often directly connected to the subjective experience itself, almost independent of content, with a desire to silence intense feelings of inner pain experienced in overwhelming psychic equivalence and teleological modes.

The mentalizing impairments associated with BPD mean that such patients are unlikely to have the capacity for reflective functioning that enables depressed patients without BPD to benefit from a mental representations approach—approaches that involve a focus on, for example, the internal working model of self and others. Patients with comorbid BPD may find the demands of such an approach unhelpful or even iatrogenic; the demands it makes may impede the development of the patient–clinician alliance and cause disruptive levels of anxiety or arousal, resulting in the use of nonmentalizing modes, particularly pretend mode. An approach focused on strengthening mentalizing that is active, structured, supportive, and interpersonal will, we believe, be of more benefit to such patients.

Treatment approach

When working with patients suffering from depression that is comorbid with BPD, the mentalizing approach is ideally used to address both problems simultaneously (Bateman & Fonagy, 2015).

Box 3.4 Treatment of BPD and depression: phase 1

- Active, supportive, validating, and interpersonally focused
- Engagement in treatment and formulation
- Focus on recovery of mentalizing
- Identification of maladaptive interpersonal cycles and interpersonal narratives.

The MBT approach to treating depression can be divided into three phases of treatment, each of which has particular aims and strategies. The core feature throughout the three phases is an unwavering focus on the patient's mind rather than his/her behavior. The clinician's interventions are primarily directed at linking interpersonal processes with the patient's mental states.

The first phase (see Box 3.4) of treatment aims at:

- *Engaging the patient in treatment* by adopting an active, supportive, and empathic therapeutic stance, providing hope and structure, and working actively together with the patient to support interpersonal change. This requires a concerted effort on the part of the clinician to help the patient identify the anxieties and defenses (i.e., the obstacles to change) that may be triggered when change is encouraged, contemplated, and/or attempted, so that the path can be cleared for the patient to experiment with more adaptive ways of relating to others.

- *Recovery of mentalizing*, particularly in severely depressed patients, using different interventions depending on the particular patient and situation (e.g., supportive techniques aimed at holding and containment, psychoeducation to provide a different perspective on symptoms and complaints, medication as appropriate, restoring sleep patterns by focusing on sleep "hygiene," encouraging activity, etc.)

- *Identifying and exploring typical maladaptive interpersonal cycles or interpersonal narratives*, the typical attachment strategies used to cope with interpersonal issues, and linking these to particular symptoms and complaints using both unstructured (e.g., in the context of a clinical interview or intake sessions) and structured methods (e.g., using attachment descriptors).

The second phase (see Box 3.5) mainly aims at:

- *Working through interpersonal issues and conflicts* by fostering mentalizing with regard to self and others. The extent to which the patient is able

---

Box 3.5 Treatment of BPD and depression: phase 2

- Working through interpersonal issues within the patient–clinician relationship
- Validation and recognition (not interpretation) of defenses
- Foster resilience by focusing on new ways of managing adversity.

---

to mentalize effectively about these issues as treatment progresses is important—particularly within the therapeutic relationship, as this provides the clinician with an "on-line" assessment of the patient's mentalizing in high-arousal conditions. The aim of focusing on this particular interpersonal relationship is to enhance and extend more broadly ("broaden and build") the patient's awareness of how his/her behavior is driven by mental states. It thus supports a mentalizing process that will hopefully become generalized beyond the specific interpersonal dynamics that are worked through during therapy.

- *Working with defenses*: this work entails recognition of the patient's defenses and their cost; validation and not interpretation of the defense to counteract inevitable shame—this helps the patient to feel more compassionate toward themselves and can lead to better regulation of anxiety and shame; recognition of the patient's strengths; and the in-session challenging of defensive behaviors. In the case of patients with significant deficits at the level of their self-representation, it will be important to recognize limits and focus primarily on more remedial work on self-representation.

- *Fostering resilience* in the face of past, current, and future adversity by actively encouraging the patient to reflect on and try out new ways of dealing with adversity, particularly new ways of relating to others and the self.

The third and final phase (see Box 3.6) aims at:

- *Working through issues around loss and separation*, as well as autonomy and identity, that are triggered by the impending end of the treatment (e.g., fears of losing the clinician, fears of relapsing, fear of failure when going back to work, etc.) by encouraging the patient to express his/her fears and wishes relating to the upcoming termination of treatment.

- *Consolidating changes and preventing future relapse* by reviewing the treatment process, examining what has been achieved, and actively exploring how the patient is going to use these achievements in the future.

Box 3.6 Treatment of BPD and depression: phase 3

◆ Careful negotiation of ending of treatment

◆ Management of separation and loss

◆ Recognition of fears about autonomy and identity

◆ Consolidation of change and relapse prevention.

Whereas the mentalizing-focused approach to depression may be implemented as a brief, time-limited treatment with more modest aims, focusing on improvements in mentalizing with regard to current interpersonal relationships (Lemma, Target, & Fonagy, 2011), depressed patients with comorbid BPD may need a longer, open-ended treatment that focuses in more detail on the links between current and past relationships and functioning.

Trauma

Comorbidity with trauma is particularly relevant to the treatment of BPD. Indeed, BPD can be considered an exemplar of complex traumatic stress disorder, insofar as its symptoms are multifaceted and it is typically intertwined with a range of comorbid disorders (see Box 3.7).

Ford and Courtois (2009) reviewed the range of proposals for characterizing complex post-traumatic stress disorder (PTSD). In this review, complex psychological trauma is defined as "resulting from exposure to severe stressors that (1) are repetitive or prolonged, (2) involve harm or abandonment by caregivers or other ostensibly responsible adults, and (3) occur at developmentally vulnerable times in the victim's life, such as early childhood or adolescence" (p. 13). They construe the multifaceted sequelae as complex traumatic stress disorders,

---

Box 3.7 BPD and trauma

◆ BPD shares features with complex traumatic stress disorder

◆ Childhood sexual abuse often has a prominent part in the histories of people with BPD

◆ Attachment trauma in BPD is conceptualized as repeated experiences of being left psychologically alone in an unbearable emotional state.

---

namely, "the changes in mind, emotions, body, and relationships experienced following complex psychological trauma, including severe problems with dissociation, emotion dysregulation, somatic distress, or relational or spiritual alienation" (p. 13). Hence, complex traumatic stress disorders potentially entail extensive comorbidity, including a range of symptoms and clinical syndromes as well as personality disorders.

Maltreatment in childhood is well established as a contributor to the emergence of PTSD, although it is neither necessary nor by itself sufficient for its development. Although childhood sexual abuse may play a particularly prominent role in the development of BPD (Paris & Zweig-Frank, 2001), it is often intertwined with a broader pattern of family disturbance. Zanarini et al. (1997) noted that "childhood sexual abuse reported by borderline patients may represent a *marker of the severity of the familial dysfunction* they experienced, as well as being a traumatic event or series of events in itself" (p. 1104, emphasis added).

Research has shown that the capacity for mentalizing is often damaged in people who have experienced trauma. For example, research has shown that children who have been traumatized find it more difficult to learn words for feelings (Beeghly & Cicchetti, 1994), while adults find it harder to recognize the intent behind facial expressions (Fonagy, Target, Gergely, Allen, & Bateman, 2003).

Allen (2004, 2012, 2013) has elaborated a complex model of trauma using the framework of mentalizing, which links trauma to attachment theory by defining it as *the experience of being left psychologically alone in unbearable emotional states*. This is potentially traumatic owing in part to the absence of social support for mentalizing. Treatment entails creating a secure attachment context conducive to mentalizing, in which emotional states that were previously unbearable can be rendered bearable. Self-compassion, mindfulness, and mentalizing all exemplify the sensitive responsiveness of secure attachment in parent–child relationships, friendships, love relationships, and "plain old therapy" (Allen, 2012). This formulation gives a "value" (of acceptance) to the psychotherapeutic approach focused on increasing the individual's capacity to mentalize. The clinician, through humble curiosity and a determination to see the world through the patient's eyes, will implicitly and explicitly engender an attitude of tolerance, compassion, and acceptance toward subjective experience, and gradually eases out the tendency we all have to berate ourselves for our feelings.

While the co-occurrence of emotion regulation and social understanding helps to ensure normal development, the disjunction of these two processes creates the background to trauma. If negative emotions normally come to be regulated through the sensitive responding of the other (e.g., an attachment figure), what happens when a sense of terror or grief in response to loss is not met by reasonably attuned comfort? When unbearable emotional states are repeatedly not reflected on, they become traumatic owing to the absence of another mind capable of reflecting on and appropriately responding to the individual's anguish.

The collapse of mentalizing in the face of trauma entails a loss of awareness of the relationship between internal and external reality (Fonagy & Target, 2000). Nonmentalizing modes of function come to the fore. In post-traumatic flashbacks, memories lose their connection with the continuity of subjectivity and are experienced with the full force of the experience of physical reality (psychic equivalence). In dissociative detachment, the failure to mentalize affect generates a feeling of unreality (pretend mode); patients report "blanking out," "clamming up," or remembering their traumatic experiences as if in a dream. Oscillating between psychic equivalence and pretend modes of experiencing the internal world is a hallmark of traumatization (see Box 3.8).

People who have been traumatized may also try to protect themselves against flashbacks through substance abuse, self-harm, or bingeing and purging (Nock, 2009; Roemer & Orsillo, 2009). Such actions typify the teleological mode. Following trauma, verbal reassurance means little. Interacting with others at a mental level has been replaced by attempts to alter thoughts and feelings through action.

Often, survivors of trauma simply refuse to think about their experience because thinking about it means reliving it. Therapy creates a situation where an appropriately sensitive individual (the therapist) is able to respond with compassion

---

Box 3.8 BPD, trauma, and nonmentalizing modes

- Psychic equivalence:
  - Loss of awareness of internal and external reality: flashbacks, avoidance behaviors, refusal to think about events and problems
- Pretend mode:
  - Dissociation: experience of unreality, blanking out, being in a "waking dream"
- Teleological mode:
  - Alter thoughts and feelings through action: drug use, alcohol, bingeing and purging, self-harm

and mindful acceptance to the subjective distress felt by the patient, and enables the patient to fully experience, express, understand, and reflect upon the subjective state from which they have constantly sought refuge.

Treatment approach

People with BPD comorbid with trauma come to treatment not simply to deal with the adversity that they have experienced. The devastation of psychic function that attachment trauma leaves in its wake impairs the capacity to cope with the ordinary vicissitudes of mental life. All the inescapable pains of life are experienced with the immediacy of an open wound unprotected by the "skin" that mentalizing provides.

The overall aim of treating traumatized patients is to help them to establish a more robust mentalizing self so that they become able to mentalize trauma and conflict, and thus to develop more secure attachments. Mentalizing provides a buffer between feeling and action—in effect, a "pause button" (Allen, 2001). Mentalizing puts the brakes on overwhelming emotions and impulsive actions, providing an opportunity for the motivations of self and other to be monitored and understood. Promoting mentalizing in this sense does not necessarily require direct processing of traumatic memories, but it does require mentalizing painful emotions and conflicts in the context of an attachment relationship. In this vein, treatment fosters mentalizing in relation to the patient's self, not just in relation to his/her trauma. It entails finding or recovering mentalizing through a developmentally appropriate process—that is, finding one's authentic psychological self through the mind of a benign attachment figure who is engaged in a reciprocal mentalizing relationship (see Box 3.9).

This kind of dyadic relationship has its challenges. The destructive behavior of the patient can elicit unbearable emotional states in the person they are with, which effectively destroys the potential for secure attachment and with it the rekindling of mentalizing. The traumatized patient may be further traumatized

---

Box 3.9 Treatment of BPD and trauma (1)

- Psychological pain of trauma is experienced without moderation from mentalizing
- Aim is to improve mentalizing to place a buffer ("pause button") between feeling and action
- New psychological self develops through the mind of an attachment figure who is engaged in a reciprocal mentalizing relationship.

(in the sense of being alone with their emotional pain) through the isolation their traumatic impact on others can generate (Allen, Fonagy, & Bateman, 2010). The clinician, who is no less likely to feel frightened and overwhelmed than the patient's family, might then be profoundly restricted in his/her capacity for compassionate understanding and might undermine rather than help the patient.

In Chapter 4, we discuss the "switch" model of understanding the relationship between attachment, mentalizing, and stress. Individuals vary in how easily their attachment system is activated by stress, which triggers a switch from controlled to automatic mentalizing. Childhood trauma may shift the switch point between the two modes of mentalizing: people with a history of trauma often respond to increases in stress/arousal that would not be high enough to inhibit controlled mentalizing in others. In light of the precariousness of mentalizing in individuals with comorbid trauma and BPD, it is important for clinicians to monitor traumatized patients' readiness to hear comments about thoughts and feelings. As arousal increases, perhaps in part in response to interpretive work with the clinician or insistence that the patient focuses on the inaccuracy of his/her thoughts, traumatized patients become unable to process talk about their mind. Hence, MBT advises caution about interpretive work for these patients until management of arousal is established. Interpretations of the patient–clinician relationship as representing aspects of the patient's past relationships at these times, however accurate they might be, are likely to be way beyond the patient's capacity to hear. The clinical priority of mentalizing treatment for trauma *must* be reducing arousal so that the patient can again think about other perspectives—that is, to mentalize.

In the aftermath of trauma, the person's sense of safety and trust in the goodness of life and of others is impaired (Janoff-Bulman, 1992). The unthinkable and/or unexpected has happened, and a fearful state of mind dominates as a result. Consequently, the mind is in a hypervigilant state, which, in turn, undermines mentalizing. Providing a safe and containing environment is therefore an essential prerequisite for treatment. There are a number of ways in which the clinician can offer this. At the most basic level, containment is expressed through establishing safe parameters within which the therapeutic process can unfold and which the patient can come to rely on. The importance of a safe, reliable frame cannot be emphasized enough, especially in the case of patients who have experienced trauma from attachment figures.

In the therapeutic situation it is also essential to establish, as far as possible, a sense of "interpersonal security" between clinician and patient that will contain the patient's anxiety (see Box 3.10). This process involves attending to the patient's experience of the therapy and responding to any anxieties or questions with genuine interest and transparency, both of which are core processes in

MBT, in the active therapeutic stance and the openness of the clinician's mental states in relation to the patient's problems and distress. Approaching the therapeutic encounter with long silences or responding to the patient's questions or anxieties with a more classical interpretive stance is likely to be unhelpful, particularly with patients who have suffered severe interpersonal trauma that has undermined their trust in other people's intentions toward them. Such an approach will only serve to escalate their anxiety and mitigate against the possibility of exploring what they may be feeling or thinking. Because of their traumatic experiences, these patients will present with considerable paranoid anxiety. The therapeutic goal is not to escalate this quality of anxiety by being opaque, but to create the best possible conditions for the patient to approach in his/her own mind what will most likely feel both disturbing and terrifying.

The central clinical task is not specific to working with the content of the traumatic events; rather, the task involves supporting a mentalizing stance in relation to the meaning and impact of the trauma (see Box 3.10). That is, the focus is primarily on the patient's mind rather than on the traumatic event. The mentalizing stance emphasizes process over content. However, when working with traumatized individuals, content is clearly important—not simply because the reality of what the patient has experienced may need to be validated by the clinician, but also because the way the event itself has been processed by the patient's mind is often part of the problem. Hence, the content of the actual traumatic event, in its affective detail, is likely to require elaboration.

Ordinarily, memories of past events are recalled as stories that change over time and that evoke manageable feelings. In the immediate aftermath of a traumatic event, most people will experience a degree of stress, and memories of the event are likely to intrude temporarily. As discussed earlier, a distinguishing

---

Box 3.10 Treatment of BPD and trauma (2)

- Detailed monitoring of arousal levels to maintain optimal mentalizing and prevent collapse into nonmentalizing modes
- Caution against asking patient to do more than his/her mental capacity allows
- Attention to patient's hypervigilance and reactivity
- Establishment of interpersonal security
- Task is to maintain a mentalizing stance in relation to the *meaning and impact* of the trauma rather than the *content* of the trauma.

feature of patients who develop PTSD is the re-emergence of psychic equiva-lence (van der Kolk & Fisler, 1996). The mind becomes a kind of "danger zone" that is best avoided. Recurring intrusive symptoms and re-enactments are com-monly observed in some patients (van der Kolk, 1989). The re-enactments per-petuate the intrusive symptoms, and the intrusive symptoms perpetuate the re-enactments (Allen, 2001); this vicious circle creates a feeling of being stuck in the traumatic past. This ongoing immersion in the past has two important consequences. First, it severs the connection between the person's pre-trauma self and post-trauma self: he/she becomes defined by the trauma as it replays itself over and over again. Any prior resilience, for example, is no longer within reach. Second, and connected to the first point, the sense of "being stuck" para-doxically represents an avoidance of thinking about the trauma in all its com-plexity and hence having to confront painful affect. The patient has only one perspective, and is haunted by it. Although the patient may feel that his/her mind is filled only with the trauma, he/she is not engaged in the kind of think-ing that involves developing a more nuanced understanding of what he/she feels and thinks. Many traumatized patients are understandably resistant to bringing to mind, and thinking about, their highly distressing experiences.

The conscious and unconscious meanings and affects that are attached to the traumatic event are a central part of the problem—and of the patient's recovery. The elaboration of meaning and affect through focused questions and observa-tions by the clinician aids the process of gradually bringing the meanings and feelings together into a coherent narrative about the self. Foa, Huppert, and Cahill (2006) identified narrative coherence as a mechanism of change in exposure treatment for PTSD. Essentially, this process involves developing a narrative about the trauma that bridges the pre- and post-trauma self and that is forward-looking (see Box 3.11).

Box 3.11 Treatment of BPD and trauma (3)

- Intrusive symptoms perpetuate "stuckness" in the past
- Pre-trauma self becomes conflated with post-trauma self, and trauma-tized self dominates
- Clinician should focus some mentalizing process on nontraumatized functioning for a more nuanced exploration of current thinking and feeling
- Reconstruction work is used to identify confusing stimuli but with a clear focus on the *current* effect on the individual's mental experience.

Reconstruction is an important component of any therapeutic process, and this is especially relevant when working with traumatized patients. One reason for this lies in the particular problems these patients have with encoding memories of traumatic events. On the one hand, patients complain of their memories intruding too much; on the other hand, paradoxically, they may also present with very fragmented memories of the traumatic incident. Intrusive symptoms frequently consist of fragmented sensory impressions, mostly visual (Brewin, Dalgleish, & Joseph, 1996; van der Kolk, 1994). Patients also may re-experience particular physiological sensations or affects, such as intense fear, without any recollection of the event itself.

Patients who present with more fragmented, confused memories of the traumatic event appear to be more likely to develop chronic PTSD. This is probably partly because they cannot intentionally retrieve the memory of trauma and process it in such a way that it can be integrated into a continuous narrative of their life before and after the event (i.e., so that it can become part of autobiographical memory). Consequently, they remain hostage to strong perceptual priming (a form of implicit memory) for stimuli that are associated with the traumatic event. They therefore have difficulty in discriminating between stimuli that were present during the trauma and other, similar stimuli. The more they feel "hounded" by the past through the intrusive symptoms they experience, the more inclined they feel to revert to various avoidance strategies to protect themselves from the painful affect. One of the most common strategies is to try to suppress thoughts about the trauma. However, this is unsuccessful, since the more one tries to suppress such intrusive thoughts, the more frequent they become (Wegner, 1994).

A core feature of the therapeutic intervention is the provision of a safe context within which the patient can be helped to bring to mind the traumatic experience along with the associated affects and the meanings ascribed to the trauma, so that these cognitive and affective components can be gradually unpacked. Working with patients who have been traumatized necessarily involves working with an event that occurred in the past. Especially when working with people who have endured attachment trauma, the time that has elapsed since the trauma may be considerable, for example, between an experience of sexual abuse in childhood and seeking help in adulthood. Although we have emphasized that it is helpful for the patient to develop a narrative about the trauma, we are not suggesting that the primary aim of therapy is to excavate the past and to retrieve repressed memories in order to develop insight. Rather, the goal of mentalizing-based therapy is to help the patient to be curious about his/her mind, and hence to focus on *current* mental states. The clinician aims to support the patient in his/her attempts to make sense of the impact the trauma has on his/her current functioning and current relationships—including the relationship with the clinician.

Inevitably, this work at times will involve revisiting early experiences, particularly when the trauma concerns abuse in childhood. Contextualizing traumatic events in a narrative about one's experiences over time is important, but it is unlikely that this will be sufficient to support change. Reconstruction of the distant past is probably best viewed as a component of the work, in the context of a more overarching focus on exploring the current implications of painful and confusing early experiences. The aim is to help the patient to develop a perspective on the past by reworking current experience (Bateman & Fonagy, 2004).

Eating disorders

High rates of comorbidity between eating disorders and personality disorders, particularly BPD, have long been observed by clinicians. Godt (2008) reported that 30% of patients with an eating disorder also meet criteria for personality disorder, with there being a particularly strong connection between BPD and bulimia nervosa. Eating disorders and personality disorders share the characteristic of vulnerability to mentalizing difficulties and strong associations with insecure attachment styles (see Box 3.12).

A mentalizing approach to this comorbidity thus seeks to target the loss of mentalizing that is common to both conditions. Patients with comorbid BPD and eating disorders clearly present a complex set of challenges, with high levels of movement from one disorder to another (Zanarini, Reichman, Frankenburg, Reich, & Fitzmaurice, 2010). Individuals with both conditions rather than an eating disorder alone are more likely to have a complicated course (Robinson et al., 2014).

Box 3.12 BPD and eating disorders

- Comorbidity of BPD and eating disorders is approximately 30%, with bulimia nervosa being most common
- Outcomes of treatment of eating disorders are poorer in the presence of comorbid BPD
- Increased vulnerability to mentalizing difficulties of self and other
- Eating disorders are understood as an expression of a disordered sense of self.

There are numerous challenges in working with eating disorders, including patients' lack of insight into the condition and its seriousness, the psychological symptoms of malnutrition, and the chemical imbalances that may ensue. There is a high risk of dropout and disrupted therapeutic relations; connected with this, it can be challenging to form a therapeutic alliance. The patient may find it difficult to accept that they have a problem, or have low motivation to change (Geller, Williams, & Sriskameswaran, 2001). Comorbid eating disorders and BPD may make these difficulties more acute because, we believe, these patients have highly vulnerable mentalizing in relation to self and other.

From the perspective of mentalizing theory, eating disorders are understood as an expression of a disordered sense of self. The solution to this incoherence is to equate the body/appearance with the subjective self in an attempt to restore a sense of coherence and pursue a sense of worth. The MBT approach is to improve mentalizing by enabling the patient to deal with his/her own mind and its affects, so that there is less retreat into the nonmentalizing modes of function in which feelings of dissatisfaction are physically embodied.

Significant associations have been found between eating disorders and attachment insecurity. Higher attachment anxiety has been significantly associated with symptom severity and poorer treatment outcome (Illing, Tasca, Balfour, & Bissada, 2010). Evidence also suggests that there is indeed a strong relationship between eating disorders and mentalizing difficulties (Kuipers & Bekker, 2012; Russell, Schmidt, Doherty, Young, & Tchanturia, 2009; Zonnevijlle-Bender, van Goozen, Cohen-Kettenis, van Elburg, & van Engeland, 2002). Skårderud has argued for the importance of impaired mentalizing in anorexia nervosa, and the relevance of MBT to its treatment (Skårderud & Fonagy, 2012). Eating disorders emerge as the consequence of an incapacity to mentalize ordinary social experience and the overwhelming emergence of prementalizing modes of function. If these impairments in mentalizing occur in conjunction with exposure to other risk factors, for example, adverse parenting (especially low contact, high expectations, and parental discord), sexual abuse, familial preoccupation with dieting, exposure to critical comments about weight or body shape from family or others, and pressure to be slim from social, occupational, or media contexts, disordered eating may ultimately arise (Fairburn & Harrison, 2003). The theoretical basis of MBT may therefore have significance for both the etiology and the treatment of eating disorders comorbid with BPD.

When considering the mentalizing processes and impairments at work in eating disorders, the psychic equivalence mode of nonmentalizing is highly relevant (see Box 3.13). Given that it conflates the internal and external worlds, psychic equivalence in eating disorders makes inner (mental) reality externally (bodily) concrete. This is a highly embodied state of mind, involving an unduly

> ## Box 3.13 BPD, eating disorders, and nonmentalizing modes
>
> ◆ Psychic equivalence:
>   - Mental reality = physical (bodily) reality
>   - Hyperembodied state: negative focus on body, looking in mirror, measuring weight/body size, fantasies related to being looked at
> ◆ Pretend mode:
>   - Disembodied state: inability to acknowledge true appearance and bodily needs
> ◆ Teleological mode:
>   - Self-worth based on physical outcomes: weight loss, purging, and excessive exercise.

negative focus on the body's exterior and an inability to distance oneself from feelings of dissatisfaction. This shows itself in, for example, repeated looking at the mirror, weighing oneself, measuring body size, and fantasies about being looked at by others. In other words, these external indices are felt over and above engagement with the experience of actually being within one's own lived body.

However, the *hyperembodied* state that arises in psychic equivalence mode is often combined with a *disembodied* state, in which there is a highly distorted relationship with the physical body. This can mean an inability to acknowledge the reality of its true appearance or its physical needs. This pretend mode of functioning can make the treatment process highly frustrating for the clinician, and the simultaneous presence of disembodied and hyperembodied mentalizing creates a highly confusing and complex picture for the clinician to grasp.

The teleological mode of nonmentalizing, in which feelings, actions, and beliefs are contingent on physical outcomes to be meaningful, is also highly relevant in understanding how the patient might respond to mentalizing breakdowns. Clearly, eating disorders are a highly teleological mode of functioning: self-worth and meaning are achievable only if concretized in the achievement of physical actions such as loss of weight, purging, or exercising excessively.

Treatment approach

The MBT approach to eating disorders aims to reduce symptoms, stimulate mentalizing, strengthen the therapeutic alliance, and prevent dropout from treatment. The mentalizing approach consists of a combination of individual sessions, group sessions, and psychoeducational groups. The basic format complies with the traditional MBT structure (see Chapters 11 and 12). It consists of a 12-month program with weekly group therapy organized as a slow open group, individual therapy that begins on a weekly basis and gradually becomes less frequent, and a limited number of psychoeducational group sessions. During therapy, the MBT clinicians are responsible for making sure that patients' physical measures are monitored (e.g., at the clinic or by the patients' general medical practitioner), consulting with the clinic physician as required. After the 12-month therapy program, patients are reassessed by a member of the clinical team and referred for further management if required. Each MBT group has a maximum of ten participants. Families and carers will be offered attendance at existing support services. Family therapy sessions may also be incorporated if required.

The focus of MBT for eating disorders is on breaks in mentalizing and the emergence of nonmentalizing modes of functioning. The approach when this happens would be to "rewind" to the moment at which mentalizing broke down, explore the emotional context, and identify the affect state between the clinician and the patient (see Chapter 6). At this point, the clinician needs to also identify his/her own contribution to the breakdown in mentalizing (see Box 3.14).

The focus of the treatment is to use this process to mentalize the relationship, but only very gently and slowly. The process requires the clinician not to assume that the patient has well-developed social-cognitive capacities, and to remain empathic and aware of the experience of disrupted mentalizing. There must

---

Box 3.14 Treatment of BPD and eating disorder

- Standard MBT structure with family support and family therapy
- Clinician responsible for monitoring weight with physician
- Focus on mentalizing and emergence of nonmentalizing modes
- Caution about assuming the patient has well-developed social-cognitive capacities
- Careful monitoring of attachment activation and therapeutic alliance
- Focus on "minding the body"—meticulous identification and exploration of concrete experiences with the body and food to reconnect them with the emotional, cognitive, and relational experiences.

also be a constant awareness of the potential for causing iatrogenic harm by overactivating the attachment system, causing further breakdowns in mentalizing.

The MBT approach seeks to allow the patient to break his/her fluctuating disembodied/hyperembodied states by a process known as "Minding the Body." This technique involves stimulating the patient to investigate his/her concrete experiences with the body and food, to reconnect them with the emotional, cognitive, and relational experiences. This involves a specific type of focus on triggers for bodily feelings, small changes in mental states that can upset the patient physically and psychologically and lead to fears and anxieties being concretized as preoccupations about food and weight. "Minding the Body" sessions might involve body awareness sessions focusing on how one senses one's feet on the floor and one's legs and seat on the chair, in order to stimulate awareness of the body and shift attention from the objectified body to the lived-in, physical body. Sessions can also involve eating together, as patients and clinicians prepare and bring in their own meal to eat together. The affects stimulated by this process can then be explored and the mentalizing breaks and fluctuations at work behind them considered.

The aim of structuring treatment across these different formats is that each one reinforces different aspects of mentalizing. The psychoeducational component seeks to stimulate curiosity, encourage the discussion of different points of view about clinical examples, and bring some flexibility to the concrete certainty associated with psychic equivalence.

The program also involves medical assessment and management, with concrete aims of symptom reduction. For patients who are underweight, this means agreements on how to restore weight, and how quickly. For patients who binge and purge, it means agreements about how to try to reduce the frequency of these behaviors. Because of the teleological stance that those with eating disorders often display, we consider written agreements to be very useful here. Similarly, clearly written formulations are used as part of the process.

The mentalizing approach is particularly pertinent to the problem of forming a therapeutic alliance, in that its explicit and continued focus is upon the current state of the therapeutic relationship as a way of modeling and experimenting with mentalizing and its fluctuations in the here-and-now. The mentalizing stance of the clinician is highly relevant here; this is perhaps particularly worth emphasizing in relation to the treatment of eating disorders, because these conditions often take a particular toll on the clinician's mentalizing. The clinician may feel aware that his/her own body is being scrutinized and judged. The physical dangers associated with eating disorders can also create considerable pressure, and therefore possibly frustration and anxiety in the clinician in the face of the patient's resistance to treatment and apparent disconnection from bodily reality. There is a high risk that the patient's symptoms and behavior will provoke strong feelings in the clinician, with the possibility of consequent over-reaction. In the face of these potential challenges to the clinician, the mentalizing stance is critical if there is to be any possibility of building a therapeutic relationship. We reiterate that the mentalizing stance does not mean that the clinician is expected *never* to experience any mentalizing difficulties: such an ideal is both unrealistic and potentially unhelpful. Rather, the clinician should use his/her own fluctuations in mentalizing as an opportunity to model how mentalizing works, to demonstrate what an interactive and context-driven process it can be, and to reflect with the patient on the therapeutic relationship.

When a patient's mentalizing is severely impaired, he/she may perceive many interventions as invasive, inauthentic, or irrelevant. If the patient is in a high state of anxiety, excessive mentalizing challenges may feel hostile or frustrating. The clinician's stance is therefore of particular importance. In a study of the factors that cause therapeutic dropout, important contributors were a perception that the treatment is too difficult, that approaches are inappropriate, and a lack of freedom and trust (Vandereycken & Devidt, 2010). The careful focus of MBT on the therapeutic alliance seeks to overcome such problems, and to use the therapeutic relationship as an opportunity to learn safely about mentalizing, to recover reflective functioning in the face of flight into nonmentalizing modes as a result of anxiety or overwhelming affect.

MBT for eating disorders in the first instance seeks to reduce symptoms. It also seeks to improve the patient's capacity to understand his/her own and other people's minds. Through careful but systematic attentiveness to mentalizing processes, improved mentalizing capacity leads to improved affect regulation, a consequence of which is that the patient is less likely to fall into entrenched nonmentalizing modes. In patients with eating disorders comorbid with BPD, mentalizing difficulties and a disordered sense of self are likely to be more strongly present. The mentalizing stance of the clinician will be critical in such cases.

References

Allen, J. G. (2001). *Traumatic relationships and serious mental disorders.* Chichester, UK: Wiley.

Allen, J. G. (2004). *Coping with trauma: A guide to self-understanding* (2nd ed.). Washington, DC: American Psychiatric Press.

Allen, J. G. (2012). *Restoring mentalizing in attachment relationships: Treating trauma with plain old therapy.* Washington, DC: American Psychiatric Press.

Allen, J. G. (2013). *Mentalizing in the development and treatment of attachment trauma.* London, UK: Karnac Books.

Allen, J. G., Fonagy, P., & Bateman, A. W. (2010). The role of mentalizing in treating attachment trauma. In E. Vermetten & R. Lanius (Eds.), *The hidden epidemic: The impact of early life trauma on health and disease* (pp. 247–256). New York, NY: Cambridge University Press.

Bateman, A., & Fonagy, P. (2004). *Psychotherapy for borderline personality disorder: Mentalization-based treatment.* Oxford, UK: Oxford University Press.

Bateman, A., & Fonagy, P. (2015). Borderline personality disorder and mood disorders: Mentalizing as a framework for integrated treatment. *Journal of Clinical Psychology*, **71**, 792–804.

Beeghly, M., & Cicchetti, D. (1994). Child maltreatment, attachment, and the self system: Emergence of an internal state lexicon in toddlers at high social risk. *Development and Psychopathology*, **6**, 5–30.

Bolton, J. M., Pagura, J., Enns, M. W., Grant, B., & Sareen, J. (2010). A population-based longitudinal study of risk factors for suicide attempts in major depressive disorder. *Journal of Psychiatric Research*, **44**, 817–826.

Brewin, C. R., Dalgleish, T., & Joseph, S. (1996). A dual representation theory of posttraumatic stress disorder. *Psychological Review*, **103**, 670–686.

Eisenberger, N. I., Lieberman, M. D., & Williams, K. D. (2003). Does rejection hurt? An fMRI study of social exclusion. *Science*, **302**, 290–292.

Fairburn, C. G., & Harrison, P. J. (2003). Eating disorders. *Lancet*, **361**, 407–416.

Foa, E. B., Huppert, J. D., & Cahill, S. P. (2006). Emotional processing theory: An update. In B. O. Rothbaum (Ed.), *Pathological anxiety: Emotional processing in etiology and treatment* (pp. 3–24). New York, NY: Guilford Press.

Fonagy, P., & Target, M. (2000). Playing with reality: III. The persistence of dual psychic reality in borderline patients. *International Journal of Psychoanalysis*, **81**, 853–874.

Fonagy, P., Target, M., Gergely, G., Allen, J. G., & Bateman, A. (2003). The developmental roots of borderline personality disorder in early attachment relationships: A theory and some evidence. *Psychoanalytic Inquiry*, **23**, 412–459.

Ford, J. D., & Courtois, C. A. (2009). Defining and understanding complex trauma and complex traumatic stress disorders. In C. A. Courtois & J. D. Ford (Eds.), *Treating complex traumatic stress disorders: An evidence-based guide* (pp. 13–30). New York, NY: Guilford Press.

Geller, J., Williams, K. D., & Sriskameswaran, S. (2001). Clinical stance in the treatment of chronic eating disorders. *European Eating Disorders Review*, **14**, 212–217.

Godt, K. (2008). Personality disorders in 545 patients with eating disorders. *European Eating Disorders Review*, **16**, 94–99.

Hudson, J. I., Arnold, L. M., Keck, P. E., Jr., Auchenbach, M. B., & Pope, H. G., Jr. (2004). Family study of fibromyalgia and affective spectrum disorder. *Biological Psychiatry*, **56**, 884–891.

Illing, V., Tasca, G. A., Balfour, L., & Bissada, H. (2010). Attachment insecurity predicts eating disorder symptoms and treatment outcomes in a clinical sample of women. *Journal of Nervous and Mental Disease*, **189**, 653–659.

Janoff-Bulman, R. (1992). *Shattered assumptions: Towards a new psychology of trauma.* New York, NY: Free Press.

Kopala-Sibley, D. C., Zuroff, D. C., Russell, J. J., Moskowitz, D. S., & Paris, J. (2012). Understanding heterogeneity in borderline personality disorder: Differences in affective reactivity explained by the traits of dependency and self-criticism. *Journal of Abnormal Psychology*, **121**, 680–691.

Kuipers, G. S., & Bekker, H. J. M. (2012). Attachment, mentalization and eating disorders: A review of studies using the Adult Attachment Interview. *Current Psychiatry Review*, **8**, 326–336.

Lemma, A., Target, M., & Fonagy, P. (2011). *Brief dynamic interpersonal therapy: A clinician's guide.* Oxford, UK: Oxford University Press.

Levenson, J. C., Wallace, M. L., Fournier, J. C., Rucci, P., & Frank, E. (2012). The role of personality pathology in depression treatment outcome with psychotherapy and pharmacotherapy. *Journal of Consulting and Clinical Psychology*, **80**, 719–729.

Levy, K. N., Edell, W. S., & McGlashan, T. H. (2007). Depressive experiences in inpatients with borderline personality disorder. *Psychiatric Quarterly*, **78**, 129–143.

Nock, M. K. (Ed.). (2009). *Understanding nonsuicidal self-injury.* Washington, DC: American Psychological Association.

Paris, J., & Zweig-Frank, H. (2001). A 27-year follow-up of patients with borderline personality disorder. *Comprehensive Psychiatry*, **42**, 482–487.

Robinson, P., Barrett, B., Bateman, A., Hakeem, A., Hellier, J., Lemonsky, F., . . . Fonagy, P. (2014). Study protocol for a randomized controlled trial of mentalization based therapy against specialist supportive clinical management in patients with both eating disorders and symptoms of borderline personality disorder. *BMC Psychiatry*, **14**, 51.

Roemer, L., & Orsillo, S. M. (2009). *Mindfulness- and acceptance-based behavioral therapies in practice.* New York, NY: Guilford Press.

Russell, T. A., Schmidt, U., Doherty, L., Young, V., & Tchanturia, K. (2009). Aspects of social cognition in anorexia nervosa: Affective and cognitive theory of mind. *Psychiatry Research*, **168**, 181–185.

Silk, K. R. (2010). The quality of depression in borderline personality disorder and the diagnostic process. *Journal of Personality Disorders*, **24**, 25–37.

Skårderud, F., & Fonagy, P. (2012). Eating disorders. In A. W. Bateman & P. Fonagy (Eds.), *Handbook of mentalizing in mental health practice* (pp. 347–384). Washington, DC: American Psychiatric Press.

Stringer, B., van Meijel, B., Eikelenboom, M., Koekkoek, B., C, M. M. L., Kerkhof, A. J., . . . Beekman, A. T. (2013). Recurrent suicide attempts in patients with depressive and anxiety disorders: The role of borderline personality traits. *Journal of Affective Disorders*, **151**, 23–30.

van der Kolk, B. (1989). The compulsion to repeat the trauma: Re-enactment, re-victimization, and masochism. *Psychiatric Clinics of North America*, **12**, 389–411.

van der Kolk, B. (1994). The body keeps the score: Memory and the evolving psychobiology of post-traumatic stress. *Harvard Review of Psychiatry*, **1**, 253–265.

van der Kolk, B. A., & Fisler, R. (1996). Dissociation and the fragmentary nature of traumatic memories: Overview. *British Journal of Psychotherapy*, **12**, 352–361.

Van Houdenhove, B., & Luyten, P. (2009). Central sensitivity syndromes: Stress system failure may explain the whole picture. *Seminars in Arthritis and Rheumatism*, **39**, 218–219.

Vandereycken, W., & Devidt, K. (2010). Why do patients drop out of therapy? *Eating Disorders Review*, **21**. Retrieved from http://eatingdisordersreview.com/nl/nl_edr_21_2_1.html

Wegner, D. M. (1994). Ironic processes of mental control. *Psychological Review*, **101**, 34–52.

Wixom, J., Ludolph, P., & Westen, D. (1993). The quality of depression in adolescents with borderline personality disorder. *Journal of the American Academy of Child and Adolescent Psychiatry*, **32**, 1172–1177.

Zanarini, M. C., Frankenburg, F. R., Dubo, E. D., Sickel, A. E., Trikha, A., Levin, A., & Reynolds, V. (1998). Axis I comorbidity of borderline personality disorder. *American Journal of Psychiatry*, **155**, 1733–1739.

Zanarini, M. C., Reichman, C. A., Frankenburg, F. R., Reich, D. B., & Fitzmaurice, G. (2010). The course of eating disorders in patients with borderline personality disorder: A 10-year follow-up study. *International Journal of Eating Disorders*, **43**, 226–232.

Zanarini, M. C., Williams, A. A., Lewis, R. E., Reich, R. B., Soledad, C. V., Marino, M. F., . . . Frankenburg, F. R. (1997). Reported pathological childhood experiences associated with the development of borderline personality disorder. *American Journal of Psychiatry*, **154**, 1101–1106.

Zonnevijlle-Bender, M. J., van Goozen, S. H., Cohen-Kettenis, P. T., van Elburg, A., & van Engeland, H. (2002). Do adolescent anorexia nervosa patients have deficits in emotional functioning? *European Child and Adolescent Psychiatry*, **2**, 28–52.

Chapter 4

Assessment of mentalizing

Some key principles in the assessment of mentalizing

Assessment of an individual's mentalizing requires an evaluation of his/her overall mentalizing strengths and weakness. This will include an evaluation of the pattern and balance of the four dimensions of mentalizing, which we discussed in Chapters 1 and 2. The complexity of mentalizing inevitably means that there are different ways in which mentalizing difficulties can manifest, depending on which elements are impaired. The importance of an accurate assessment of the mentalizing process is underscored by the fact that a different treatment approach and focus is required for different mentalizing impairments.

Mentalizing, and the language of mentalizing, is a fundamental part of who we are. So most of us can sound *as if* we are mentalizing even though we are not actively engaged in thinking in a reflective way about mental states, simply by using well-worn phrases ("canned" mentalizing language). However, name-checking and stating a feeling or thought does not necessarily mean that the speaker is actually engaging with that thought or feeling. If, for example, I say "He is angry," I may have in mind the other person's angry facial expression or bodily attitude rather than contemplating their mental state, let alone the reasons for him feeling that way. Thus, the assessment of mentalizing has to look beyond what may be "canned" mentalizing language, and instead focus on the individual's capacity to meet different mentalizing challenges.

Mentalizing is highly responsive to context. An individual may be quite an adept and stable mentalizer in most interpersonal situations, except where powerful emotions or the activation of attachment-related ideas undermine the capacity to understand or even pay attention to the feelings of others. Therefore, the assessment of mentalizing needs to take into account the ways in which an individual's mentalizing is affected by different triggers—how he/she might respond to stress or arousal in different situations and in different relationships, with particular attention to attachment relationships.

The assessment of mentalizing involves first of all identifying individuals whose mentalizing is so poor that the precise nature of their mentalizing difficulties is hard to identify. It is difficult to establish the quality of mentalizing in an individual who, for example, fails to respond meaningfully to questions about how they feel and what it is they are thinking about. When this is not the case (i.e., in an individual whose mentalizing capacities are impaired, but to a lesser extent), the assessment of mentalizing consists of identifying one of a number of non-mutually exclusive forms of mentalizing failure.

The purpose of assessing the quality of mentalizing is twofold: first, it can help the clinician create a focus for therapy. Second, in conjunction with an assessment of interpersonal relationships, it can provide the clinician with an understanding of the particular relational contexts within which an individual's mentalizing problems need to be addressed.

It must always be borne in mind that mentalizing failure does not always look the same. An example is that of the so-called *borderline empathy paradox* (Dinsdale & Crespi, 2013). It has long been observed that people with borderline personality disorder (BPD) are not necessarily unable to mentalize; they may in some respects and in certain situations show normal or even superior mentalizing skills. Individuals with BPD commonly excel in one particular form of mentalizing: intuitive empathy. The contrast between obvious competence in intuitive empathy and drastic impairment in other areas of mentalizing is commonly referred to as the "empathy paradox". The experience of "borderline empathy" will be familiar to many clinicians who have noted a patient's particularly perceptive insight. The insightfulness often displayed by individuals with BPD will, however, often not be accessible during times of interpersonal stress and activation of the attachment system.

Failure to recognize the unevenness and complexity of an individual's mentalizing capacities can lead to the apparently iatrogenic effects often described in unsuccessful therapeutic encounters for BPD (Higgitt & Fonagy, 1992). Clinicians working with BPD patients usually learn to recognize that exceptional interpersonal sensitivity should not be taken as an indication of psychological mindedness (Bateman & Fonagy, 2006); it is better seen as analogous to the so-called "savant syndrome" (Treffert, 2014), where the dramatic absence of a capacity enables the brain to excel in an alternative domain, albeit one that is quite restricted (see Chapter 2 for further discussion of this issue). Being astute at judging subjective states by interpreting facial expressions may not mean that the individual has a similar level of understanding when reasoning about mental states is called for. However, some clinicians may misjudge this, leading them to address issues at a level of complexity that is simply beyond the patient's capacity to process (Fonagy & Bateman, 2006). Similarly, as we have seen, individuals with antisocial personality disorder (ASPD) may appear to be quite proficient in cognitive mentalizing and in the mentalizing of other people's cognitive and emotional states, and so may give an impression of sophisticated social understanding, yet have little sense of the emotional impact of their actions on others (Viding & McCrory, 2012).

Unstructured clinical assessment of mentalizing

There is no single technique for the assessment of mentalizing and so a number of approaches will be discussed here. In general, though, the assessment of mentalizing should take place in the context of routine history taking. A comprehensive assessment of mentalizing requires at least one, and preferably two to three, detailed clinical interviews. There are specific classes of questions (see Box 4.1) that might prove particularly helpful; in addition, eliciting situational descriptions of a problematic or successful interpersonal event can provide valuable information (see Box 4.2 for an example of a situational event).

Such interviews should review the patient's attachment history, with particular attention to past and current relationships, and they should include clear demand questions that explicitly probe mentalizing in the context of *past and current* attachment relationships as well as with regard to the *context and the way* patients experience their symptoms and complaints. Without such probing, initial assessment of patients may leave assessors (and clinicians) with the misleading impression that they are working with an individual who has relatively high psychological mindedness, who is eminently suitable for insight-oriented psychotherapy.

Box 4.1 Questions that can reveal the quality of mentalizing

- You described how your parents were with you—do you have any idea why they acted as they did?
- Do you think what happened to you as a child explains the way you are as an adult?
- Can you think of anything that happened to you as a child that created problems for you?
- As a child did you ever feel that you were not wanted?
- In relation to losses, abuse, or other trauma, how did you feel at the time and how have your feelings changed over time?
- How has your relationship with your parents changed since childhood?
- In what important ways have you changed since childhood?

Box 4.2 An example of a situational event

"Last night Rachel and I had an argument about whether I was doing enough around the house. She thought I did not do as much as her and that I should do more. I said I did as much as my work obligations allow. Rachel got angry and we stopped talking to each other. In the end I agreed to do the shopping from now on. But I ended up feeling furious with her."

The accounts patients give of their symptoms and complaints, in turn, provide an important additional opportunity for gauging the potential for either temporary or more global failures of mentalizing, as well as patients' ability to recover from such lapses of mentalizing. For instance, most BPD patients show partial failures of mentalizing in the context of talking about self-harm or suicide, from which they can subsequently recover in the remainder of the interview. Some patients, however, are completely unable to give an account of such experiences, and become overwhelmed (often observed in patients with a history of severe trauma) or caught up in excessively lengthy accounts of their symptoms (often observed in patients with obsessive–compulsive or somatoform disorders). Importantly, the assessor needs to see past "canned" or "borrowed" accounts of symptoms, complaints, or the nature of problems more generally. These accounts have often been learned from other professionals, patients, family and friends, or the Internet.

In the first phase of assessment interviewing, the assessor should try to get a good impression of the patient's general mentalizing abilities. This involves a global assessment across the four mentalizing dimensions (see Boxes 4.3–4.6). The prevalence and nature of prementalizing modes should be assessed (see later for more on this topic). Patients with the most severe impairments in mentalizing often seem to be the ones who make most use of distorted mentalizing to fend off painful feelings or realities, and to seduce, manipulate, or control others. For instance, a borderline patient's hypersensitivity to emotional states in others, generating a high proclivity for emotional contagion, often leads to vicious interpersonal cycles, marked by attributions of hostile intent, induction of guilt and shame, impulsive outbursts of aggression, and subsequent rejection by others (Fonagy & Luyten, 2009). Individuals with ASPD often build on their insensitivity to the internal emotional states of others while having the cognitive insight to be able to engender trust in others, to detect their sensitivities and, for example, seduce them to buy or sell goods, or to feel compassion, but they may also use these capacities to (sometimes deliberately) undermine others' mentalizing capacities.

Box 4.3 Internally and externally focused mentalizing

- Awareness of internal and external features of the self and others, and the relationship between the two
- Sensitivity to external and internal features of the self and others
- Ability to perceive and to self-correct initial impressions based on external features (e.g., "I immediately saw on his face that he couldn't be trusted"; "I didn't like the way he talked, and therefore I can never like him") and to let others correct these impressions.

Box 4.4 Mentalizing with regard to self and others

- Presence of egocentrism, that is, the capacity to see others in terms of self, versus degree of control/inhibition of own perspective
- Liability to emotional contagion (self–other diffusion with regard to mental states) versus defensive separation from the mental states of others
- Response to contrary moves, particularly flexibility to move between self and other perspectives
- Ability to integrate embodied knowledge with more reflective knowledge of self and others.

Box 4.5 Cognitive and affective mentalizing

- Cognitive focus: tendency to see "mind-reading" as an intellectual, rational game
- Tendency for either cognitive or affective hypermentalizing or pseudomentalizing
- Affective focus: tendency to become overwhelmed by affect when thinking about states of mind
- Ability to engage in *mentalized affectivity* and *embodied mentalizing*, that is, to integrate cognitive knowledge and affective knowledge about the self and others.

Box 4.6 Automatic and controlled mentalizing in specific contexts and relationships

+ Are there *global* impairments in mentalizing (e.g., marked automatic mentalizing based on distorted assumptions about the self and others), versus more *partial* difficulties?

+ Are there marked discrepancies between mentalizing in non-stressful versus stressful conditions, or are mentalizing levels approximately equally high or low in both conditions?

+ What is the optimal stress level for adequate mentalizing?

+ Are there differences related to self–other and context, particularly attachment relationships (e.g., gross imbalances with regard to mentalizing about self and others, or between one attachment figure and another)?

+ How extensive is the failure of mentalizing under stress?

+ Time to recovery of mentalizing (e.g., relatively quick versus slow)

+ Ability to self-correct and be corrected by others when under high stress levels

+ Is there a sense of sufficient and realistic security in relation to the assessor or clinician (e.g., patients may feel very stressed and/or constantly on their guard, or alternatively may show an unrealistic sense of security, as if they have known their clinician for many years)?

+ Are there specific attachment relationships that lead to impairments in mentalizing?

Structured assessment of mentalizing

Much of the original work on mentalizing was inspired by the use of the Reflective Functioning Scale (RFS; Fonagy, Target, Steele, & Steele, 1998), a broad measure of mentalizing that can be scored from transcripts of interviews such as the Adult Attachment Interview (AAI) (Hesse, 2008; Main, Hesse, & Goldwyn, 2008) or the Child Attachment Interview (Shmueli-Goetz, Target, Fonagy, & Datta, 2008) (see Table 4.1 for details of the scoring system). Although the RFS was originally developed to score general mentalizing aggregated across different context and attachment experiences (as is the case with the AAI), it can also be used to score mentalizing with regard to specific issues or symptoms (e.g., anxiety attacks) (Rudden, Milrod, Meehan, & Falkenstrom, 2009; Rudden,

Table 4.1 Reflective Functioning Scale scoring of reflective functioning (RF) in interview transcripts

Score	Description of RF	
9	**Full or Exceptional**	
	Interviewee's answers show exceptional sophistication, are surprising, quite complex or elaborate, and consistently manifest reasoning in a causal way using mental states	**Moderate to high RF**
7	**Marked**	
	Interviewee's answers contain numerous statements indicating full RF, which show awareness of the nature of mental states, and explicit attempts at teasing out the mental states underlying behavior	
5	**Definite or Ordinary**	
	Interviewee shows a number of instances of RF, even if prompted by the interviewer rather than emerging spontaneously	
3	**Questionable or Low**	
	Some evidence of consideration of mental states throughout the interview, albeit at a fairly rudimentary level	**Negative to limited RF**
1	**Absent but not Repudiated**	
	RF is totally or almost totally absent	
−1	**Negative**	
	Interviewee systematically resists taking a reflective stance throughout the interview	

Milrod, Target, Ackerman, & Graf, 2006) and specific attachment figures and relationships (Diamond, Stovall-McClough, Clarkin, & Levy, 2003), or in relation to specific experiences of trauma (Ensink et al., 2015). The validation of the Reflective Functioning Questionnaire (a self-report questionnaire) is currently underway (Fonagy & Ghinai, 2008; Perkins, 2009), and a version for adolescents is already available (Ha, Sharp, Ensink, Fonagy, & Cirino, 2013). Meehan, Levy, Reynoso, Hill, and Clarkin (2009) have also developed a clinician-rated multidimensional RFS, and Vrouva and Fonagy (2009) have reported preliminary data concerning the validity of a Mentalizing Stories for Adolescents test.

Relationship-specific assessments of mentalizing include measures of parental mentalizing, such as a modified RFS that can be scored on the Parent

Development Interview (Slade, 2005; Slade, Bernbach, Grienenberger, Levy, & Locker, 2004) or on an adapted version of the Working Model of the Child Interview (Schechter et al., 2005). The Maternal Mind-Mindedness Scale, which can be scored on different types of narrative material (Meins & Fernyhough, 2006), also examines aspects of parental mentalizing. Furthermore, the validation of a self-report Parental Reflective Functioning Questionnaire (Luyten et al., 2009) is currently underway and, in addition, several experimental models have been developed to assess (relationship-specific) mentalizing in children and adolescents (Sharp & Fonagy, 2008). A recent review of reflective function measures gives further details (Katznelson, 2014).

However, the assessment of mentalizing is by no means limited to these instruments and scales: there are a wide variety of measures of social cognition that tap into the different mentalizing dimensions. Without attempting to be exhaustive, Table 4.2 provides an illustrative overview of measures that assess aspects of the dimensions (see also Sharp & Fonagy, 2008). A selection of these measures can form part of either a standard assessment battery or a battery that can be adapted for specific patients or populations. For instance, clinicians working primarily with individuals with ASPD might want to include measures that assess the cognitive and affective aspects of mentalizing (Bateman & Fonagy, 2008), whereas those working with BPD patients might want to primarily assess the extent of mentalizing impairments with regard to self and others (Fonagy & Luyten, 2009). Hence, the measures listed in Table 4.2 may help both clinicians and researchers in developing mentalizing profiles. Moreover, the overview of measures in Table 4.2 might assist researchers and clinicians in selecting instruments when they wish to test hypotheses about specific mentalizing impairments in specific patients or patient groups.

With few exceptions, most of the measures listed in Table 4.2 primarily assess controlled mentalizing, although some of these measures (e.g., the AAI-RFS) include an assessment of more automatic mentalizing, or can be adapted to assess less controlled mentalizing (e.g., using stress and/or affective priming procedures, or using eye tracking or electroencephalography to tap into less controlled aspects of mentalizing). Moreover, while some of these measures assess mentalizing retrospectively ("off-line"), others assess mentalizing "on-line," that is, in real time as social interactions evolve. These latter methods are currently relatively cumbersome. As noted earlier, the assessment of the extent of loss of mentalizing under stress, particularly in social interactions, may be clinically most relevant. Hence, there is a need to develop and validate brief, easy-to-use measures to assess this key feature of mentalizing. Most of the measures listed in Table 4.2 depend upon the individual integrating cognition and affect in performing the tasks or completing the measures.

Table 4.2 Illustrative list of measures assessing the dimensions of mentalization

	Self–Other		Cognitive–Affective		Internal–External		Automatic–Controlled	
	Self	Other	Cognitive	Affective	Internal	External	Automatic	Controlled
Questionnaires								
Beliefs about Emotions Scale (Rimes & Chalder, 2010)	x	(x)	x	x	x			x
Toronto Alexithymia Questionnaire (Bagby, Parker, & Taylor, 1994)	x		x	x	x			x
Kentucky Mindfulness Scale – Describe and Act with Awareness subscales (Baer, Smith, & Allen, 2004)	x		x	x	x		(x)	x
Mindful Attention Awareness Scale (Brown & Ryan, 2003)	x		x	x	x		(x)	x
Levels of Emotional Awareness Scale (Lane, Quinlan, Schwartz, & Walker, 1990)	x	x	x	x	x			x
Psychological Mindedness Scale (Shill & Lumley, 2002)	x	x	x	x	x			x
Interpersonal Reactivity Index – Perspective Taking Subscale (Davis, 1983)		x	x	x	x			x
Empathy Quotient (Lawrence, Shaw, Baker, Baron-Cohen, & David, 2004)	x	x	x	x	x		(x)	x
Mayer–Salovey–Caruso Emotional Intelligence Test (Salovey & Grewal, 2005)	x	x	x	x	x	x	(x)	x
Reflective Functioning Questionnaire (Fonagy & Ghinai, 2008)	x	x	x	x	x	(x)		x
Parental Reflective Functioning Questionnaire (Luyten et al., 2009)	x	x	x	x	x	(x)		x
Mentalizing Stories for Adolescents (Vrouva & Fonagy, 2009)		x	x	x	x	(x)		x

Interviews/narrative coding systems

	1	2	3	4	5	6	7
Adult Attachment Interview–Reflective Functioning Scale (Fonagy, Target, Steele, & Steele, 1998)	x	x	x	x	(x)	(x)	x
Parent Development Interview–Reflective Functioning Scale (Slade, Aber, Berger, Bresgi, & Kaplan, 2002)	x	x	x	x	(x)	(x)	x
Working Model of the Child Interview–Reflective Functioning Scale (Grienenberger, Kelly, & Slade, 2005)	x	x	x	x	(x)	(x)	x
Toronto Structured Interview for Alexithymia (Bagby, Taylor, Parker, & Dickens, 2006)	x		x	x		(x)	x
Mental States Measure and Grille de l'élaboration Verbale de l'Affect (Bouchard et al., 2008)	x	x	x	x	(x)	(x)	x
Metacognition Assessment Scale (Carcione et al., 2007)	x	x	x	x		(x)	x
Intentionality Scale (Hill, Fonagy, Lancaster, & Broyden, 2007)	x	x	x	x	(x)	(x)	x
Internal State Lexicon (Beeghly & Cicchetti, 1994)	x	x	x	x		(x)	x

Experimental/observational tasks

	1	2	3	4	5	6	7
Reading the Mind in the Eyes Test (Baron-Cohen, Wheelwright, Hill, Raste, & Plumb, 2001)		x	x	x	x		x
Reading the Mind in the Voice Test (Golan, Baron-Cohen, Hill, & Rutherford, 2007)		x	x	x	x		x
Reading the Mind in Films Task (Golan, Baron-Cohen, & Golan, 2008)		x	x	x	x		x
International Affective Picture System (Lang, Bradley, & Cuthbert, 2008)		x	x	x	x		x
NimStim Set of Facial Expressions (Tottenham et al., 2009)	x	x	x	x	x		x
Face Morphs (Bailey et al., 2008)	x	x	x	x	x	(x)	x

(Continued)

Table 4.2 (Continued)

	Self–Other		Cognitive–Affective		Internal–External		Automatic–Controlled	
	Self	Other	Cognitive	Affective	Internal	External	Automatic	Controlled
Dynamic Body Expressions (Pichon, de Gelder, & Grèzes, 2009)		x	x	x		x	(x)	x
Electromyography of facial mimicry (Sonnby-Borgström & Jönsson, 2004)	(x)	x	(x)	x		x	x	
Affect Labeling (Lieberman et al., 2007)		x	x	x		x		x
Movie for the Assessment of Social Cognition (Dziobek et al., 2006)		x	x	x	x	x	(x)	x
Trust Task (King-Casas et al., 2008)	(x)	x	x	x	x			x
Interoceptive Sensitivity (Barrett, Quigley, Bliss-Moreau, & Aronson, 2004)	x		x	x	x			x
Empathy for Pain in Others (Hein & Singer, 2008)	(x)	x	x	x	x	x	x	x
Manipulating Body Consciousness (Brass, Schmitt, Spengler, & Gergely, 2007; Lenggenhager, Tadi, Metzinger, & Blanke, 2007)	x	x		x	x	x	x	x
Animated Theory of Mind Inventory for Children (Beaumont & Sofronoff, 2008)		x	x	x	x	x	(x)	x
Maternal Mind-Mindedness (Meins & Fernyhough, 2006)	x	x	x	x	x	(x)	(x)	x
Maternal Accuracy Paradigm (Sharp, Fonagy, & Goodyer, 2006)		x	x	x	x	(x)	(x)	x
Strange Stories Task (Happé, 1994)		x	x	x	x			x
Projective measures								
Projective Imagination Test (Blackshaw, Kinderman, Hare, & Hatton, 2001)	(x)	x	x	x	x	x	(x)	x

Note: x = applicable; (x) = partly applicable

Creating a mentalizing profile

After conducting assessment interviews, the clinician should draw up a *mentalizing profile* (see Figure 4.1). This involves locating the individual's style of mentalizing on each of the different dimensions, and then considering the relationship between these different ways of functioning on each dimension: that is, do they cause mentalizing difficulties to snowball, or do they compensate for each other? Boxes 4.3–4.6 give an indication of what balanced (i.e., good) mentalizing looks like along these dimensions and indicate with examples when the balance has been lost in favor of one or the other pole of each dimension.

This stage of the assessment process should also involve considering how quickly and easily the individual is triggered to switch between controlled and automatic mentalizing (see Chapter 1), and how long it takes them to recover controlled mentalizing after the switch has happened. This necessarily requires quite a detailed assessment of the individual's relational context, with special attention paid to their attachment history and possible use of secure versus hyperactivating and deactivating attachment strategies. Assessors should be aware of the extent to which specific attachment relationships might increase the sensitivity of the switch from controlled to automatic mentalizing, and to

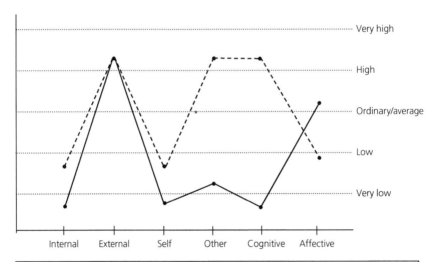

Fig. 4.1 Prototypical mentalizing profiles for BPD and ASPD.

what extent the individual is able to self-correct mentalizing lapses and to allow responses from the assessor (and, more generally, attachment figures) to help restore mentalizing.

The four dimensions provide an important guide and structure for assessment, as they set out how, in the course of a full assessment, consideration must be given to the patient's attention to internal and external features of the self and others, for their own internal states as well as those of others, and for the integration of cognitive and affective features involved. For instance, the assessor may ask questions such as "Why did you think he looked so angry at you?" or "You have been telling me how you felt toward her, but how do you think she feels?" or "You have been telling me now what you thought in this situation, but how did you feel?" Such switching of perspectives from self to other, or challenging the patient's mentalizing by counterfactual responses (e.g., suggesting an explanation that is the opposite of the patient's own explanation), may reveal important discrepancies among the patient's mentalizing abilities, particularly pseudomentalizing or psychic equivalence. For example, some patients whose thinking is imbalanced in the direction of focusing on affect rather than cognition, and is dominated by psychic equivalence, may be totally unable to switch from their own perspective to that of any other. Or, if dominated by cognition, the patient may be surprised if asked how they *felt* as opposed to what they *thought* or were "*supposed to feel*" in a particular situation. Finally, challenging patients' perspectives may lead to uncovering pseudomentalizing when patients readily agree with a change of perspective offered to them if their mentalizing is trending toward the automatic pole of the implicit–explicit mentalizing dimension.

What does good mentalizing look like?

As we shall explain, while poor mentalizing may be readily categorized into one of several types, good mentalizing takes but one form. To help with the assessment of mentalizing quality, we have developed a simple scoring chart ("Checklist for the clinical assessment of mentalizing"). A copy of the chart and the interpretations of the scores are available online at http://annafreud.org/training-research/mentalization-based-treatment-training/checklist/.

In completing the checklist, the assessor is simply asked to reflect on the interview he/she has just conducted and note compelling examples of categories of mentalizing on the chart, ticking either the "strong evidence" or "some evidence" column as appropriate. Each of the four themes is to be scored.

Here we consider several contexts within which the assessor may note high-quality mentalizing. We have listed these as simple statements of description, but across an actual assessment the clinician would be looking for evidence of these traits emerging through discourse rather than simply responding to the patient's self-descriptive statements that they possess such attributes.

1 In relation to other people's thoughts and feelings:

   a *Opaqueness*—acknowledgement in commentary that one often does not know what other people are thinking, yet not being completely puzzled by what happens in the minds of others (e.g., "What happened with Chris made me realize that we can often misunderstand even our best friends' reactions").

   b *Absence of paranoia*—not considering the thoughts of others as in themselves a significant threat and having in mind the possibility that minds can be changed (e.g., "I don't like it when he feels angry but mostly you can cajole him out of it by talking with him about it").

   c *Contemplation and reflection*—a desire to reflect on how others think in a relaxed rather than compulsive manner (e.g., during the interview the person actively contemplates the reasons why someone he/she knows well behaves as they do).

   d *Perspective-taking*—acceptance that the same thing can look very different from different perspectives based on individual history (e.g., a description of an event that was experienced as a rejection by one person and a genuine attempt made to identify how it came about that they misunderstood it as rejection).

   e *Genuine interest* in other people's thoughts and feelings—not just for their content, but also for their style (e.g., the person appears to enjoy talking about why people do things).

   f *Openness to discovery*—the person is naturally reluctant to make assumptions about what others think or feel.

   g *Forgiveness*—acceptance of others, conditional on understanding their mental states (e.g., the person's anger about something dissipates once they understand why the other person had acted in the way they did).

   h *Predictability*—a general sense that, on the whole, the reactions of others are predictable given knowledge of what they think and feel.

2 Perception of own mental functioning:

   a *Changeability*—an appreciation that one's views of and understanding of others can change in line with changes in oneself.

   b *Developmental perspective*—understanding that with development one's views of others deepen and become more sophisticated (e.g., the person acknowledges that as they grew up they began to understand their parents' actions better).

c *Realistic skepticism*—a recognition that one's feelings can be confusing.

d *Acknowledgement of preconscious function*—a recognition that at any one time one may not be aware of everything that one feels, particularly in the context of conflict.

e *Conflict*—awareness of having incompatible ideas and feelings.

f *Self-inquisitive stance*—a genuine curiosity about one's thoughts and feelings.

g *An interest in difference*—an interest in the ways minds unlike the person's own work (e.g., a genuine interest in children's minds).

h *Awareness of the impact of affect*—insight into how affects can distort one's understanding of oneself or others.

3 Self-representation:

a *Advanced pedagogic and listening skills*—the patient feels that they are able to explain things to others and are experienced by others as being patient and able to listen.

b *Autobiographical continuity*—a capacity to remember oneself as a child and evidence the experience of a continuity of ideas.

c *Rich internal life*—the person rarely experiences their mind as empty or content-less.

4 General values and attitudes:

a *Tentativeness*—on the whole, a lack of absolute certainty about what is right and what is wrong, and a preference for complexity and relativism.

b *Moderation*—a balanced attitude to most statements about mental states in both oneself and others that comes from accepting the possibility that one is not in a privileged position in regard to either one's own mental state or that of another person, and sufficient self-monitoring to recognize flaws (e.g., "I have noticed that sometimes I overreact to things").

What does nonmentalizing look like?

Poor mentalizing or nonmentalizing may be indicated by a wide range of possible signs. Box 4.7 lists some typical examples. Some key indicators pertain to the style of the narrative as well as its content and the attitudes implicit in the patient's accounts.

Box 4.7 What does nonmentalizing look like?

+ Excessive detail, to the exclusion of motivations, feelings, or thoughts
+ Focus on external social factors (e.g., the school, the local council, the housing office, the neighbors)
+ Focus on physical or structural labels (tired, lazy, clever, self-destructive, depressed, short fuse)
+ Preoccupation with rules and responsibilities, "shoulds" and "should nots"
+ Denial of involvement in problem
+ Blaming or fault-finding
+ Expressions of certainty about the thoughts or feelings of others.

Nonmentalizing is most commonly revealed in the content of the narrative. For example, in preference to talking about mental states, patients might focus on general external factors, social institutions, the physical environment, the government, or the management of the organization where they work, rather than the individuals who are involved and whose mental state is pertinent to the narrative. A preoccupation with rules and roles, obligations and responsibilities, as if these were adequate explanations of behavior rather than created to "short-circuit" mentalizing, may characterize such narratives. In other patients, a sparse narrative characterized by a denial of involvement indicates a reluctance to mentalize and look at one's own and others' intentions in a meaningful way.

Nonmentalizing is also revealed in a bias toward generalizations and labeling. For example, explanations of behavior may go around in circle—most commonly, behavior is regarded as being accounted for by a diagnosis or a personality, for example, "I blew up at him because I have such a short fuse" or "I failed at these exams because I am very self-destructive."

Not all nonmentalizing is identifiable in terms of content. It is also evident in style and at an implicit level. Nonmentalizing style may be excessively sparse or excessively detailed. If it is excessively detailed, the patient may describe events in such depth that the narrative obscures the states of mind of the participants—for example, by including endless side-stories or excessive description of physical detail.

At an implicit level, nonmentalizing is easy to see, but may also be easily overlooked. An individual may express inappropriate certainty about the thoughts and feelings of others, and speak as if they had no doubt that their model of the mind of another person was the only true perspective. Similarly, a lack of curiosity about motives betrays nonmentalizing. In others, an attitude of blaming and fault-finding indicates a wish to short-circuit the genuine possibility of understanding.

Extremely poor mentalizing revealed during the assessment process

The response of some individuals to attempts to assess their mentalizing may compromise its adequate assessment. In response to probing questions about mental state attributions, the patient may be overtly hostile, actively evasive (e.g., by changing the subject or refusing to answer the question), or even show nonverbal reactions such as walking out or starting a telephone conversation in the middle of the assessment. Somewhat less extreme—but equally unhelpful, from the point of view of an adequate assessment—responses come from individuals who fail to give adequate elaboration in response to probes about mental states. To questions about why a given person might feel in a specific way, the answer "I don't know" may be accurate, but may also communicate "I don't want to think about it."

At other times, a failure of elaboration is indicated by an absence of integration or complete confusion. Slightly less pervasive are inappropriate responses such as complete non sequiturs, gross assumptions about the interviewer's intentions, or focusing on the literal meaning of words. We view all these challenges to an adequate assessment of mentalizing as responses to the threat that mentalizing can represent. Someone whose experience has been traumatic in relation to thinking about thoughts and feelings may understandably resist being forced to think in this way. In all such instances, we code mentalizing as "poor."

Inevitably, clinicians will wonder whether a person with such limited capacities for mentalizing is treatable in MBT or, for that matter, any other form of treatment. Yet such a person is in desperate need. Their relationships are often volatile, short-lived, and characterized by suspicion of others' motives; their level of anxiety is high in everyday interactions; and their emotions are either absent or severely dysregulated. We do not have empirical evidence that this group of patients is less treatable than others in MBT. However, the clinical presentation suggests that the initial emphasis of treatment needs to be on forming a therapeutic alliance that includes a sense of hope that change is possible. Sensitive work needs to be done on building up trust in the therapeutic relationship and helping the patient define some restricted but achievable goals early in treatment. Some quick "wins" can cement the patient–clinician relationship. Empathic validation rather than challenge needs to be the main focus of interaction for some time (see Chapters 8 and 9 for discussion of these types of intervention).

Generalized versus partial difficulties

Very poor mentalizing or nonmentalizing is typically relatively easy to identify. It is more challenging to judge the extent or degree of concrete understanding or pseudomentalizing at the expense of genuine balanced mentalizing. We consider interpersonal understanding to be severely nonmentalizing if the problems are generalized and the individual consistently misses mentalizing meanings—for example, if the individual's preferred explanations for interpersonal interactions are consistently seen in physical terms, either in terms of who did what (external) or of a physical condition, such as illness, tiredness, or hunger (internal) that explains events. Systematic distortion of emotion awareness is a further indication of generalized difficulties. For example, a patient may react to sadness or anxiety on someone's part as though it indicated aggression. Rigidity of communication and relationships is a further indicator of quite generalized problems, such as an expectation that relationships cannot and will not change and that interactions with particular individuals will always be in a particular "key." The manipulative use of specific communications and relationships in general is another hallmark of generalized difficulties.

By contrast, we talk about mentalizing difficulties as being *partial* when difficulties in mentalizing emerge around particular thoughts, feelings, and situations. Commonly, the ability to mentalize breaks down when a patient is reminded of a traumatic situation by a particular person, and mentalizing then becomes difficult or impossible in relation to that person, who is associated with the trauma. Linked to this, particular mood states can interact with trauma in some individuals. Thus, depression can make a person's thoughts and feelings about him/herself appear concrete and unmentalized. In general, high arousal and also intense attachment feelings can temporarily lower the capacity to mentalize. A fleeting thought of unacceptability or inadequacy can become "as if" it was objective reality. Interactions with particular individuals may interrupt mentalizing. This could happen in relation to particular topics that arouse emotion; alternatively, mentalizing can fail in relation to a particular individual because they remind the patient of an ambivalently regarded figure.

In assessing mentalizing, we note in relation to each type of mentalizing problem whether the difficulty appears to be generalized or partial (see Box 4.8). In our experience, partial problems are often easier to reverse, although this is by no means invariably the case and many partial problems of mentalizing can be resistant to clinical interventions.

Box 4.8 Generalized versus partial difficulties in mentalizing

Generalized poor mentalizing or nonmentalizing

- Consistently misses mentalizing
- Interactions consistently seen in physical terms (internal, e.g., illness; external, e.g., who *did* what)
- Systematic distortion of emotion awareness
- Rigidity of communication and relationships
- Manipulative use of specific communications and relationships.

Partial forms of poor mentalizing

- Limited to particular thoughts, feelings, and situations (context-dependent)
- Particular mood states can interact with trauma to undermine mentalizing
- Triggered chiefly by arousal but also depression and even intense attachment
- The ability to mentalize breaks down around the idea of trauma
- Interactions with particular individuals can disrupt mentalizing.

The switch model of mentalizing

Useful to understanding partial mentalizing difficulties is what we have termed the "switch model" of understanding the connection between attachment, mentalizing, and stress (Fonagy, Luyten, & Strathearn, 2011) (see Table 4.3). The idea is that in response to stress, an individual's attachment system is activated. In this state of mind, the person's mentalizing switches to automatic, rather than being controlled. This is an almost universal human process that encourages us to seek reassurance at moments of need. However, there is considerable variation between individuals in terms of how easily their attachment systems are activated, how strongly they tend to switch into automatic mentalizing at the expense of their controlled mentalizing capacity, and how quickly they are able to recover controlled mentalizing. According to the "switch model," individuals with a hyperactive attachment strategy (anxious/resistant) will switch into automatic mentalizing more quickly and will take longer to restore controlled mentalizing.

Table 4.3 Attachment strategies, arousal, and the "switch" from controlled to automatic mentalizing

Attachment strategy	Threshold for switch	Strength of automatic response	Recovery of controlled mentalizing
Secure	High	Moderate	Fast
Hyperactivating	Low: hyperresponsive	Strong	Slow
Deactivating	Relatively high: hyporesponsive, but failure under increasing stress	Weak, but moderate to strong under increasing stress	Relatively fast
Disorganized	Incoherent: hyperresponsive, but often frantic attempts to downregulate	Strong	Slow

Disorganized attachment, which, like anxious/resistant attachment, is commonly associated with BPD (Choi-Kain & Gunderson, 2008), will similarly be hyperresponsive to stress, although this might be made incoherent by frantic attempts to suppress the stress response; however, the switch to automatic mentalizing will, again, happen quickly and be long-lasting. An individual who is securely attached will have a relatively high threshold in terms of how much stress is needed for their mentalizing to switch from controlled to automatic in the face of stress, and controlled mentalizing will be restored relatively quickly. A deactivating (avoidant) attachment strategy usually creates relatively high resistance to the switch, but these individuals' mentalizing will show increasing vulnerability to switching as stress levels increase. However, after switching, controlled mentalizing will be recovered relatively quickly.

The tendency to retain high levels of mentalizing even when faced with stressful circumstances is associated with secure attachment; it is similarly associated with the relatively quick restoration of mentalizing capacities after normal mentalizing has been knocked off course. As mentioned previously, lapses in mentalizing are part of normal functioning. A genuinely balanced mentalizing capacity is characterized by being able to appropriately switch from automatic to controlled mentalizing, the tendency to be able to maintain mentalizing even in stressful conditions, and relatively swift recovery from breakdowns in mentalizing when they occur.

The capacity to continue to mentalize even under considerable stress is associated with the so-called *broaden and build cycles* of attachment security described by Fredrickson (2001). These strategies serve to develop feelings of secure attachment, personal agency, and affect regulation ("build"), and lead one into different and more adaptive environments ("broaden") (Mikulincer & Shaver, 2007). High levels of mentalizing, therefore, are typically associated with resilience in the face of stressful conditions, and the ability to take a different perspective as a result of adversity. What is more, individuals who are strong mentalizers also show a good capacity for relationship-recruiting, that is, they are able to become attached to others who are caring and helping (Hauser, Allen, & Golden, 2006) and can assist in the effective co-regulation of stress and adversity (Luyten, Mayes, Fonagy, & Van Houdenhove, 2015).

The ability to "broaden and build" in the face of stress has been found to be less compatible with attachment hyperactivation and deactivation strategies. These strategies also constrain other behavioral systems that promote resilience, such as exploration, affiliation, and caregiving. Typically, hyperactivation and deactivation strategies lead individuals to experience difficulties in entering and maintaining lasting relationships—including relationships with mental health clinicians. Individuals using these strategies also tend to demonstrate lower than normal interest in or capacity to explore their own or other people's internal world.

The nature of each individual's "switch point" also depends on the mentalizing abilities of the relationship partner; again, this demonstrates how mentalizing is shaped by what is going on around us. Some relationships might reinforce mentalizing strengths: after all, were this not the case, what would be the point of psychotherapy? Conversely, some relationships trigger and exacerbate mentalizing difficulties, which can cause a downward spiral in mentalizing. Mentalizing develops within attachment relationships, and throughout life it is closely tied to relationships.

Overall, an accurate assessment of mentalizing will take context into account and will not focus exclusively on a single relationship (see also Choi-Kain & Gunderson, 2008). Clinicians should be particularly aware of how mentalizing skills fluctuate considerably in different situations or relationships, for example, when thinking about the relationship with one's mother versus one's father or one's partner. Hence, in assessing mentalizing, assessors should attempt to grasp the patient's wide relational context, and explore relationships that patients do not spontaneously describe or only briefly touch on. Finally, as noted, the assessment should consider the patient's capacity to co-regulate stress in the context of the relationship to the assessor, and to restore mentalizing when it becomes impaired during the assessment.

In the course of treatment, patients frequently experience dramatic temporary failures of mentalizing (when the "switch" has been triggered). When a patient shouts "You are trying to drive me crazy" or "You hate me" the likelihood is that the thoughts and feelings of the person they are shouting at, or indeed those of bystanders, are no longer clearly perceived. In truth, all of us (not just patients with personality disorder) are capable of such temporary failures. Three factors prevent these episodes from impacting more widely on our lives, none of which is available to individuals with chronic difficulties in achieving mentalizing:

1 A self-correcting mechanism rules out improbable attributions

2 The brevity of the episode

3 Perhaps most important, the normally corrective response of the other person with whom one is interacting.

None of these mechanisms works adequately for individuals with BPD, for whom context-specific, temporary failures of mentalizing can turn into a serious disruption that lasts hours rather than minutes. When we act in an atypical manner, cues from the social context help us to readjust our sense of other people. Individuals with BPD might not have access to this, as they are often not able to accurately perceive and attend to the subtle changes in other people's attitudes toward them. As we have seen, they are also less likely or less able to test the accuracy of an initial impression. Not only can they often be insensitive to the normalizing social context, but the social context is often less normalizing toward them because their reactions, born of the temporary failure of mentalizing, are less typical as far as others are concerned. Finally, as is often pointed out, they find it hard to inhibit impulses and thus to limit the duration of an outburst.

In the course of assessment, the clinician may inadvertently trigger such a context-specific failure of mentalizing. In many instances, the trigger for this might be of apparently little relevance. A combination of the patient's emotional arousal and the intensification of the attachment relationship is probably sufficient cause. However, the context within which this occurs can be important in that it points to issues or themes where the patient is unable to maintain a consistent level of mentalizing. Commonly, these contexts concern a particular relationship (i.e., being with a particular person), a particular location where this has happened before, or a particular subject or issue. The relevant aspect of such observations is noting that a particular context may need to be gradually approached, as the loss of mentalizing clearly undermines the possibility of adequately processing whatever prior experiences are raised by a relationship, a location, or a theme.

Assessment of the prementalizing modes

The switch from controlled to automatic mentalizing often also involves the re-emergence of prementalizing modes of thinking about internal states: that is, the *psychic equivalence, pretend,* and *teleological* modes of representing the internal world of oneself and others (see Chapter 1).

These modes are particularly likely to emerge in individuals with a history of trauma. Typically, these individuals will, for self-protective reasons, shut off mentalizing to avoid thinking about traumatic experiences (often in combination with acts of self-harm or substance abuse), and/or they may recreate unpleasant or frightened states of mind in others (e.g., by starting to shout, or humiliating or threatening others). This latter strategy may be used by individuals with ASPD as a means of deliberately controlling others and/or undermining their capacities for thinking and mentalizing.

The assessment of mentalizing should first and foremost take into account the different levels of arousal involved in triggering an individual's switches in mentalizing. This requires exploring mentalizing in different arousal contexts, and the assessor may need to actively probe and challenge the mentalizing process. This work must be undertaken carefully and sensitively. Individuals with a history of trauma are often easily overwhelmed, whereas, in contrast, it often takes considerable effort to gauge the mentalizing abilities of individuals with narcissistic features. Moreover, the fact that the assessment of mentalizing takes place in the context of a new attachment relationship with the assessor is important, and the responses of individuals to this new attachment relationship, and its influence on mentalizing, should be closely monitored. Do individuals show little interest in what the assessor thinks or feels? Or, conversely, are they hypervigilant with regard to the assessor's responses? In addition, the extent to which the individual is able to use the assessor to regulate arousal levels during the assessment, and thus is able to co-regulate stress in the context of the exploration of his/her internal world, provides important clues with regard to his/her mentalizing abilities "when the going gets tough." A second important implication is that individual differences in the use of secondary attachment strategies (i.e., avoidant and resistant as opposed to secure strategies) should be closely monitored.

Finally, as noted, clinicians should tailor their interventions to the specific impairments in mentalizing associated with the different attachment strategies. More specifically, evidence suggests that in individuals who primarily use hyperactivating strategies, the emphasis in treatment should be on the supportive aspects of the treatment setting, and clinicians should strive to scaffold these patients' mentalizing abilities as much as possible, particularly early in treatment (Blatt, 2008). Moreover, the clinician should closely monitor the balance between closeness and distance, as coming too close may easily lead to self–other confusion and undermine the patient's mentalizing abilities, while being too distant may lead to feelings of rejection and early dropout (Fonagy & Luyten, 2009). In patients who primarily use deactivating strategies, the integration of cognitive and affective mentalizing will take center stage, and will particularly involve bringing these patients into contact with their emotions, specifically as they emerge in the therapeutic relationship. The danger here is that patients will drop out when they start to realize that treatment involves a new attachment relationship—which challenges their deactivating approach. Another important pitfall is that the clinician assumes too readily that the patient has sufficient capacity for insight, and gets lost in intellectualized accounts of the nature of the patient's problems.

Pseudomentalizing

The biggest challenge in recognizing mentalizing is being able to distinguish it from pseudomentalizing. In pseudomentalizing, a person's overt consideration of mental states lacks some of the essential features of mentalizing outlined earlier. Thus, pseudomentalizing may be revealed by a tendency to express absolute certainty without recognizing the inherent uncertainty that "knowing" someone else's mind entails.

We have linked pseudomentalizing to the nonmentalizing *pretend mode*. This mode of experiencing one's own mind, developmentally expectable in children 2–3 years of age, is thought to be representational in a very limited sense. The young child is capable of representational thought as long as no link is made between the thought and external reality. Thus, while 2–3-year-olds can engage in "pretend" games or fantasy, they are not yet able to integrate this experience with physical reality. If challenged about their belief (e.g., whether the chair they are pushing around, treating it as a tank, is a tank or not), their play is disrupted, as they are unable to conceive of the mental state of pretending. Similarly, an adult who is pseudomentalizing appears to be capable of conceiving of and even reasoning with mental states, but only as long as these have no connection with actual reality.

Genuine mentalizing is rarely entirely self-serving. When someone makes statements about their own or others' states of mind that are entirely consistent with the individual's self-interest or preferences, one may suspect pseudomentalizing. At other times, pseudomentalizing is quite easy to recognize because the statements made about mental states are improbable, based on little evidence, are likely to be inaccurate, and yet are nevertheless asserted with great confidence.

Most pseudomentalizing falls into one of three categories (see also Box 4.9):

1 Intrusive
2 Overactive
3 Destructively inaccurate.

Box 4.9 What does pseudomentalizing look like?

Intrusive pseudomentalizing

- Opaqueness of minds is not respected
- Extends knowledge of thoughts and feelings beyond a specific context
- Presents knowledge of thoughts and feelings in an unqualified way
- Presents thoughts and feelings with a richness and complexity that is unlikely to be based on evidence
- When challenged, defaults to nonmentalizing accounts.

Overactive form of pseudomentalizing

- Idealization of insight for its own sake
- Thoughts about other felt by them as confusing and obscure.

Destructively inaccurate pseudomentalizing

- Denial of objective realities that undermines the subjective experience
- Cast in terms of accusations
- Denying someone's real feelings and replacing them with a false construction.

This categorization is given as a heuristic to help identify pseudomentalizing, not as a way of classifying individuals, as the categories tend to overlap.

Intrusive pseudomentalizing

Intrusive pseudomentalizing arises when the separateness or opaqueness of minds is not respected. The individual believes they "know" how or what another person feels or thinks. Often, elements of what is claimed may be accurate and appropriate, and it is in subtle differences or changes in emphasis that pseudomentalizing is revealed. Quite commonly this occurs in the context of relatively intense attachment relationships where the individual who is pseudomentalizing expresses what their partner is feeling but extends this beyond a specific context or presents it in an unqualified way. Mostly, mental states are described and elaborated with such richness and complexity that it is improbable that they could be based on evidence. When challenged in the course of an assessment, (e.g., "How do you know that he feels inadequate and rivalrous in relation to you?"), the account becomes clearly nonmentalizing and refers to personality traits or makes unsupportable claims about intuition ("I just know . . .").

Overactive pseudomentalizing

The overactive form of pseudomentalizing is characterized by excessive energy being invested in thinking about how people think or feel. Overactive pseudomentalizing is an idealization of insight for its own sake. There is little relationship between what is elaborated as a person's internal reality and the genuine concerns of that individual.

The person about whom such mentalizing is undertaken is most likely not even aware of it, as using mentalizing in the service of improved communication is not part of the motivation for pseudomentalizing. But, even if the person being thought about is aware, he/she is likely to find the thoughts about him/her confusing and obscure. The pseudomentalizing individual may be surprised by this and express frustration about the lack of interest the person shows about the understanding he/she has arrived at. The absence of enthusiasm is unlikely to lead to a questioning of the accuracy or validity of the mentalizing enterprise but is likely instead to be attributed to resistance or deliberate self-serving denial.

Destructively inaccurate pseudomentalizing

In essence, the first and second categories of pseudomentalizing are both, strictly speaking, "inaccurate" ways of thinking about someone else's mind. However, often they are plausible even if unlikely to be true. In contrast, the third type of pseudomentalizing, destructively inaccurate pseudomentalizing, is characterized by the denial of objective reality that undermines the subjective experience of the person described. Often, such pseudomentalizing is cast in terms of accusations, such as "You provoked me," "You were asking me to hit you." The inaccuracy is in denying someone's real feelings and replacing them with a false construction. A concerned mother might be told by her daughter, "You would be glad if I was dead." At the extreme, mental state attributions can be quite bizarre: "You are trying to drive me crazy," "I think you are in league to try to destroy me." This type of destructively inaccurate pseudomentalizing shades into the category of *misuse of mentalizing* when the inaccuracy serves the goal of one person using mentalizing to control another.

Indications of pseudomentalizing should be noted in the course of the assessment and looked at in conjunction with the assessment of the overall quality of mentalizing. All forms of poor mentalizing and pseudomentalizing may also be context-specific. Pseudomentalizing can occur only in the context of a specific attachment relationship, or only in a particular thematic context. In these cases we would consider the evidence for pseudomentalizing to be limited. Such evidence of limited pseudomentalizing should reduce the overall rating of mentalizing by one category. In other words, if there is some evidence of pseudomentalizing, mentalizing that would otherwise be scored as "good" becomes "moderate." If the evidence for pseudomentalizing is strong, the overall assessment of mentalizing should be reduced by two categories: in this case, "good" mentalizing is to be rated "poor," and "very high" mentalizing becomes "moderate."

Concrete understanding

Concrete understanding—which is associated with the psychic equivalence mode—is the most common category of nonmentalizing. It often reflects a general failure to appreciate internal states (see Box 4.10). The developmental corollary of concrete understanding is a psychic equivalence mode of experiencing subjectivity. This mode, which is also typical of 2–3-year-old children, treats mental state experiences overly seriously. There is no distinction between the status assigned to a thought or belief and that assigned to physical reality. The internal is equated with the external. For example, a child's fear of ghosts generates as real an experience as the presence of a real ghost might be expected to. Similarly, in the case of concrete understanding, mental states are deprived of their special status and are treated as if equivalent to the concretely accessible physical world.

The patient in this mode fails to make connections between thoughts and feelings on the one hand, and actions of the self and others on the other hand. He/she shows a general lack of attention to the thoughts, feelings, and wishes of others. Behavior is commonly interpreted in terms of the influence of situational or physical constraints rather than feelings and thoughts. Prejudice and other types of generalizations are common, as are tautologous and circular explanations of behavior. Descriptions or categorizations are taken as explanations; (e.g., "He does nothing all day because he is just lazy"). While concrete explanations are mostly incorrect, this is not always the case. However, in these instances concrete explanations are extended beyond the range within which they should be appropriately used. They can be offered at the wrong level of discourse; for example, a mentalized account searching for internal motives is asked for but a physical account is given in response. In explaining a violent outburst, for instance, the patient might refer to the oppressive character of the room he was in (poor air conditioning, overheated) but does not refer to the

Box 4.10 Concrete understanding

General indicators

- Lack of attention to the thoughts, feelings, and wishes of others
- Influence of the situational or physical
- Predisposition to massive generalizations and prejudice
- Circular explanations
- Concrete explanations are extended beyond the range within which they could be appropriately used.

Stylistic indicators

- Speak in absolute terms (e.g., "He always . . . ")
- Style of blaming or fault-finding
- Exaggerated characterizations and "black-and-white" thinking
- Attributions in terms of unchangeable personal characteristics
- Unnecessarily detailed descriptions
- Inflexible and rigid, sticking to the first reasonable account of behavior available
- Absence of reflection—resonance immediately triggers action.

Typical content of concrete mentalizing

- Psychologically quite implausible frames of reference
- Assumptions of motives based on physical appearance
- Thoughts and motives often misinterpreted
- Arbitrarily established ideas accepted without question
- Unquestioned attribution of malevolent intent
- Superficial or concrete understanding of behavior
- Difficulties in emotion recognition
- Problems in recognizing the impact of one's thoughts, feelings, and actions on others
- Overgeneralizing from single instances of expression on the part of others to a general and more extreme state.

impact this had on him (felt trapped, suffocated, reminded of being held down as a child when being punished, etc.).

There are subtle stylistic indications of concrete mentalizing. The concrete mentalizer will speak in absolute terms: "You always . . . ," "You never . . . ," "You totally . . . ," "It's always the same, they [a group, e.g., healthcare professionals] are all like that." Such generalizations short-circuit the need to acquire information about any specific state of mind. There is frequently a blaming or fault-finding quality to concrete mentalizing, which is similarly born out of a reluctance to explore complex mentalistic reasons for events. Obviously, such a bias is often, although not invariably, self-serving. Self-blame is another sign of concrete understanding. Splitting, or "black-and-white" thinking, is a further characteristic; this is another form of generalization that closes down the possibility of complexity. Other shortcuts are provided by focusing on the other's unchangeable personal characteristics, such as race, intelligence, or cultural background. Burying substance in detail is another stylistic strategy; excessively long and detailed descriptions of the sequence of events in interpersonal encounters can replace economical and mentalistic explanations.

A hallmark of concrete understanding is an apparent absence of flexibility. The limitations of understanding thoughts or feelings make the individual inflexible, such that he/she opts for and rigidly sticks to the first apparently reasonable account he/she can find. The natural process of working through a range of possibilities and discarding those that are implausible is simply not accessible. The individual should be thought of as being engaged in a constant struggle to relate thoughts and feelings to reality. This in itself is an aversive experience that leads to a deep sense of alienation and a feeling of not being understood. Acting without thinking is not simply a failure of inhibition; it is a failure of a normal mechanism that acts as a buffer between perception and action. Normally, resonance with another's state of mind starts a process of reflection and response selection. In a patient whose understanding of states of mind is extremely concrete, resonance immediately triggers action.

In terms of content, a concrete account often indicates that the person is at a loss when faced with a need to find a mental state-based explanation. They may resort to psychologically quite implausible frames of reference—mysticism, star signs, the supernatural—or confused accounts of unconscious interpersonal communication. Commonly, a generic reference is made to "just knowing" or general intuition. Concrete understanding, as the term suggests, is based on appearance—a physical state of affairs is often misinterpreted, a shut door inevitably means rejection—and there is a lack of questioning in relation to such interpretations. At the more extreme, more generalized end of the spectrum of difficulties, fleeting thoughts that might briefly cross all our minds become established ideas that are accepted without question. In this context, preoccupation with grievances and taking revenge may be particularly painful. The unquestioned attribution of malevolent intent to another person, supported by the assumption of intrinsic malevolence, can trigger ferocious rage.

As we have seen, a range of factors act together to generate these and other indicators of concrete understanding. While the most powerful is the superficial or concrete understanding of behavior, other consequences of mentalizing failure also play a part. For example, difficulties in emotion recognition may send the person off on a "wild goose chase" of trying to understand a reaction that was not there in the first place, say, an angry reaction. The difficulty in observing one's *own* thoughts and feelings generates obvious problems in recognizing the impact that one's thoughts, feelings, and actions have on others. If a person does not know they are feeling angry, for instance, they may have considerable difficulty in understanding others' reactions to the chronically hostile stance they unknowingly present. Inadequately conceptualizing mental states may lead a person to overgeneralize from single instances of expression of intent on the part of others. For example, a modest expression of liking someone might, for the patient, be distorted and heard as feeling deep affection or even love. The bias is understandable and obviously self-serving. The lack of limitations upon it that would normally be introduced by social cognition is what requires explanation.

Enactment

A hallmark of working with individuals with personality disorder is that "treatment" rarely begins and ends in the consulting room. As we know, things happen. It is unusual for a treatment not to involve conflict between the clinician and the patient about what actions the patient engages in with others or in relation to the clinician, or indeed in relation to their own best interest. Sometimes these actions lead the clinician to consider the patient "provocative," "manipulative," or "controlling." These kinds of actions are rarely neutral and mostly they provoke general anxiety in the clinician, which may manifest as worries on behalf of the patient, or indeed on the clinician's own behalf in terms of the reputational damage the patient's actions may inflict. Some actions are "diagnostic," such as self-harm, suicide attempts, or violent, aggressive acts. At other times, the actions involve violent conflict that does not reach the level of physical aggression but is nevertheless unusual in its ferocity and apparently uncontrolled quality. Actions that involve the clinician as a subject of either an aggressive attack or exaggerated affection are reported as difficulties that clinicians commonly encounter. More common, but less recognized, is the situation in which the clinician is not directly subject to an action but something is demanded of him/her, such as writing letters of support or making telephone calls to the patient outside normal working hours. At the mild end, this can consist of pressure to reply to e-mails from the patient; at the more burdensome end it can involve visiting the patient in hospital or at home.

What all these situations have in common is:

- An awareness on the part of the clinician that something is or was not quite right
- Puzzlement on the part of the clinician as to how he/she should act in relation to the patient's actions, often accompanied by anxiety
- A sense of urgency about something needing to be done quickly and effectively, to "deal" with the situation
- A deep, often conscious realization that, however the clinician responds, there is no appropriate action—whatever he/she does will be associated with major long-term consequences and ultimately nothing good will come of it.

The following is a real clinical example that was reported to us in supervision.

The patient, in the process of being relatively successfully treated by a good community mental health team, made the claim that her progress was being obstructed by the state of her apartment. The patient explained that although she was feeling better and more "centered," when she returned home, her "new-found balance" was lost because she had been unable to tidy her apartment for a considerable time because of her illness. Indeed, the apartment had become chaotic and dirty, and it was now beyond the client's capacity to make good: "How can I fully recover if every time I go home, I'm confronted by the results of my illness? I can never find anything—I spend all my time searching for things that I know must be there somewhere. The shambles at home drives me mad—it just forces me to remember how bad things had been and still could be." The patient requested that the apartment should be deep-cleaned by the hospital trust. The team considered the request and, after reflection, turned it down. They considered the request to be an "enactment" and that complying with it carried risks. The patient wrote to the chief executive of the Health Trust making the same request, writing lucidly and eloquently about how her progress was being curtailed by her physical environment while expressing gratitude for the helpfulness of the mental health team in other areas. The chief executive was sympathetic and asked the team to arrange the deep clean. The arguments mounted by the team to dissuade the chief executive were met with a brief note to the team leader, "Please arrange!" Reluctantly, the team agreed, and the deep clean was arranged. While the patient's mental state appeared not to benefit—in fact, if anything, it slightly deteriorated—the unanticipated consequence was a weekly e-mail correspondence from the patient to the chief executive in relation to aspects of her care. After a while, the chief executive tired of this and wrote to the team: "Please stop this."

This example illustrates that enactment—as with all other expressions of poor mentalizing—cannot and should not be tackled head on. Mentalizing will never be an adequate response to nonmentalizing. It simply does not address the patient's need. In this example, the issue is all too clear: the patient's teleologically driven wish for a clean and tidy home environment was only very loosely coupled to the need to experience oneself and one's subjectivity in a coherent and predictable way. If the real worry is not being able to "find" thoughts and feelings in one's mind in a predictable way, tidying up one's home, however comforting, is not really relevant. Enactments are an indication of nonmentalizing in the teleological mode. Engaging with enactments forces the patient to stay in a poorly mentalizing domain. Directly addressing the reasons that may lie behind the patient's actions is not helpful either. Explaining to the patient that her wish for a clean and well-ordered home was just a symbolic expression of her dissatisfaction with her subjective state of confusion was unlikely to have been helpful.

So how do we understand the frequent need to "act out" on the part of individuals with BPD or ASPD? Translating experiences into action is primarily an interpersonal process. The action is a signal that mentalizing is momentarily vulnerable and any kind of reflection is unhelpful. The action has no meaning at the time it is performed. Any attempt to create meaning flies in the face of a nonmentalizing process and reflects the *clinician's* need for a tidy, organized subjective world rather than addressing the patient's experience. Our understanding of such outcome-oriented behavior is that it is the clinician's subjective reaction that the patient is trying to direct, and that the purpose of this is to relieve the patient of feelings that are difficult to tolerate. In people with ASPD, engendering anxiety and/or helplessness in one's partner may be a way of making feelings in oneself more tolerable: the feeling is now outside the patient, therefore it is not something that the patient feels. As clinicians, we may feel controlled or manipulated, but responding along these lines misses the patient's point: they need us to feel frightened or helpless in order to be able to tolerate the feeling we have engendered in them. Clinicians with a psychoanalytic background may be tempted to name these feelings for the patient in an attempt to persuade them to own them. This again misses the point: enactments and the teleological thinking that drives them occur precisely because these feelings *cannot* be tolerated or owned. A patient of one of us (PF) came in dripping with blood following an act of self-cutting in the washroom in the clinic before the session: the sight was alarming and generated distinct squeamishness. The temptation was to express horror, sharing the experience of shock and distress, and to attribute malign intent to the patient in creating this situation. Within MBT, the principal clinical obligation is to help the patient recover mentalizing when encountering nonmentalizing. In this case, in the context of self-harming, expressing concern is a natural human reaction. But in the context of MBT it should be followed by genuine curiosity about what was going on for the patient before the event happened. Of course, it is important to be able to genuinely listen to a genuine response to a genuine enquiry: with blood dripping on the floor, this is hard to achieve! Enactments are difficult to manage precisely because they impose powerful constraints on the clinician's capacity to mentalize. Our advice is to ensure that the therapist's own mentalizing is intact before addressing the nonmentalizing of the patient. To put it metaphorically, the patient may not feel the need for a bandage, but the clinician needs the patient to have one before he/she can perform in his/her role.

Misuse of mentalizing

A substantial proportion of individuals with severe personality disorder appear to have an almost excessive capacity to mentalize. This impression is created by the patient's determination to use mentalizing to control the behavior of another individual, often in a manner that is detrimental to them. Mind-reading is helpful in enabling the patient to "press other people's buttons" and get them to react in ways that are advantageous to the patient. The reaction called for is often apparently negative (e.g., provoking the other so as to elicit anger) but in the broader context can be seen as self-serving (e.g., the patient feels that he/she is "in the right," vindicated as a victim of the unjustified overreaction of the person being provoked). At other times, the same person may use their mentalizing abilities to seduce or reassure, anticipating the needs or concerns of the person they are interacting with (see Box 4.11).

All this might give the impression of someone with extraordinary mentalizing capacities. However, in these individuals the reading of the mind of another person often comes at the expense of the capacity to represent their own mental state. There is a massive imbalance between the capacity to mentalize others and to see oneself accurately. A further imbalance may be observed between the ability to be sensitive to what people know or believe (thoughts, beliefs, and knowledge) and their emotional states and affective experiences. At the extreme end of this continuum, the person may know how someone else feels but cannot resonate with this feeling. This can, of course, give them apparent freedom to cause distress in others.

Box 4.11 Misuse of mentalizing

General indicators

- Use mentalizing to control the behavior of another individual
- Often used in a manner that is detrimental to those "mentalized"
- Apparently almost excessive capacity to mentalize, at the expense of the capacity to represent own mental state
- Knowledge of how someone else feels without being able to resonate with this feeling.

Mild misuse

- Limited intention to control the mind of the other
- Empathic understanding of the other
- Distortions of the other's feelings or a misrepresentation of one's own experience
- Manipulative intent relevant to a complex set of social relationships
- Unlikely to involve psychological abuse.

Attempts to induce specific thoughts and feelings in another person

- Use knowledge of others' feelings in a sadistic way
- Inducing guilt, anxiety, or shame
- Engendering unwarranted loyalty
- Almost universal in the psychotherapeutic treatment of individuals with BPD.

Deliberate undermining of a person's capacity to think

- Most readily achieved by generating arousal
- Invariably aversive
- Physical threats, shouting, and/or abusive language
- Humiliating or threatening humiliation, for example, by suicidal threats.

(Continued)

Box 4.11 What is mentalizing? (Continued)

Trauma and maltreatment

- Self-protective shutting off of mentalizing to protect from malevolent intent of attachment figure
- Recreate a vacuous or panicked state of mind in others
- Traumatogenic misuse of mentalizing turned against the self—substance misuse, self-cutting, and dissociation.

The misuse of mentalizing needs to be assessed in terms of its severity. At the milder end of this type of problem are individuals who use their understanding of mental states in a detrimental and self-serving way but with only limited intentions to control the mind of the other. Even empathic understanding of the other may be used manipulatively in self-serving ways. Often, this kind of misuse of mentalizing involves exaggeration or distortion of others' feelings or a misrepresentation of one's own experience. While the experience of not being accurately understood is likely to be aversive, the creation of that sense of being misperceived is not likely to be the aim of the misuse of mentalizing. More commonly, there is a manipulative intent relevant to a complex set of social relationships. For example, a parent may overreact to a child's mild sadness and claim that the child is deeply distressed about something in order to cause difficulties for an ex-partner as part of a custody dispute. An ostensibly empathic understanding of the child's "upset" serves as ammunition in a relationship battle. Very rarely does this form of misuse of mentalizing amount to psychological abuse.

A more complex set of problems arises when there is an apparent attempt to induce specific thoughts and feelings in another person. At the extreme, there are antisocial individuals who use knowledge of others' feelings in a sadistic way. This kind of manipulation is characteristic of so-called psychopaths, who may use their mentalizing capacities to engender trust in another person in order to then be able to exploit them. This type of elaborate control of someone's behavior is rare. More commonly, the misuse of mentalizing involves inducing guilt, anxiety, or shame, or sometimes engendering unwarranted loyalty, as part of establishing control over the other person. This type of misuse of mentalizing is encountered almost universally in the psychotherapeutic treatment of individuals with BPD, whereby the clinician is induced to experience mental states that are the patient's own.

A special form of this coercive misuse is a deliberate undermining of a person's capacity to think. For someone whose mentalizing capacity is poor, the presence of another person who is capable of thought may often be deeply threatening. There are relatively easy ways of undermining mentalizing, which is achieved most readily by generating arousal. These are invariably aversive experiences for the "victim." Physical threats, shouting, abusive language, or simply overtaxing the listener's attentional capacities may all serve to block his/her mentalizing. More subtly, patients may induce a failure of mentalizing in the other by humiliating them or threatening humiliation. For example, suicidal threats by a patient may create anxiety in a clinician as well as implying professional failure (shame) and thus serve to partially or fully arrest the clinician's capacity to adequately contemplate the mental state of the patient.

A further special issue concerning the misuse of mentalizing relates to trauma and maltreatment. Children often respond to an abusive adult's hostile intent toward them by inhibiting their own capacity to think about mental states: contemplating the state of mind of their abuser (who is often an attachment figure, e.g., a parent) is often simply too painful. Not surprisingly, exploring the issue of trauma in adult survivors of maltreatment frequently causes a loss of mentalizing. More pertinent in this context is the need of traumatized individuals to recreate a vacuous or panicked state of mind in others around them in order to relieve themselves of such unbearably painful states. Even more frequently, the trauma-induced misuse of mentalizing may be turned against the self. Stopping oneself from thinking may be achieved in various ways, including substance misuse, self-harm, or seeking an extreme version of pretend mode functioning in a state of dissociation.

Summary

A thorough assessment of mentalizing involves investigating the different dimensions of mentalizing, in varying stress conditions, and across different relationships. This includes how the patient mentalizes in relation to the assessor. It may require some probing to locate the patient's mentalizing limits and also to see beyond "canned" impressions of mentalizing. Overall, the assessment of mentalizing should fulfill the following aims:

1 Provide a map of important interpersonal relationships and their connections to key problem behaviors

2 Assess the quality of mentalizing in these contexts

3 Delineate significant attempts at undermining mentalizing

4 Assess whether difficulties in mentalizing are generalized or partial

5 In either case, assess whether pseudomentalizing or concrete understanding predominates

6 Any tendency to misuse mentalizing needs to be considered separately.

References

Baer, R. A., Smith, G. T., & Allen, K. B. (2004). Assessment of mindfulness by self-report. *Assessment*, **11**, 191–206.

Bagby, R. M., Parker, J. D. A., & Taylor, G. J. (1994). The twenty-item Toronto Alexithymia Scale – I. Item selection and cross-validation of the factor structure. *Journal of Psychosomatic Research*, **38**, 23–32.

Bagby, R. M., Taylor, G. J., Parker, J. D. A., & Dickens, S. E. (2006). The development of the Toronto Structured Interview for Alexithymia: Item selection, factor structure, reliability and concurrent validity. *Psychotherapy and Psychosomatics*, **75**, 25–39.

Bailey, C. A., Pendl, J., Levin, A., Olsen, S., Langlois, E., Crowley, M. J., & Mayes, L. C. (2008). *Face morphing tutorial: From models to morphs*. Unpublished manual. New Haven, CT: Yale Child Study Center.

Baron-Cohen, S., Wheelwright, S., Hill, J., Raste, Y., & Plumb, I. (2001). The "Reading the Mind in the Eyes" Test revised version: A study with normal adults, and adults with Asperger syndrome or high-functioning autism. *Journal of Child Psychology and Psychiatry*, **42**, 241–251

Barrett, L. F., Quigley, K. S., Bliss-Moreau, E., & Aronson, K. R. (2004). Interoceptive sensitivity and self-reports of emotional experience. *Journal of Personality and Social Psychology*, **87**, 684–697.

Bateman, A., & Fonagy, P. (2008). 8-year follow-up of patients treated for borderline personality disorder: Mentalization-based treatment versus treatment as usual. *American Journal of Psychiatry*, **165**, 631–638.

Bateman, A. W., & Fonagy, P. (2006). *Mentalization based treatment for borderline personality disorder: A practical guide*. Oxford, UK: Oxford University Press.

Beaumont, R., & Sofronoff, K. (2008). A new computerised advanced theory of mind measure for children with Asperger syndrome: The ATOMIC. *Journal of Autism and Developmental Disorders*, **38**, 249–260.

Beeghly, M., & Cicchetti, D. (1994). Child maltreatment, attachment, and the self system: Emergence of an internal state lexicon in toddlers at high social risk. *Development and Psychopathology*, **6**, 5–30.

Blackshaw, A. J., Kinderman, Hare, D. J., & Hatton, C. (2001). Theory of mind, causal attribution and paranoia in Asperger syndrome. *Autism*, **5**, 147–163.

Blatt, S. J. (2008). *Polarities of experience: Relatedness and self definition in personality development, psychopathology, and the therapeutic process*. Washington, DC: American Psychological Association.

Bouchard, M.-A., Target, M., Lecours, S., Fonagy, P., Tremblay, L.-M., Schachter, A., & Stein, H. (2008). Mentalization in adult attachment narratives: Reflective functioning, mental states, and affect elaboration compared. *Psychoanalytic Psychology*, **25**, 47–66.

Brass, M., Schmitt, R. M., Spengler, S., & Gergely, G. (2007). Investigating action understanding: Inferential processes versus action simulation. *Current Biology*, **17**, 2117–2121.

Brown, K. W., & Ryan, R. M. (2003). The benefits of being present: Mindfulness and its role in psychological well-being. *Journal of Personality and Social Psychology*, **84**, 822–848.

Carcione, A., Dimaggio, G., Falcone, M., Nicolo, G., Procacci, M., & Semerari, A. (2007). *Metacognition Assessment Scale (MAS) 3.1*. Rome, Italy: Centro di Psicoterapia Cognitiva.

Choi-Kain, L. W., & Gunderson, J. G. (2008). Mentalization: Ontogeny, assessment, and application in the treatment of borderline personality disorder. *American Journal of Psychiatry*, **165**, 1127–1135.

Davis, M. H. (1983). Measuring individual differences in empathy: Evidence for a multidimensional approach. *Journal of Personality and Social Psychology*, **44**, 113–126.

Diamond, D., Stovall-McClough, C., Clarkin, J. F., & Levy, K. N. (2003). Patient-therapist attachment in the treatment of borderline personality disorder. *Bulletin of the Menninger Clinic*, **67**, 227–259.

Dinsdale, N., & Crespi, B. J. (2013). The borderline empathy paradox: Evidence and conceptual models for empathic enhancements in borderline personality disorder. *Journal of Personality Disorders*, **27**, 172–195.

Dziobek, I., Fleck, S., Kalbe, E., Rogers, K., Hassenstab, J., Brand, M., . . . Convit, A. (2006). Introducing MASC: A Movie for the Assessment of Social Cognition. *Journal of Autism and Developmental Disorders*, **36**, 623–636.

Ensink, K., Normandin, L., Target, M., Fonagy, P., Sabourin, S., & Berthelot, N. (2015). Mentalization in children and mothers in the context of trauma: An initial study of the validity of the Child Reflective Functioning Scale. *British Journal of Developmental Psychology*, **33**, 203–217.

Fonagy, P., & Bateman, A. (2006). Progress in the treatment of borderline personality disorder. *British Journal of Psychiatry*, **188**, 1–3.

Fonagy, P., & Ghinai, R. A. (2008). *A self-report measure of mentalizing: Development and preliminary test of the reliability and validity of the Reflective Function Questionnaire (RFQ)*. Unpublished manuscript. London, UK: University College London.

Fonagy, P., & Luyten, P. (2009). A developmental, mentalization-based approach to the understanding and treatment of borderline personality disorder. *Development and Psychopathology*, **21**, 1355–1381.

Fonagy, P., Luyten, P., & Strathearn, L. (2011). Borderline personality disorder, mentalization, and the neurobiology of attachment. *Infant Mental Health Journal*, **32**, 47–69.

Fonagy, P., Target, M., Steele, H., & Steele, M. (1998). *Reflective functioning scale manual*. London, UK: University College London.

Fredrickson, B. L. (2001). The role of positive emotions in positive psychology. The broaden-and-build theory of positive emotions. *American Psychologist*, **56**, 218–226.

Golan, O., Baron-Cohen, S., & Golan, Y. (2008). The "Reading the Mind in Films" Task [Child Version]: Complex emotion and mental state recognition in children with and without autism spectrum conditions. *Journal of Autism and Developmental Disorders*, **38**, 1534–1541.

Golan, O., Baron-Cohen, S., Hill, J., & Rutherford, M. (2007). The "Reading the Mind in the Voice" Test–Revised: A study of complex emotion recognition in adults with and without autism spectrum conditions. *Journal of Autism and Developmental Disorders*, **37**, 1096–1106.

Grienenberger, J. F., Kelly, K., & Slade, A. (2005). Maternal reflective functioning, mother–infant affective communication, and infant attachment: Exploring the link between mental states and observed caregiving behavior in the intergenerational transmission of attachment. *Attachment and Human Development*, **7**, 299–311.

Ha, C., Sharp, C., Ensink, K., Fonagy, P., & Cirino, P. (2013). The measurement of reflective function in adolescents with and without borderline traits. *Journal of Adolescence*, **36**, 1215–1223.

Happé, F. G. E. (1994). An advanced test of theory of mind: Understanding of story characters' thoughts and feelings by able autistic, mentally handicapped and normal children and adults. *Journal of Autism and Developmental Disorders*, **30**, 129–154.

Hauser, S. T., Allen, J. P., & Golden, E. (2006). *Out of the woods. Tales of resilient teens.* Cambridge, MA: Harvard University Press.

Hein, G., & Singer, T. (2008). I feel how you feel but not always: The empathic brain and its modulation. *Current Opinion in Neurobiology*, **18**, 153–158.

Hesse, E. (2008). The Adult Attachment Interview: Protocol, method of analysis, and empirical studies. In J. Cassidy & P. R. Shaver (Eds.), *Handbook of attachment: Theory, research, and clinical applications* (2nd ed., pp. 552–598). New York, NY: Guilford Press.

Higgitt, A., & Fonagy, P. (1992). Psychotherapy in borderline and narcissistic personality disorder. *British Journal of Psychiatry*, **161**, 23–43.

Hill, J., Fonagy, P., Lancaster, G., & Broyden, N. (2007). Aggression and intentionality in narrative responses to conflict and distress story stems: An investigation of boys with disruptive behaviour problems. *Attachment and Human Development*, **9**, 223–237.

Katznelson, H. (2014). Reflective functioning: A review. *Clinical Psychology Review*, **34**, 107–117.

King-Casas, B., Sharp, C., Lomax-Bream, L., Lohrenz, T., Fonagy, P., & Montague, P. R. (2008). The rupture and repair of cooperation in borderline personality disorder. *Science*, **321**, 806–810.

Lane, R. D., Quinlan, D. M., Schwartz, G. E., & Walker, P. A. (1990). The levels of emotional awareness scale: A cognitive-developmental measure of emotion. *Journal of Personality Assessment*, **55**, 124–134.

Lang, P. J., Bradley, M. M., & Cuthbert, B. N. (2008). International affective picture system (IAPS): Affective ratings of pictures and instruction manual (Technical Report No. A-8). Gainesville, FL: University of Florida.

Lawrence, E. J., Shaw, P., Baker, D., Baron-Cohen, S., & David, A. S. (2004). Measuring empathy: Reliability and validity of the Empathy Quotient. *Psychological Medicine*, **34**, 911–919.

Lenggenhager, B., Tadi, T., Metzinger, T., & Blanke, O. (2007). Video ergo sum: Manipulating bodily self-consciousness. *Science*, **317**, 1096–1099.

Lieberman, M. D., Eisenberger, N. I., Crockett, M. J., Tom, S. M., Pfeifer, J. H., & Way, B. M. (2007). Putting feelings into words: Affect labeling disrupts amygdala activity in response to affective stimuli. *Psychological Science*, **18**, 421–428.

Luyten, P., Mayes, L., Fonagy, P., & Van Houdenhove, B. (2015). The interpersonal regulation of stress: A developmental framework. Manuscript in preparation.

Luyten, P., Mayes, L. C., Sadler, L., Fonagy, P., Nicholls, S., Crowley, M., . . . Slade, A. (2009). *The Parental Reflective Functioning Questionnaire-1 (PRFQ-1).* Leuven, Belgium: University of Leuven.

Main, M., Hesse, E., & Goldwyn, R. (2008). Studying differences in language usage in recounting attachment history: An introduction to the AAI. In H. Steele & M. Steele (Eds.), *Clinical applications of the Adult Attachment Interview* (pp. 31–68). New York, NY: Guilford Press.

Meehan, K. B., Levy, K. N., Reynoso, J. S., Hill, L. L., & Clarkin, J. F. (2009). Measuring reflective function with a multidimensional rating scale: Comparison with scoring reflective function on the AAI. *Journal of the American Psychoanalytic Association*, **57**, 208–213.

Meins, E., & Fernyhough, C. (2006). *Mind-mindedness coding manual*. Unpublished manuscript. Durham, UK: Durham University.

Mikulincer, M., & Shaver, P. R. (2007). *Attachment in adulthood: Structure, dynamics and change*. New York, NY: Guilford Publications.

Perkins, A. (2009). *Feelings, faces and food: Mentalization in borderline personality disorder and eating disorders*. (DClinPsych dissertation). Guilford, UK: University of Surrey.

Pichon, S., de Gelder, B., & Grèzes, J. (2009). Two different faces of threat. Comparing the neural systems for recognizing fear and anger in dynamic body expressions. *Neuroimage*, **47**, 1873–1883.

Rimes, K. A., & Chalder, T. (2010). The Beliefs about Emotions Scale: Validity, reliability and sensitivity to change. *Journal of Psychosomatic Research*, **68**, 285–292.

Rudden, M., Milrod, B., Target, M., Ackerman, S., & Graf, E. (2006). Reflective functioning in panic disorder patients: A pilot study. *Journal of the American Psychoanalytic Association*, **54**, 1339–1343.

Rudden, M. G., Milrod, B., Meehan, K. B., & Falkenstrom, F. (2009). Symptom-specific reflective functioning: incorporating psychoanalytic measures into clinical trials. *Journal of the American Psychoanalytic Association*, **57**, 1473–1478.

Salovey, P., & Grewal, D. (2005). The science of emotional intelligence. *Current Directions in Psychological Science*, **14**, 281–285.

Schechter, D. S., Coots, T., Zeanah, C. H., Davies, M., Coates, S. W., Trabka, K. A., . . . Myers, M. M. (2005). Maternal mental representations of the child in an inner-city clinical sample: Violence-related posttraumatic stress and reflective functioning. *Attachment and Human Development*, **7**, 313–331.

Sharp, C., & Fonagy, P. (2008). The parent's capacity to treat the child as a psychological agent: Constructs, measures and implications for developmental psychopathology. *Social Development*, **17**, 737–754.

Sharp, C., Fonagy, P., & Goodyer, I. (2006). Imagining your child's mind: Psychosocial adjustment and mothers' ability to predict their children's attributional response styles. *British Journal of Developmental Psychology*, **24**, 197–214.

Shill, M. A., & Lumley, M. A. (2002). The Psychological Mindedness Scale: Factor structure, convergent validity and gender in a non-psychiatric sample. *Psychology and Psychotherapy: Theory, Research and Practice*, **75**, 131–150.

Shmueli-Goetz, Y., Target, M., Fonagy, P., & Datta, A. (2008). The child attachment interview: A psychometric study of reliability and discriminant validity. *Developmental Psychology*, **44**, 939–956.

Slade, A. (2005). Parental reflective functioning: An introduction. *Attachment and Human Development*, **7**, 269–281.

Slade, A., Aber, J. L., Berger, B., Bresgi, I., & Kaplan, M. (2002). *The Parent Development Interview – Revised*. Unpublished manuscript. New Haven, CT: Yale Child Study Center.

Slade, A., Bernbach, E., Grienenberger, J., Levy, D., & Locker, A. (2004). *Addendum to Fonagy, Target, Steele & Steele Reflective Functioning Scoring Manual for use with the Parent Development Interview.* Unpublished manuscript. New York, NY: City College.

Sonnby-Borgström, M., & Jönsson, P. (2004). Dismissing-avoidant pattern of attachment and mimicry reactions at different levels of information processing. *Scandinavian Journal of Psychology*, **45**, 103–113.

Tottenham, N., Tanaka, J. W., Leon, A., C., McCarry, T., Nurse, M., Hare, T. A., . . . Nelson, C. (2009). The NimStim set of facial expressions: Judgments from untrained research participants. *Psychiatry Research*, **168**, 242–249.

Treffert, D. A. (2014). Savant syndrome: Realities, myths and misconceptions. *Journal of Autism and Developmental Disorders*, **44**, 564–571.

Viding, E., & McCrory, E. J. (2012). Why should we care about measuring callous-unemotional traits in children? *British Journal of Psychiatry*, **200**, 177–178.

Vrouva, I., & Fonagy, P. (2009). Development of the Mentalizing Stories for Adolescents (MSA). *Journal of the American Psychoanalytic Association*, **57**, 1174–1179.

Part 2

Mentalizing practice

Chapter 5

Structure of mentalization-based treatment

Introduction

The overall aim of MBT is to develop a therapeutic process in which the mind of the patient becomes the focus of treatment. The objective is for the patient to find out more about how he/she thinks and feels about him/herself and others, how that dictates his/her responses to others, and how "errors" in understanding him/herself and others may lead to actions in an attempt to retain mental stability and to attenuate incomprehensible feelings. The clinician has to ensure that the patient is constantly reminded of this goal, that the therapy process itself is not mysterious, and that the patient understands the underlying focus of treatment. This cannot be assumed even if the patient has undertaken the MBT-Introductory (MBT-I) course (see Chapter 11).

The mentalizing process can only be developed if the structure of treatment is carefully defined. The overarching structure in MBT consists of the assessment process followed by MBT-I, and then MBT-Individual plus MBT-Group (see Figure 5.1).

It is important to remember that the assessment process itself is an intrinsic part of the trajectory of treatment and *not* something dislocated from the whole treatment process. It forms part of the initial sessions and is a significant aspect of engaging the patient in treatment itself. Because of its importance, assessment is dealt with separately, in Chapter 4.

Trajectory of treatment

The trajectory of treatment has a number of main phases, with a beginning, a middle, and an end. The overall aim of the initial phase is assessment of the patient's mentalizing capacities and personality function, contracting and engaging the patient in treatment, and identifying problems that might interfere with treatment. Specific processes include giving a diagnosis, providing psychoeducation, establishing a hierarchy of therapeutic aims, stabilizing social and behavioral problems, reviewing medication, defining a crisis pathway, and agreeing outcome monitoring (see Figure 5.2).

Structure of treatment

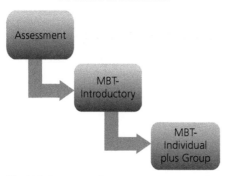

Fig. 5.1 Structure of treatment.

During the middle sessions, the aim of all the active therapeutic work is to stimulate a more robust mentalizing ability within the context of emotional arousal and attachment relationships. The more specific technical aspects of this phase of treatment are discussed in later chapters.

In the final stage, preparation is made for ending treatment. This requires the clinician to focus on the feelings of loss associated with ending treatment and how to maintain gains that have been made, as well as developing, in conjunction with the patient, an appropriate follow-up program tailored to his/her

Trajectory of treatment

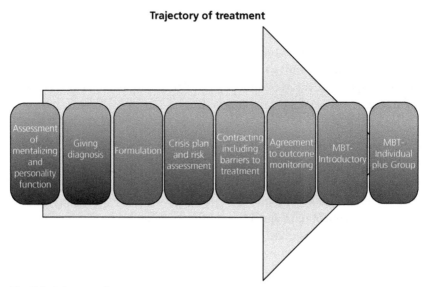

Fig. 5.2 Trajectory of treatment.

particular needs. The view often expounded by protagonists of particular models of therapy that patients with severe personality disorder improve adequately following 12–18 months of treatment to the extent that they require no further support is fanciful, and remains part of research mythology rather than realistic clinical practice.

Initial phase

Assessment of mentalizing

The assessment of patients' mentalizing capacity is discussed in Chapter 4.

Giving the diagnosis and introducing the approach

Mental health professionals have expressed a great deal of anxiety about giving a patient a diagnosis of personality disorder. Fears are rightly expressed about pejorative overtones, judgmental attitudes, blaming the patient, attacking the very "soul" of the individual, and stigmatizing the patient for life.

> One of our patients complained that even after treatment, when she no longer met criteria for a personality disorder, medical staff treated her with suspicion and uncertainty as soon as they saw her notes, despite her obvious ability to interact with services appropriately.

Despite these potential drawbacks, we firmly believe that it is both necessary and constructive to give the patient an appropriate diagnosis. But how does one give the diagnosis in such a way that it is beneficial and helpful? This is less of a problem with patients who show characteristics of non-comorbid borderline personality disorder (BPD), although even then it may be difficult. But it becomes more problematic if the patient meets criteria for borderline, narcissistic, paranoid, or antisocial personality disorder and also has a major psychiatric disorder such as depression. We cannot hide behind the failings of nosology, pass responsibility and blame on to inadequate diagnostic systems, or simply say that we do not believe in diagnosis. Even if we do not believe in categorical diagnostic systems, someone else in the mental health service is likely to have given the patient a diagnosis or simply to have told the patient that their needs cannot be met within the normal service "because they have a personality disorder which is untreatable." Uncertainty and doubt about the value of diagnosis may be appropriate, but avoidance and lack of clarity are likely to induce the patient to distrust the competence of the practitioner, making the development of a therapeutic alliance more difficult.

Let us assume that you are taking a categorical approach to personality and have concluded that a patient has BPD. In our experience, the best approach is to be direct and explanatory, bearing in mind that you want to stimulate the patient's capacity to reflect on him/herself and on your perspective about him/her. There are many ways to go about this and we do not presume to have the correct answer. You, the reader, may have a better way of explaining the diagnosis and, if so, you should keep to what you do. However, from the perspective of MBT, the primary purpose of giving the diagnosis is to stimulate the patient to consider all aspects of him/herself and to reflect on your thoughts about him/her, while you demonstrate your capacity to consider his/her problems.

When giving the diagnosis it is necessary to check out the patient's understanding of what you are saying frequently. It is anti-mentalizing on the part of the clinician to make assumptions about how much or how little the patient knows. If you assume too much you will induce defensiveness, but if you assume too little you may well be challenged as patronizing. It is equally anti-mentalizing—that is, undermining to the patient's mentalizing—to "make sure that the patient has understood what you are saying." The point is not to "tell" the patient what you know and to demonstrate the extent of your knowledge, but to stimulate reflection. The mentalizing clinician finds out what the patient has understood about what the clinician is saying. In principle, you are trying to find out whether what you have in your mind about the patient actually corresponds to a state of mind that he/she recognizes. You are not trying to persuade the patient of your viewpoint.

Opening a "dialogue about diagnosis"

You may wish to begin with a clear statement of your diagnosis, but in general it is best to move toward the diagnosis sensitively, asking the patient about what sort of person he/she feels that he/she is. Some questions that can be used as part of this process are summarized in Box 5.1.

Eventually, the diagnosis should be broached:

> Trying to put together everything that you have told me, I think that you have borderline personality disorder. Have you ever heard this term?

Box 5.1 Establishing a diagnosis

- How would you describe yourself as a person?
- What makes you an individual?
- How would someone else describe you?
- What sort of person are you in close relationships?
- What are your best features as a person?

If the patient has some prior knowledge of the disorder, then ask what he/she understands about BPD from what he/she has learned about it previously. More specifically, try to access his/her underlying feelings about talking and thinking about him/herself as "having a diagnosis." For some patients the process may stimulate anxiety; for others, it is a relief to be told that what has been happening to them over a period of years is well recognized by mental health professionals and part of a known psychological problem. Yet others may find it dehumanizing and demeaning. So, the clinician must ensure that his/her attitude is thoughtful and sensitive, and at times reassuring. In particular, the discussions should be illustrated by relevant examples from the patient's story to exemplify what is actually meant. Equally, the judicious use of clinical examples from the clinician's previous experience may alleviate tension by temporarily taking the focus away from the patient him/herself.

In our experience, once the diagnosis has been broached in a sensitive manner the subject becomes less of a philosophical conundrum and more of a stimulus to understand what the patient's underlying problems actually are. This requires a dialogue about our understanding of the development of BPD, giving an explanation—and at this point a conflict arises for the mentalizing clinician. On the one hand, it goes against the spirit of mentalizing to promote our understanding of the disorder as a vulnerability to loss of mentalizing within the context of attachment relationships (because in doing so we are in danger of taking over the patient's own understanding), but on the other hand, it is important that the patient understands the mentalizing focus of treatment and our reasons for taking this particular approach. It is therefore important for the clinician to present this as an understanding, rather than a "fact."

Giving an explanation

Psychoeducation

Psychoeducation is perfectly in keeping with our model. Hence, an introductory program, which normally lasts 12 weeks but can sometimes be shorter, is part of the treatment pathway (see Chapter 11). In the assessment, the clinician starts off this process by explaining the possible causes of BPD, the psychological problems and difficulties in maintaining a mentalizing mind that are a consequence of BPD, the goals of treatment, and how group and individual therapy are used in MBT to stabilize mentalizing in the context of attachment relationships. Nevertheless, the primary method used to help a patient appreciate the process of therapy is not through "education" but by engaging him/her in the work itself during the initial sessions. The clinician listens carefully to the way in which the patient talks about him/herself and others, identifies features that suggest mentalizing strengths, highlights emotional competencies, and, when these positive aspects of mentalizing occur, uses them to explain the therapy process.

> You sound like you really understood what happened then. Increasing your ability to do that even when you are upset, hurt, or having other feelings is the focus of treatment. In treatment we will come across a lot of experiences that you have, both here and outside, which we won't understand. One of the main tasks of therapy is for us to explore those times so that we can make sense of what might have been going on in your mind at the time.

An attachment understanding of borderline personality disorder

Our understanding of BPD, outlined in Chapter 2, is discussed with the patient at the end of the assessment process. To this extent, the patient is prepared for the introductory group sessions, that is, MBT-I (see Chapter 11).

In discussing the origins of BPD there is a danger of oversimplifying the causes on the one hand, and on the other of becoming excessively complicated. Some patients feel patronized if clinicians give explanations that appear trite and might react by becoming angry. Others feel overwhelmed by the information, often becoming perplexed. It is therefore important that the clinician gauges the patient's knowledge and capacity to focus on new concepts carefully before embarking on explanations. In our experience it is becoming increasingly common to find that higher-functioning patients have sought information on the Internet before coming for treatment, and so the clinician should first explore what the patient knows about the disorder—"Maybe you have already read something about BPD yourself?" It is essential that "giving the model" does not mimic a classroom in which the clinician, as a "teacher," imparts information that needs to be "learned" by the patient. Some individuals will want to treat the exercise like a school lesson, but this commonly indicates that their mentalizing has been switched off and teleological functions are in the ascendant. Patients with BPD often feel cared about according to concrete outcomes, so imparting information in the manner of a teacher can be converted into a signal that to these patients indicates "real" care. For the most part it is best to allow the patient to consider each aspect of the developmental model in terms of his/her own life and to consider its relevance to him/her. Rather than giving a long and complicated explanation, the clinician should give simple and short accounts of each aspect of the model, preferably in terms of the patient's own history and current problems. The explanation must be tailored to the individual him/herself to stimulate a reappraisal of the patient's own understanding of his/her problems and, in the furtherance of mentalizing, each problem area should be linked to the treatment program.

CLINICIAN: It sounds like you and your Mum just did not see eye to eye and that you felt that she didn't really understand things. But you didn't give up trying to let her know that you were unhappy. Even when you were a teenager, it sounds like you wanted her to recognize that you were in trouble, for example, asking her to come to the school when you were expelled and to the hospital when you took an overdose. What is your understanding of why she didn't seem to respond?

PATIENT: She was just a horrible woman. [A nonmentalizing explanation, because it is a descriptor, an absolute, and lacks elaboration and reflection on mental content.]

CLINICIAN: I suspect that it might have been more complicated than that, and in the treatment we will help you explore that a bit more. One feature of treatment is that we ask patients to reconsider some of their personal explanations of events and especially how they understand things now. In the group therapy you will have a chance to hear other people's understanding of your problems, which will help you reappraise your own understanding. One possibility is that you will begin to feel that people here don't understand, and you must let us know if that is the case. We all bring our past experiences to present situations, and you have told me that you have never really trusted anyone so you may be constantly on the lookout to see if we understand. So, talk to your individual clinician about this and perhaps let the group know if you feel that they are misunderstanding what you are trying to tell them.

Treatment program

Historically, there have been two variants of MBT. The first studies of MBT were undertaken in the context of a day (partial) hospital program in which patients attended initially 5 days per week. The maximum length of time in this program was 18–24 months. For entrance to the day (partial) hospital program, patients were required to show a number of clinical and descriptive features, including high risk to self or others, repeated hospital admissions interfering with adaptations to everyday living, severe daily substance misuse, fragmented mentalizing, inadequate social support, and unstable housing. Patients who showed some capacity for everyday living and who had stable social support and adequate accommodation were more likely to be treated within an intensive outpatient program (see following paragraphs), particularly if their vulnerability to loss of mentalizing processes was confined mostly to close emotional relationships.

The day (partial) hospital program (Bateman, 2005; Bateman & Fonagy, 1999) is no longer offered in the United Kingdom, although some services in Europe continue to offer this more intensive treatment. All patients in the United Kingdom are treated in outpatient programs (MBT-OPD), of which the best researched is an 18-month intensive outpatient treatment consisting of a weekly individual session of 50 minutes and a weekly group session of 75 minutes (MBT-IOP) (Bateman & Fonagy, 2009).

There were a number of reasons for the change from the day hospital to the outpatient program. First, our research suggested that those patients whom we thought required more intensive treatment, for example, those with more than one personality disorder, who were at risk to themselves or others, and had serious drug misuse engrained in their daily function, did equally well in the outpatient program. Second, the clinicians found that managing this group of individuals as outpatients did not elevate their own anxiety to unacceptable levels. Finally, the lower level of interaction between patients and clinicians increased the pressure on the patients to maintain a higher level of self-efficacy. The outpatient program was also more cost-efficient.

Further programs aiming to help people with BPD have been developed over the past few years. In some of these, patients are offered less intensive treatment than MBT-IOP, for example, group MBT or individual MBT alone. On the other hand, a slightly higher-intensity treatment, MBT-HIOP, also now exists. MBT-HIOP is MBT-IOP plus an additional element if warranted, such as an expressive therapy. Currently, there are no data to support these variants of the original mentalizing approach, but many services for people with personality disorder attempt to allocate patients to treatment according to the severity of their symptoms. However, at present, there is no agreed measure of severity of personality disorder, so it is impossible to assign patients to one program or another according to a universally agreed severity score. This may change with the current proposal for the 11th revision of the International Classification of Diseases (ICD-11), which suggests that personality disorders be organized according to severity, ranging from mild to moderate to severe (Tyrer et al., 2011; Tyrer, Reed, & Crawford, 2015). So far, there is no clarity about how severity will be assessed by clinicians. Our data suggest that allocation of patients to programs of different intensity should be done according to levels of comorbidity for personality disorders as an indicator of severity, risk, and instability of social circumstances (Bateman & Fonagy, 2013).

Mentalizing programs

What is important in all the programs is the interrelationship of the different aspects of the program, the working relationship between the different clinicians, the continuity of themes between the groups, and the consistency with which the treatment is applied over a period of time. Such nonspecific aspects probably form the key to effective treatment, and the specificity of the therapeutic activities remains to be determined.

It will come as no surprise to the reader that integration within the program is achieved through our focus on mentalizing. All of the constituent parts of the MBT program have an overall aim of increasing mentalizing and within a framework that encourages exploration of minds by minds, even if the route to this goal is via expressive techniques such as artwork and writing.

Intensive outpatient program

In MBT-IOP, patients are offered one individual session (50 minutes) and one group session (75 minutes) per week. This is not an "a la carte" but a "fixed" menu. We clarify at the outset of treatment that the two aspects of the program, that is, the group and individual sessions, are not divisible, and that frequent absence from one will lead to a discussion about continuation in treatment. It is not our policy to simply discharge a patient because of nonattendance. But it is our guiding principle that if someone does not attend one aspect of the program on a regular basis this has to be discussed with him/her in the next session he/she attends, whether it is the individual or group session. It is more common for patients to fail to attend the group than the individual session; nonattendance in the group thus requires the individual clinician to explore the patient's underlying reasons for absence in the next individual session. Only when it appears to be impossible to help the patient to return to the group is the question of discharge from the program raised. It is not possible to suggest an exact point at which this should be considered for a nonattending patient, but in our clinical experience patients are told at the beginning of treatment that persistent and prolonged absence from the any aspect of the program will lead to discharge to our low-maintenance outpatient clinic for further consideration of treatment. Return to the program remains possible after this, but only following further work on the patient's underlying anxieties.

This fairly rigorous stance about attendance is taken because many patients find the individual sessions more acceptable than the group sessions and attend the former and not the latter. On occasions, this has understandably stimulated patients and others to ask why we have group sessions at all. "The group is no good"; "I don't get anything out of it" may become the refrain and eventually the individual clinician is challenged to explain the purpose of the groups. This question should not be avoided by the clinician but understood from a perspective of mentalizing, with some judicious further explanation about the importance of the group work. Of course, the reason for group therapy should have already been explained toward the end of the assessment.

Why group work?

Some patients are reluctant to participate in group therapy and their lack of enthusiasm surfaces as soon as group therapy becomes a reality. The patient may have apparently accepted the inevitability of group work in the assessment interviews but have done so only to access individual therapy. This must be addressed as soon as treatment starts. People with BPD have a reduced capacity to keep themselves in mind or to recognize that others have them in mind when listening to the problems of others, which accounts, to some degree, for their anxiety about groups and their oscillations between over- and under-involvement with others. As they become involved with someone else's problems they lose themselves in their own mind and in the mind of the other and, when they do so, they begin to feel alone and "self-less," which in turn leads to rapid distancing from the other person to save themselves.

The clinician needs to have a convincing reason for group therapy and a way of discussing it with the patient that does not become patronizing or frightening but is encouraging and explanatory. It is best if a team of clinicians providing MBT can develop their own understanding about the reason for group therapy within a mentalizing framework, so that a consistent explanation is given that is in keeping with the overall approach (see later in this chapter for some discussion of the mentalizing team).

Many clinicians explain group therapy by talking about the ability of people to function within groups in society and how group therapy can be used to practice this exceptionally complex skill, which requires a high level of mentalizing. In many ways, the capacity to function well within constantly changing social situations and within social groups is a peculiarly human attribute, and many people with BPD decompensate when "the going gets tough." For these individuals, social interactions create anxiety, misunderstandings abound, and mental collapse is inevitable, often leading to "flight or fight." So, to explain group therapy, we first discuss the conscious anxieties the patient has about groups and link them to the patient's own experiences when mixing with friends or others in social situations. We try to understand the feelings the patient has about groups, for example, anxieties about having to share with others when feeling that they have always been deprived of attention, or being concerned that others will not be interested in their problems. But primarily we discuss the power of group therapy to stimulate the capacity of the patient to manage anxiety within highly charged circumstances while maintaining mentalizing. It is in the group that patients can truly practice balancing emotional states evoked in a complex situation and their ability to continue mentalizing. The group requires patients to hold themselves in mind while trying to understand the minds of a number of others at the same time.

Here is an explanation (condensed from a whole session) about the reason for group therapy given to a patient. We make no claims that it is a perfect explanation, but it does contain the essential components: suggesting that the purpose is to consider one's own mind and the minds of others within a dynamic process.

> Groups can be very difficult for all of us, but they remain the context in which we lead our lives. All of us meet with other people and have to function in relation to others, sometimes suppressing our feelings and ideas because we know that they may cause offence or lead to reactions that we don't want. Negotiating all this is part of our everyday life. We also have to learn how to say things while remaining true to ourselves. The purpose of our groups is to work all this out and to learn that we can discuss things, even personal things about ourselves or our feelings toward others, without causing disturbing reactions in others and while feeling that we have expressed what we mean. We need to be able to say how much we feel for someone or how we value their support and friendship. Doing all this requires us to understand not only our own motives and needs but also the reactions of others to what we are saying. We also need to be able to think about others' responses and to change our own way of thinking accordingly, otherwise we simply insist that others take on our views. One problem we all have is respecting different views. We try to focus on this process in the groups. We hope that if you have a problem discussing things in the group you will be able to talk to your individual clinician about it, which will help you feel stronger to talk about it in the group.

Formulation

The initial formulation is made by the individual clinician after the first few sessions and after discussion with the treatment team. It is then given in written form to the patient for further consideration. The aims and important aspects of the formulation are outlined in Box 5.2.

If formulations are to be openly discussed, developed, and redeveloped, the team members must be able to work together with honesty and consideration of each other, and refrain from excessive competition within the group and rivalry between individuals. Each team member must develop the skill of discussing the formulation with patients without overstimulating their emotional states. For all patients, reading a frank account of how someone else thinks they may have become who they are evokes considerable turmoil, and its significance to the patient should not be underestimated.

> A patient who read her formulation along with the complete medical notes was overwhelmed by the information. On reading the transfer letter from her former psychiatrist and psychotherapist she became upset because former feelings of rejection, which she had experienced when they had talked to her about referring her for specialist treatment, were reawakened. She felt abandoned and tricked by the transfer of care and that they had not told her the real reasons for referral, which were that they could not

---

Box 5.2 Aims of formulation

- Aims:
  - Organize thinking for therapist and patient—each sees different minds
  - Model a mentalizing approach in a formal way (explicit, concrete, clear, and exampled)—do not assume that the patient can do this
  - Model humility about the nature of truth
- Management of risk:
  - Analysis of components of risk in intentional terms
  - Avoids overstimulation through formulation
- Beliefs about the self:
  - Relationship of these to specific (varying) internal states
  - Historical aspects placed into context
- Central current concerns in relational terms:
  - Identification of attachment patterns—what is activated?
  - Challenges that are entailed
- Positive aspects:
  - When mentalizing worked and had the effect of improving a situation
- Anticipation for the unfolding of treatment:
  - Impact of individual and group therapy.

---

cope with her and were concerned about her level of risk. In short, she believed that the information in the letters suggested that they were frightened of her. There was some merit in this, but it was clearly not the complete story. Balancing her feelings of rejection was an appreciation that they had taken great care to document everything that had happened and put in a considerable amount of thought about her. Nevertheless, the experience of reading her medical notes followed by the formulation led her to feel overwhelmed, and she cut herself despite seeing a member of the team shortly after reading the notes to discuss her reactions.

In the formulation, the initial goals should be clearly stated and linked to the aspects of treatment that will enable the patient to attain them. There should be a brief summary of the joint understanding that has developed between the patient and clinician, with a focus on the underlying causes of the patient's problems in terms of loss of mentalizing. The formulation should also include longer-term goals in terms of the patient's social and interpersonal adjustment, which are likely to be important indicators of improved mentalizing. Finally, it is necessary to identify the attachment strategies of the patient (Choi-Kain, Fitzmaurice, Zanarini, Laverdiere, & Gunderson, 2009) and explicitly work jointly to establish them as important for treatment.

Example of a formulation

Ms. A is 22 years old and has difficulties relating constructively to others and persistent doubts about herself. She has tried to harm herself on a number of occasions and was referred following an overdose of her antidepressant medication that resulted in admission to the intensive care unit. She has not been able to work over the past year, but prior to this was working part-time as a secretary. She is the oldest of four children and experienced her mother as strict, rigid, and controlling. She was closer to her father, who often agreed with her that her mother was a "difficult woman." She was sent away to school, in part because of uncontrollable behavior, where she was bullied and at the age of 8–11 regularly sexually abused by an older boy. She informed the school, who did not believe her, but never told her parents.

She now sees herself as being dependent on others' approval. Without it she rapidly becomes insecure. This applies to many of the relationships she has had in the past, which have been characterized by seeking approval, to the extent of trying to do what the other person wants even if she herself does not want to do it. This has extended to her sexual relationships, in which she has been abused by two men whose wishes to inflict pain have been gratified by her passive compliance.

Despite these areas of developmental and interpersonal difficulty she managed to complete school and gain a number of higher examination passes. However, when she went to university she found that after a term she could not go back, much to her mother's scorn. She obtained employment as a secretary but this broke down over a year ago, for reasons that are unclear. Ms. A just woke up one morning and felt that she could not go to work.

Engagement in therapy

Ms. A is likely to engage in therapy initially, partly because she recognizes that she has problems but also because she will be eager to please and to seek our approval.

It is possible that if she feels she is not getting adequate recognition or feels that others have not given her enough attention (e.g., not being given enough time in the group) she may suffer in silence initially but then stop coming. The group clinicians will try to be alert to this.

Her anxieties in relationships and tendency to engage with others within a passive role may make her vulnerable to exploitation by others. This includes other members of her group, and the individual clinician should be aware that this might become an important dynamic within the individual sessions.

Relationship difficulties (Individual plus Group)

Ms. A finds it difficult to make her wishes and desires clear to others and sometimes does not actually know what they are.

She tends to accept that her wishes are those of the other person and she cannot separate the two. Alternatively, in an attempt to establish her own wishes she withdraws.

She recognizes a tendency to devalue others, especially when she feels she has failed them in some way. This was explored in the assessment as being a way to manage feelings of rejection.

These solutions are unsatisfactory and she feels angry, misunderstood, and neglected, although her behavior becomes passive and accepting of the other person.

Other problem areas (Group)

Ms. A tries to listen so carefully to others that she tires easily. This may be more apparent in the group sessions when she tries to listen to everybody.

She feels that she has to do something useful for other people and to provide a solution to their problems, and this may be represented by her becoming the helper in the groups.

Her inability to show anger and anxieties in relation to others costs her a lot of energy and adds to her feeling of being tired and listless.

She recognizes that she becomes quiet and withdrawn when feeling excluded and that this has been a long-term characteristic. She tends to blame others for this, seeing them as "jerks," "snobs," etc.

Self-destructive behavior (Individual)

Alcohol and cannabis are used on an intermittent basis but on average 2–3 evenings per week. She tends to wake late after cannabis use or alcohol binges, and this might interfere with therapy and so will need to be a focus of early sessions of Individual Therapy

Self-laceration of wrists and thighs occurs on an almost daily basis. Ms. A recognizes that this occurs in relation to bewildering feelings with high levels of tension and often when she experiences difficult interactions with others—focus of early sessions of Individual Therapy. Consider any links with alcohol and cannabis use.

Mentalizing

Concrete mentalizing

Ms. A tends to judge people based on what they do and makes assumptions without checking them out. She has not spoken to her current closest friend for 2 weeks because the friend failed to ring her at a prearranged time. She feels that it indicated that her friend did not care about her.

If people do not agree with her suggestions about what they should do to solve their problems she believes that they don't like her.

Antireflective mentalizing

Ms. A avoids disagreement and she acquiesces to other people's opinions. She withdraws when difference arises and avoids any conflict.

In the assessment she was aware that she actively avoided certain areas—she often reacted to things by saying "Maybe" or "So whatever," and when this was pointed out she agreed that it usually meant that she did not want to talk about something.

Sensitive mentalizing

Ms. A has spent a lot of time thinking about her problems and feels ashamed that she was unable to go back to university after the first term and that she was no longer able to work. She recognizes that this shame is in keeping with her mother's opinion of her as a failure, and this causes her tremendous distress.

She is able to understand what is in the mind of others a lot of the time, but when she becomes anxious she finds that she loses her clarity of mind and becomes uncertain. Her only way of managing this is to withdraw. She is also aware that she is oversensitive to the opinions of others but doesn't know what to do about it.

She wants to be able to develop relationships in which she feels there is a mutual sharing. She has found that when she has been able to explain her underlying feelings this has made a difference to her relationships. Although she has not spoken to her closest friend since her failure to phone at the agreed time, she realizes that she is being unforgiving and has left her friend a message.

The written formulation is given to the patient for discussion during the individual session on the basis that the clinician's understanding of the patient is a jointly developed hypothesis about the patient's problems and that this understanding can be influenced by the patient him/herself, leading to a reformulation as additional evidence accumulates. If the patient disagrees with aspects of the formulation it is incumbent on the clinician to consider the reasons for the underlying disagreement and to modify his/her own opinion accordingly, if appropriate, and to demonstrate that he/she has done so. A briefer formulation than the example given here is preferable for many patients. Indeed, the example here could be summarized before it is given to the patient and even given an "executive summary" as an aide-memoire for both clinician and patient (see Box 5.3).

Review and reformulation

All patients in MBT programs have a review with the whole treatment team every 3 months. The group clinician, the individual clinician, the psychiatrist, and other relevant mental health professionals meet with the patient to discuss progress, problems, and other aspects of treatment. Practitioners meeting together jointly with the patient does not just ensure that everyone's views are

---

Box 5.3 Formulation: executive summary

- Attachment strategies and interpersonal problems:
  - Vulnerability factors from past experience
  - Current use of alcohol and drugs
  - Dependent, anxious with others, avoidant, and devaluing
  - Defers to others and vulnerable to exploitation
- Impulsivity and emotional problems:
  - Self-destructive behavior, high risk of self-harm
  - Anxiety
- Mentalizing process:
  - Concrete, antireflective, sensitive.

taken into account and integrated into a coherent set of ideas; it also ensures that mentalizing, as manifested through the discussion of the different viewpoints that may be expressed in the meeting, is modeled as a constructive activity that furthers understanding. These regular reviews lead to a reformulation, which can then form the basis of ongoing treatment. If required, they can also become more than a review about progress or lack of it and be used to address significant impairments to treatment.

Review of medication

As part of good medical practice, all patients should have their medication reviewed on a regular basis. This review can take place in the "review and reformulation" meeting. Many patients are now referred after prolonged treatment with medications, and over 50% are taking various combinations of antipsychotics, antidepressants, mood stabilizers, anxiolytics, and hypnotics (Zanarini, 2004). Medication is reviewed at the beginning of treatment by the team psychiatrist, but rarely is the prescription changed immediately unless it is obviously dangerous or inappropriate. Medication is reviewed regularly and altered only by agreement when the team and the psychiatrist know the patient better. As a general protocol we follow the guidance on use of medication in BPD outlined in the UK National Institute for Health and Clinical Excellence guidance for the treatment of BPD (2009) and provide the patient with information about the recommendations made in this guidance.

Crisis plan

Developing a crisis plan with a patient is possibly one of the most effective general therapeutic strategies for people with BPD, although a recent study has thrown this clinical opinion into doubt (Borschmann, Henderson, Hogg, Phillips, & Moran, 2012). Nevertheless, all patients with BPD will experience crises during treatment, and so it is necessary for the clinician and patient to outline what to do in the event of a crisis. Here we will discuss only the practical aspects of developing a plan. From a mentalizing perspective, it is not appropriate to "give" the patient a plan but more fitting to stimulate identification of a pathway that will help the patient to access help when he/she needs it, in the hope that this will prevent serious self-destructive acts. The format described here is used both in MBT and in structured clinical management for people with BPD (Bateman & Krawitz, 2013). At its core is a responsibility shared between the patient and clinician to manage crises.

What signals does the patient have that a crisis is emerging?

Ask the patient to describe at least three examples of crises that have led to self-destructive behavior and/or contact with services. Taking each in turn, spend time attempting to work out early warning signs:

◆ Was there a particular feeling?

◆ Was there a behavioral change?

◆ Were thought patterns different?

Even if a patient cannot answer these questions, the task of attending to what was happening is in itself therapeutic. Empathize with the patient who does not know what happens and finds that his/her feelings go "from zero to a hundred" in milliseconds—"It just happens and there is nothing that I can do." Even if this is the case, the clinician needs to work with the patient to find some early warning signs, as this aspect of the crisis plan is one of the basic strategies for focusing mentalizing on the precursors of self-harm.

Patients are asked to rate their crises on an "escalator," with 0 at the bottom of the escalator = in control; 1 and 2 = defined by patient and clinician; and 3 at the top of the escalator = crisis point or out of control. The clinician uses clarification techniques, frequently coaxing the patient to rewind their mental processes to points before their loss of control, thereby helping them to identify triggers and the effect they have on their internal states. In other words, the patient is asked to work methodically on answering the question "What makes me vulnerable?" Jointly, the points on the escalator are defined in increasing detail.

What can the patient do and not do?

The patient identifies when they could have re-established self-control and what could prevent them from moving on to the next stage toward a crisis. How do you stop the escalator? How do you get off or walk back down against the direction of movement? Strategies that have been helpful in managing emotional crises in the past are identified, for example, leaving a provocative situation, telephoning someone if trapped in a feeling of loneliness, or distracting the mind by engaging in an action task such as cooking. The clinician also tries to stimulate the patient to reflect on how others might observe each stage (i.e., signals for others) and what others could or should not do that might be helpful (see next section). Significant others are invited to sessions to work out this part of the crisis plan jointly.

What can other people do and not do?

How do others know that a crisis is emerging? What might they do to help? Taking in turn the examples of crises that the patient has provided, the clinician asks him/her to consider what practical and emotional responses of others would have been helpful and to identify those that are unhelpful. Someone else being aware of what *not* to do might have more traction in a crisis than attempting actively to do something useful. For example, partners may be advised to avoid confrontation, side-step disagreement, and to minimize defensiveness when the patient with BPD is emotional and anxious. This is not the same as simply asking others to accept unwarranted personal attacks. Partners need to choose the time for discussion; an emerging crisis in people with BPD is not one of them. After the patient has carefully defined what his/her partner or others can do when he/she feels vulnerable and in danger of reaching the top of the escalator, discuss how he/she can pass on this information to them.

What can services do and not do?

In general terms, it is important to minimize the usefulness and effectiveness of services in a crisis. Certainly, medical emergency health services are not well organized to manage patients with BPD, and personnel are poorly trained to understand the severity of the condition. Sadly, the same can be said for many mental health emergency services, and the patient is well advised to keep away from poor-quality mental health emergency services if at all possible. Again, the crisis plan may not so much be about what the services can do, but what they should try *not* to do. For example, crisis presentation is a time when clinicians commonly change medication, when it is, in fact, the least sensible time to alter a prescription. A statement in the crisis plan such as "Even if I demand it, please be careful about changing my medication in a crisis. I can consider this later when I am calmer" will help professionals act responsibly rather than out of their own ill-considered panic and need to do something.

The crisis plan is a work in progress, and each time certain points become clearer they are added to the plan. *The clinician is required to revisit the crisis plan whenever a crisis occurs.* When agreed actions or psychological techniques fail to stop movement "up the escalator," they are re-evaluated. In this way the clinician continuously maintains the patient's own responsibility for dealing with painful and possibly overwhelming emotions while at the same time strengthening his/her ability to do so, with clinician support.

Having identified possible self-help interventions and the role of the MBT treatment team during office hours, the feasibility of implementation of the plan 24 hours, 7 days a week needs to be considered. Many crises will occur in the evenings, at night, or at weekends, when only emergency services are available. The clinician outlines the emergency system that is available to the patient, emphasizing that emergency teams will have access to the crisis plan and will attempt to help the patient manage an acute situation until he/she is able to discuss the problem with the MBT treatment team on the next working day. The patient and the team may organize an emergency appointment the following working day, which lasts no more than 20 minutes and is focused entirely on the crisis, how to stabilize the situation if it recurs, and reinstating psychological and behavioral safety for the patient and others. Further work on the crisis should be done within the group and individual sessions.

The lack of availability of MBT clinicians outside office hours requires the person with BPD to develop his/her own strategies in advance and implement them without the immediate involvement of an "expert" in the emotional turmoil. Having an agreement within the treatment contract of an emergency session the next day with a member of the team if the crisis has been contained without serious consequence helps to bolster the patient's resolve, maintains responsibility with the patient, and gradually increases the patient's confidence to manage increasingly complex situations. Each crisis is discussed in detail at the emergency meeting that follows and, if necessary, the crisis plan is reworked.

Contracts

Clarification of some basic "rules" and giving guidance

We follow the common "principles of engagement" that are applied when treating patients in any health service. We have a commitment to implement the treatment program professionally and with interpersonal respect, just as patients have an obligation to attend to their difficulties within the boundary of the treatment outline. There are particular "principles" we follow about violence and the use of drugs and alcohol, and we offer guidelines about sexual relationships between patients—that is, that they interfere with the treatment of both people involved. These principles are discussed in more detail in our description of the program in our original book on MBT and BPD (Bateman & Fonagy, 2004). The question here is how the clinician explains the "principles" to the patient.

It is wise to be straightforward about general "principles" and guidelines of treatment, to have a leaflet or information sheet about them, and to make them as clear as possible so that both patient and clinician understand them fully. It is inadequate simply to state "rules" or to give guidance without giving reasons. A discussion about why the principles are necessary must take place and be explored with the patient. Some patients will accept the principles without question, but others will apparently agree with them while privately ignoring them or at least feeling that "the rules don't apply to them." Still others, perhaps more commonly those with antisocial personality disorder, will actively challenge "rules," seeing them as authoritarian, unenforceable, and excessively restrictive. Whatever the patient's reaction, the clinician must discuss the underlying reasons for the principles and explore the patient's response. So, what are the underlying reasons?

First, there is a general point that anything that reduces mentalizing is antithetical to the treatment program. Drugs and alcohol alter mental states and interfere with the exploration of mental states, and as such, negate the overall aim of treatment. Sexual relationships involve the "pairing" of minds, which will alienate others within the group. Violence controls minds through fear, closing them down rather than opening them up. So, we suggest to the patient that anything that is likely to reduce their interest in the whole group, alienate them from the group, prevent them reflecting on themselves, or close down the minds of others is not recommended. Second, we explain that there is some overlap between the areas of the brain responsible for mentalizing and those that are affected by drugs and alcohol and even sexual relationships. This surprises many patients. We have found that the best way to explain this is to point out that when anyone is excited, in love, or smoking cannabis there is often no space in their mind for other people. The person in love does not reflect but becomes preoccupied with their loved one, the person "high" on cannabis becomes self-centered and may even be, in an altered state of consciousness, unaware of others around, and the person who is violent or threatening has his/her mind taken over altogether and attempts to close down the minds of others. Our view about the overlap between the neurobiological systems responsible for addiction and those driving attachment relationships is discussed in more detail elsewhere (Bateman & Fonagy, 2006; Insel, 2003).

Finally, we also know from empirical data that BPD symptoms can improve over time, but this natural progression can be influenced by factors such as substance misuse, which prevents patients taking advantage of positive social and interpersonal circumstances and decreases the likelihood of a natural remission (Zanarini, Frankenburg, Reich, & Fitzmaurice, 2012). The patient should be made aware of this.

Individual contracts

Principles apply to a whole group, protect the integrity of an overall treatment program, and define boundaries of professional involvement. *Contracts* tend to be individualized and specific, often targeting particular areas likely to cause problems in treatment. We are not great proponents of draconian contracts likely to lead to discharge when their conditions are not fulfilled. Fluctuating mentalizing capacity means that a patient who agrees to a contract at one point may not actually have the same competence in a different context, or have access later on to the state of mind he/she was in when he/she agreed the contract. It is important to remember that effective mentalizing requires a patient to understand his/her state of mind at any given time, to be able to project him/herself into the future and recognize his/her likely emotional state at that time, to reflect on his/her state of mind in the past, and to consider his/her possible state of mind in many different contexts. Agreeing a contract relevant to future time requires all these capacities. Patients whose BPD is severe do not retain these abilities over time, and so can do only one of two things when faced with a contract—they can either agree the contract without hesitation, attributing little meaning to it and giving it only cursory importance, or challenge it as being a further way to test them that is likely to lead to humiliating failure. The hesitant patient who is wary of agreeing a contract because he/she realizes that he/she may not be able to fulfill his/her obligations may well have a higher capacity to mentalize than someone who simply signs the contract straight away. Doubt at entry to treatment may be a good prognostic feature rather than an indication of a lack of motivation. It is important for the clinician to engage with this uncertainty and ensure that the contract does not induce a sense of failure in the patient if it is broken.

There are a number of dangers associated with issuing contracts. Too often they become punitive and unachievable, and place the clinician in a "therapeutic corner" where there is limited flexibility. Clinicians often introduce contracts to put pressure on an individual to control behaviors that interfere with treatment. We have some sympathy with this view, but have found that in patients with severe personality disorder this use of contracts is of limited effectiveness—particularly in improving attendance and reducing self-harm and suicide attempts, which are the most common reasons given for issuing contracts. Under these circumstances the patient is being asked to control the very behavior for which he/she is seeking treatment, and he/she is likely to fail. Disorganized behavior outside treatment is mirrored within treatment, so discharge of patients who fail to attend consecutive sessions due to chaotic lifestyles, and preventing an early return to treatment, will simply perpetuate their poor engagement in services. Some patients, particularly those with antisocial and narcissistic features, may even be triumphant about defeating contractual strictures and relish their "untreatability" as they challenge treatment boundaries. Finally, contracts with negative consequences are unenforceable within statutory health services, although, of course, it is important not to keep offering a treatment that is manifestly failing. Under these circumstances it is necessary to suggest alternative help.

Outcome monitoring

MBT now incorporates routine outcome monitoring of treatment, and this has become an integral part of the model. Evidence suggests that individual clinicians can have a substantial impact on patient outcomes independent of the treatment method, and this may be of particular importance in routine clinical practice. In any psychotherapy treatment, around 5–10% of patients will have a negative outcome; between-clinician differences may account for this (Hansen, Lambert, & Forman, 2002). In one study of psychotherapy (Luborsky, McLellan, Woody, O'Brien, & Auerbach, 1985), the outcome effect size across clinicians for patients with drug addiction (many of whom were likely to have had personality disorder) ranged between 0.13 and 0.79. In the US National Institute of Mental Health trial of treatment for depression, no differences were found between treatments when differences between clinicians were accounted for (Elkin, Falconnier, Martinovich, & Mahoney, 2006). Furthermore, some clinicians are able to retain patients in treatment more effectively than others, suggesting the existence of distinct differences in clinicians' ability to repair therapeutic ruptures.

A classic analysis by Luborsky, Chandler, Auerbach, Cohen, and Bachrach (1971) identified a number of clinician characteristics that influenced the prognosis of therapy across 161 studies of different groups of patients. These included (1) experience, (2) attitude and interest patterns, (3) empathy, and (4) similarity between the clinician and patient. These parameters have stood the test of time (Ackerman & Hilsenroth, 2003), and there is no reason to believe that they are any less important in the treatment of patients with BPD. Indeed, there are indications that clinician effects may be of particular importance in the treatment of people with BPD, who may be especially sensitive to therapeutic interventions and, when treated by less skilled clinicians, may be left worse off at the end of treatment than when they began (Fonagy & Bateman, 2006). However, such descriptions of clinicians are of little value in the context of quality improvement initiatives in clinical services as they fail to offer tangible goals—either to clinicians and managers, or to patients—that are likely to improve services. Clearly, individual clinicians who are more likely to have negative outcomes need support and practical assistance to enhance their outcomes, rather than to be stigmatized.

Fortunately, in the area of generic psychotherapeutic work, a method based on intensive outcome monitoring of ongoing treatments has been developed and applied, which apparently serves to create an "early warning" of negative outcomes and provide a means of supporting modifications of ongoing interventions (Okiishi, Lambert, Nielsen, & Ogles, 2003; Okiishi et al., 2006). Randomized controlled trials have demonstrated the value of such an approach in reducing negative outcomes by over 50% and leading to improvements in patient satisfaction and treatment alliance (Shimokawa, Lambert, & Smart, 2010). It is possible that a combination of improved therapeutic alliance and moderation of the wish to disengage from therapy accounts for the improvements observed. This patient-focused research aims to evaluate patients' response to treatment throughout the course of therapy. Feedback is provided to clinicians on patients' progress. This allows clinicians to make treatment decisions based on patients' distress rather than simply trusting in the treatment itself. Providing feedback to clinicians on a regular basis has been shown to improve patient retention in treatment and to improve outcomes if clinical support is given to clinicians whose patient(s) are deviating from the expected course (Okiishi et al., 2006). Clinicians need feedback to be able to identify which patients are not on track. Research shows that they are notoriously poor at predicting which of their patients will do badly. Hannan and colleagues (2005) interviewed 40 clinicians and asked them early in treatment to predict which of their 550 patients would deteriorate. They identified only 1 of the 40 patients who eventually deteriorated. In addition, they were even poor at recognizing that a patient was currently showing deterioration and consistently rated them as doing better when they were not.

There is no reason why such benefits of clinician feedback should not accrue in the treatment of BPD, although previous work on outcome monitoring has focused on short- rather than medium- or long-term psychotherapy, and has avoided patient groups with a primary diagnosis of personality disorder. Identifying the trajectory of patient change during treatment and the impact of clinician feedback and provision of clinical support when a patient is deviating from the expected course of change has not been investigated with patients with BPD. If clinicians could monitor the trajectory of patient progress and have rapid access to information suggesting that change is not taking place at the expected rate, clinical services offering complex psychotherapeutic treatments for BPD may also be improved. The variability of outcomes observed in the treatment of BPD suggests that clinician effects may be particularly important for this group. In a trial of dialectical behavior therapy for BPD (Feigenbaum et al., 2012), all of the patients of one clinician dropped out despite significant attempts by the team to retain them in treatment. Gunderson and colleagues (1997) found that ratings of the patient–clinician alliance by clinicians treating patients with BPD was predictive of subsequent dropout. Lingiardi, Filippucci, and Baiocco (2005) also showed that early evaluations of the therapeutic alliance are good predictors of dropout in patients with personality disorders and that clinicians evaluate their alliances with patients with BPD significantly more negatively than their alliances with patients with other personality disorders. A trial of MBT (Bateman & Fonagy, 2009), using general linear modeling to map the progress of individual patients over time, also suggested that there was a statistically significant variability in the rate of clinical improvement, some of which could be accounted for by clinician identity. The longer length of treatment provided for patients with BPD makes research into these sources of variance mandatory. Treatment lengths of 12–18 months make it imperative to identify such patients early in treatment, even if only on the basis of personal cost for the patient and clinician, let alone the financial cost to services, to see if problems can be addressed at an early stage.

In conclusion, variability in outcomes is a significant factor in service provision. Using actual treatment outcomes based on the effects of individual clinicians to improve patient outcome would dramatically influence the delivery of effective care and give an opportunity to manage and improve outcomes in specific clinics. So, all patients engaged in MBT are now asked to complete brief weekly monitoring questionnaires, and they and their clinicians have full access to the scores over time. The patient has to be inducted into this process at the beginning of treatment so that it becomes an area of interest for both patient and clinician. In effect, both "mentalize" about the change, good or bad, in the scores. Improvement is of equal interest to deterioration—what might be the explanation for this change, how has the change come about, is there something happening in therapy that is useful or harmful? Current measures in use include symptoms, quality of life, social adjustment, interpersonal function, service use, suicidality and self-harm, reflective function, and therapeutic alliance (scored independently by the patient and the clinician). In addition, a goals-based outcome measure is completed every 3 months to ensure that the formulation and goals are revisited methodically and the treatment focuses on areas of importance to the patient.

Process

It is in the middle phase that the hard work for the patient takes place. For the clinician, this phase may appear easier because by the time the initial phase has been negotiated many of the crises will have subsided, the patient's level of engagement in treatment will be clear, the patient's motivation may have increased, and his/her capacity to work within individual and group therapy may be more apparent. This allows an increasing focus on process rather than management. In addition, the clinician may have a better understanding of the patient's overall difficulties and so have a more robust image of him/her in mind, while the patient will have also become aware of the clinician's foibles and way of working.

While this somewhat rosy picture may be the case for some patients and clinicians, for others the treatment trajectory may continue to be disrupted. A primary task of clinicians is to repair ruptures in the therapeutic alliance and to sustain their own and patients' motivation while maintaining a focus on mentalizing. The mentalizing techniques associated with the middle phase form the core of this book. Here we will mention the need to develop and to sustain good team morale for the MBT treatment team by building in supervision and paying heed to feelings engendered in the clinicians.

The mentalizing team

This section borrows heavily on the summary of team work included in the manual of structured clinical management for BPD (Bateman & Krawitz, 2013) and on the team working recommended in adolescent mentalization-based integrative treatment (AMBIT—see http://www.annafreud.org/services-schools/services-for-professionals/ambit/).

The characteristics of a mentalizing team are summarized in Box 5.4.

United mind

A commonality of purpose in a team and coherent responses to a wide variety of clinical situations can come about if a team functions with one mind while its members retain their own individuality. To do this, a team needs to follow some basic principles. First, respect for each other has to be apparent and worked on rather than assumed. Second, the team needs constantly to define and redefine its aims with each patient; these aims have to be consistent with the overall aims of the treatment process. Third, the team must emphasize communication between its members. All members hold equal responsibility for ensuring that information, ideas, and plans are shared appropriately. Finally, leadership and support structures need to be agreed upon. All members have to be committed to working within these structures—mavericks are welcome but loose cannons will destroy a team, and it may never recover. The identified team leader does not have to be the permanent leader of team discussions. Well-functioning teams show flexible processes rather than strict hierarchical structures, and the leader of

---

Box 5.4 The mentalizing team

- United mind with a commonality of purpose
- Respect for themselves and others
- Ability to develop and adhere to coherent clinical plans
- Good team morale
- Effective leadership.

a discussion may be someone identified at the beginning of a team meeting or, for example, be chosen on a rotational basis.

Respect

Respect means that each team member gives appropriate regard to other team members' feelings, opinions, and experience. All clinicians are aware that people with BPD can evoke contradictory feelings, and this inevitably becomes apparent between team members. One team member may be enraged with a patient while another feels highly protective; patients may engage one member of the team by outlining—perhaps exaggerating—the shortcomings of another clinician in the team. For the unwary, this can have a seductive quality, as criticism of a "rival" promises the potential of clinical "riches" in becoming special to a patient. Sometimes the criticisms of a colleague reported in a clinical session by a patient are highly accurate and may even hit sensitive differences between members of the team. Of course, this cuts both ways, and the same patient may be reversing the criticisms when seeing another team member. An explicit and collective refusal by team members to be drawn into these subtly subversive conversations improves the chances of effective team functioning. Integrating the views of the patient and the reciprocal reactions of the clinicians to the patient's perspective is a key function of the team. Valuing another view, however different from your own, maintains the respect required to facilitate an integrated view of a patient's psychological function.

Team morale

Maintaining good team morale is essential to prevent "burnout" and to minimize inappropriate emotional responses to patients and other clinicians. It is remarkable how apparent the underlying atmosphere can be in a treatment facility, even if entering it for only a short time. The atmosphere of a unit is likely to be instrumental in the effectiveness of interventions and the outcome for patients. Bearing in mind that MBT treatment programs involve multiple clinicians providing individual and group psychotherapy and crisis support, it is easy to see that problems can arise between clinicians and that, if unresolved, they are likely to interfere with the implementation of treatment.

Team morale refers to the overall sense of safety and the prevailing attitude in the team. Positive, hopeful, and enthusiastic attitudes in the team are likely to instill similar feelings in patients and stimulate involvement in a therapeutic process. Negative, anxious, and hopeless attitudes will fuel despair and mirror many of the inner feelings of patients, who may begin to feel that what is inside is now outside; their psychic equivalence is confirmed.

Team morale is maintained by ensuring that the focus of treatment for the patient—namely mentalizing—also becomes the heart of the interaction between clinicians. The clinicians have to be able to practice what they preach and stick to a mentalizing stance when discussing their own viewpoints with each other. Splitting is more frequently described in the treatment of patients with BPD than most other psychiatric disorders, but it is less often recognized as a problem of the team rather than the patient. Clinicians who disagree have to work together toward integration and synthesis. But the interaction of the clinicians cannot be left to chance, and so case discussion between clinicians is built into the timetable to maintain morale and to ensure that clinicians adhere to the mentalizing model.

In the day (partial) hospital program that is now practiced in the Netherlands, brief team meetings are arranged on a daily basis to discuss clinical issues as they arise within the groups and individual sessions. The leaders of the discussion about the groups are, of course, the group clinicians; responsibility for integration of the team perspective in the overall treatment of each patient lies with the individual clinician.

In MBT-IOP, the individual and group clinician must meet, or at least talk, between sessions so that prior to each session, whether an individual or a group session, the clinician knows what has happened in the other treatment session. These discussions take place in a meeting held shortly after each group or individual session in which the clinician reports the session. Differences in opinion should be aired and resolved if possible, and each clinician should try to understand the perspective of his/her co-clinician. Inevitably, some differences arise, and these are discussed in a larger consultation/supervision meeting, which occurs weekly. It is here that views are discussed and integrated and strategies are agreed for use in the group and individual sessions. This ensures that clinicians keep to the mentalizing model, because in our experience it is easy to be diverted from the model and for clinicians to revert to their base technique, whether dynamic or cognitive in orientation.

Clinical planning

Successful planning needs organizational support for team meetings and an explicit statement to all team members about the emphasis in practice on taking into account different clinical perspectives. The team members organize themselves around the problems of the patient and begin a process of integrating different ideas and clinical suggestions. Often this can be done with the patient, who, detached from the emotional intensity of team interactions, may be able to benefit from observing others discuss alternative ideas about help, which gradually coalesce into a practical and meaningful plan to which everyone can commit.

One patient informed a member of the team that she brought a knife to sessions as she felt unsafe on the streets and felt more secure in therapy sessions with the knife in her bag. The clinician was concerned—not only because carrying an offensive weapon is illegal but also for her own safety in the session. It was a concern to the team for exactly the same reasons, and team members expressed worries that the clinician would not be able to focus on the patient's treatment while she was so concerned that the patient was carrying a knife. The team was uncertain what to do, so they organized a meeting of the whole team with the patient to discuss the matter. An array of opinions were expressed, ranging from discharging the patient unless she promised not to carry knives to sessions to more protective comments about the patient's anxieties. The process of discussion enabled the patient to realize that the states of mind she was evoking in the team were untenable for continuing treatment, and she agreed never to bring weapons to sessions. The process of discussion allowed all participants to believe that her statement was an accurate reflection of change rather than a mere glib and superficial statement with no basis in future reality.

Team meetings

Many teams follow an agreed protocol in clinical meetings (see Box 5.5), and we outline here some suggestions for this protocol based on work with young people with emerging personality disorder. First, it is important that the clinicians who want to discuss a clinical problem make this known at the beginning of the meeting. It is surprising how often people bring up some complex clinical problem just before a meeting finishes! Second, the clinician who wants to discuss a problem identifies or "marks" the task. Third, the clinician states his/her case. Fourth, there is a general discussion, which enables all team members involved in the treatment of the patient to offer their perspective. Team members who are not involved "mentalize the discussion" by ensuring that all views are respected and that the emotional support the clinician needs is addressed. Finally, the team "returns to task" to answer the initial questions posed by the clinician.

Box 5.5 Structure of team meeting

- Identify and "mark" the task
- State the focus for discussion
- Discuss the team members' perspectives on the focus
- Return to task to link the discussion with the focus
- Define practical and clinical actions.

Identifying and marking the task

Once team members have expressed a wish to discuss a clinical problem and the order of discussion has been agreed, the team must help the clinician to explicitly identify the problem and what he/she wants out of the discussion. Too often, clinicians and teams revert to story-telling. While this has merits, particularly in helping clinicians ventilate their feelings and feel validated, it is unlikely to lead to practical and effective ongoing treatment planning. This is why marking the task is necessary. This is the responsibility of the presenting clinician. In the earlier example, the clinician identified her concerns about the patient carrying a knife and marked the task as being how to manage this practically and how she processed her fearfulness in the session. Additional examples of marking a task are:

> I would like to discuss the level of risk of this patient and decide on how to address it.
> I would value discussing how to increase this patient's level of motivation for treatment and what I can do—or even do less of—to improve his attendance.
> I am anxious before seeing this patient. During the session I am very careful about what I say. I feel reticent about challenging her and I would like to think more about that.

Stating the case

The clinician then briefly presents the clinical problem without interruption. The veto on interruption is important because too many diversions from the task will prevent effective presentation of the problem as the clinician experiences it. Equally, the clinician has to ensure that the presentation of the problem does not drift into story-telling but focuses on the identified task.

Discussing and mentalizing the process

Once the clinician has completed his/her presentation, the meeting is open to the team for comments and perspectives. Importantly, any team member who is not involved in the care of the patient acts as the guardian of the mentalizing process of the discussion, listening carefully for "absolutes" and extreme views (e.g., "She is just ...," "Clearly he is ... ") and quickly identifying them explicitly. Teams can easily and yet imperceptibly fall into a group process that demonizes patients with BPD, seeing the problem as the fault of the patient when in fact it is a problem within the team or the treatment plan. Organizing a team discussion so that dispassionate members of the team act as "sentinels" of the process is necessary to prevent this.

Return to task

The chair of the meeting takes charge of returning the team to task. Often this is best done by summarizing much of the discussion and linking it to the problem identified initially. An effort is required at this point to define clear practical actions. It is helpful to remember the START criteria around any planned task. The five aspects of START are *Space* (where?), *Time* (when?), *Authority* (who has authority?), *Responsibility* (who has responsibility?), and *Task* (what actions need to be done?).

Final phase

It is now known that people with BPD naturally improve over time, and that they do so to a greater extent than was formerly believed (Zanarini, Frankenburg, Hennen, Reich, & Silk, 2005; Zanarini, Frankenburg, Hennen, & Silk, 2003). However, the improvement is primarily in impulsive behavior and symptoms of affective instability. While this seems to be good news on the surface, the same data also suggest that interpersonal and social/vocational functioning remains impaired. Complex interpersonal interaction, intricate negotiation of difficult social situations, vocational functioning, and interaction with systems may improve less even with treatment. The patient with BPD who no longer self-harms may still lead a life severely curtailed by his/her inability to form constructive relationships with others. Patients remain incapacitated in how they live their lives unless they develop constructive ways of interacting with others. The focus of the final phase of MBT is on the interpersonal and social aspects of functioning, provided the symptomatic and behavioral problems are well controlled, and on integrating and consolidating earlier work. The goals of the final phase are summarized in Box 5.6.

The final phase starts at the 12-month point when the patient still has a further 6 months of treatment. In keeping with the principles of dynamic therapy, we consider the ending of treatment and associated separation responses to be highly significant in consolidation of gains made during therapy. Inadequate

---

Box 5.6 Goals of final phase

+ Increase patient's responsibility and independent functioning
+ Facilitate patient's negotiation about the future, for example, with outside organizations
+ Consolidate and enhance social stability
+ Collaboratively develop a follow-up treatment plan
+ Enhance patient's understanding of the meaning of ending treatment
+ Focus on affective states associated with loss.

negotiation by the clinician of the experience of leaving and/or inadequate processing of the ending on the part of the patient may provoke in the patient a re-emergence of earlier ways of managing feelings and a concomitant decrease in mentalizing capacities. The consequence is a reduction in social and interpersonal function.

It is important that the clinician maintains an awareness of time throughout the trajectory of treatment. The unconscious is timeless, making it easy for both patient and clinician to "forget" about time when working closely together. It may fall to another member of the team to point out to the clinician that time is passing faster than anticipated and that it is time to raise the issue of ending.

> When a clinician mentioned to a patient that he had been in treatment for a year and that there were 6 months left, the patient fell silent and eventually responded by saying that he might as well leave now—"I can't see my feelings changing during that time and so I might as well get it over and done with. What is the point of the next 6 months if finishing is going to be hanging over my head?" The clinician recognized this as a collapse in mentalizing in the face of anxiety, demonstrated by the difficulty the patient had in seeing himself as different in the future. "It is a bit of a shock, isn't it, but I am intrigued that you can't see yourself or your feelings about our relationship as being any different at that time." The clinician then explored the patient's immediate shock about having only a further 6 months in treatment and the fears associated with the loss of the clinician and treatment support.

Entrenchment of negative reactions can be avoided by allowing the patient to take the lead in leaving—setting the date, putting forward his/her own plans for what he/she is to do after discharge, negotiating contingency plans—with the clinician judiciously supporting him/her in reasonable endeavors such as returning to education, obtaining part-time employment, or doing voluntary work.

Follow-up

Responsibility for developing a coherent follow-up program and for negotiating further treatment is given to and shared by the patient and individual clinician. No specific follow-up program is routinely offered in MBT. Most patients ask for further follow-up, which may be a measure of the success of treatment but, equally, can be a way for some patients to avoid finishing treatment and an indicator of our failure to adequately address the anxieties associated with ending. Some patients may have had a "career" over many years of interacting with mental health services; to leave this behind requires a radical change in lifestyle, which may not be fully embedded by the end of 18 months. For patients with severe personality disorder who have a history of many years of failed treatments, multiple hospital admissions, and inadequate social stability, it is unlikely that they will be able to walk away from services, never to return, after the 18 months of MBT, irrespective of the success of the treatment. Most patients require further support as they adapt to a new life. To refuse appropriate help to them would "spoil the ship for a hap'orth of tar."

Various follow-up programs are available: group therapy, couple therapy, outpatient maintenance treatment, college/educational counseling associated with return to education, and, rarely, further individual therapy. These treatment programs are not fully integrated into the specialist treatment programs because all patients are considered in their own right for follow-up and have to apply for further treatment alongside other patients referred to the unit. We attempt to minimize the waiting time for further treatment once the form of further help has been discussed, but there may be a gap between ending the specialist program and entering the follow-up phase. This is the reality of the statutory provision of treatment in the United Kingdom and patients have to adapt to the vagaries of the National Health Service, like all other citizens, if they are to access treatment from this source, whether psychological or physical, in a constructive manner. The ability to use services appropriately offers obvious benefit to a patient who may either have been refused treatment in the past or failed to have his/her physical health taken seriously. In addition, the constructive use of services leads to considerable cost-offset to health systems.

Outpatient maintenance of mentalizing

Many patients choose intermittent follow-up appointments rather than further formal psychotherapy. This is organized within the treatment team. Senior clinicians who have known the patient and who are known to the patient offer individual appointments on a 4–6-weekly basis for 30 minutes per appointment. The purpose of these meetings is clearly specified, as summarized in Box 5.7.

During follow-up appointments, the clinician continues to use mentalizing techniques exploring the underlying mental states of the patient and discussing how understanding themselves and others is leading to resolution of problems,

---

Box 5.7 Goals in follow-up phase

+ Maintain gains in mentalizing that have been made
+ Stimulate further rehabilitative changes
+ Support for return to education or employment
+ Negotiation of further interpersonal and social problems.

enabling them to reconcile differences, and helping them to manage problematic interpersonal areas and intimate relationships. The follow-up contract is flexible and the patient can request an additional appointment if there is an emotional problem that cannot easily be managed. In general, however, the trajectory over follow-up is to increase the time between appointments over a 6-month period to encourage greater patient self-determination. How long a patient is seen in this manner is dependent on the clinician and patient and should be agreed between them. Some patients elect to be discharged relatively early during follow-up on the basis that they can call and request an appointment at any time in the future. We offer this option in our own clinical service. Other patients prefer to make an appointment many months ahead, which provides adequate assurance within their own mind that we continue to have them in mind, giving them greater confidence and self-reliance to negotiate the stresses and strains of everyday life.

References

Ackerman, S. J., & Hilsenroth, M. J. (2003). A review of therapist characteristics and techniques positively impacting the therapeutic alliance. *Clinical Psychology Review*, **23**, 1–33.

Bateman, A. (2005). Day hospital treatment of borderline personality disorder. In M. C. Zanarini (Ed.), *Borderline personality disorder* (pp. 281–304). Boca Raton, FL: Taylor & Francis.

Bateman, A., & Fonagy, P. (1999). Effectiveness of partial hospitalization in the treatment of borderline personality disorder: A randomized controlled trial. *American Journal of Psychiatry*, **156**, 1563–1569.

Bateman, A., & Fonagy, P. (2004). *Psychotherapy for borderline personality disorder: Mentalization-based treatment*. Oxford, UK: Oxford University Press.

Bateman, A., & Fonagy, P. (2006). Mentalizing and borderline personality disorder. In J. G. Allen & P. Fonagy (Eds.), *Handbook of mentalization-based treatment* (pp. 185–200). Chichester, UK: John Wiley & Sons.

Bateman, A., & Fonagy, P. (2009). Randomized controlled trial of outpatient mentalization-based treatment versus structured clinical management for borderline personality disorder. *American Journal of Psychiatry*, **166**, 1355–1364.

Bateman, A., & Fonagy, P. (2013). Impact of clinical severity on outcomes of mentalisation-based treatment for borderline personality disorder. *British Journal of Psychiatry*, **203**, 221–227.

Bateman, A., & Krawitz, R. (2013). *Borderline personality disorder: An evidence-based guide for generalist mental health professionals*. Oxford, UK: Oxford University Press.

Borschmann, R., Henderson, C., Hogg, J., Phillips, R., & Moran, P. (2012). Crisis interventions for people with borderline personality disorder. *Cochrane Database of Systematic Reviews*, **6**, CD009353.

Choi-Kain, L. W., Fitzmaurice, G. M., Zanarini, M. C., Laverdiere, O., & Gunderson, J. G. (2009). The relationship between self-reported attachment styles, interpersonal dysfunction, and borderline personality disorder. *Journal of Nervous and Mental Disease,* **197**, 816–821.

Elkin, I., Falconnier, L., Martinovich, Z., & Mahoney, C. (2006). Therapist effects in the National Institute of Mental Health Treatment of Depression Collaborative Research Program. *Psychotherapy Research,* **16**, 144–160.

Feigenbaum, J. D., Fonagy, P., Pilling, S., Jones, A., Wildgoose, A., & Bebbington, P. E. (2012). A real-world study of the effectiveness of DBT in the UK National Health Service. *British Journal of Clinical Psychology,* **51**, 121–141.

Fonagy, P., & Bateman, A. (2006). Progress in the treatment of borderline personality disorder. *British Journal of Psychiatry,* **188**, 1–3.

Gunderson, J. G., Najavits, L. M., Leonhard, C., Sullivan, C. N., & Sabo, A. N. (1997). Ontogeny of the therapeutic alliance in borderline patients. *Psychotherapy Research,* **7**, 301–309.

Hannan, C., Lambert, M. J., Harmon, C., Nielsen, S. L., Smart, D. W., Shimokawa, K., & Sutton, S. W. (2005). A lab test and algorithms for identifying clients at risk for treatment failure. *Journal of Clinical Psychology,* **61**, 155–163.

Hansen, N. B., Lambert, M. J., & Forman, E. M. (2002). The psychotherapy dose-response effect and its implications for treatment delivery services. *Clinical Psychology: Science and Practice,* **9**, 329–343.

Insel, T. R. (2003). Is social attachment an addictive disorder? *Physiology & Behavior,* **79**, 351–357.

Lingiardi, V., Filippucci, L., & Baiocco, R. (2005). Therapeutic alliance evaluation in personality disorders psychotherapy. *Psychotherapy Research,* **15**, 45–53.

Luborsky, L., Chandler, M., Auerbach, A. H., Cohen, J., & Bachrach, H. M. (1971). Factors influencing the outcome of psychotherapy: A review of quantitative research. *Psychological Bulletin,* **75**, 145–185.

Luborsky, L., McLellan, A. T., Woody, G. E., O'Brien, C. P., & Auerbach, A. (1985). Therapist success and its determinants. *Archives of General Psychiatry,* **42**, 602–611.

National Institute for Health and Clinical Excellence. (2009). *Borderline personality disorder: Treatment and management. Clinical guideline 78.* London, UK: National Institute for Health and Clinical Excellence. http://www.nice.org.uk/nicemedia/pdf/CG78NICEGuideline.pdf

Okiishi, J., Lambert, M. J., Nielsen, S. L., & Ogles, B. M. (2003). Waiting for supershrink: An empirical analysis of therapist effects. *Clinical Psychology and Psychotherapy,* **10**, 361–373.

Okiishi, J. C., Lambert, M. J., Eggett, D., Nielsen, L., Dayton, D. D., & Vermeersch, D. A. (2006). An analysis of therapist treatment effects: Toward providing feedback to individual therapists on their clients' psychotherapy outcome. *Journal of Clinical Psychology,* **62**, 1157–1172.

Shimokawa, K., Lambert, M. J., & Smart, D. W. (2010). Enhancing treatment outcome of patients at risk of treatment failure: Meta-analytic and mega-analytic review of a psychotherapy quality assurance system. *Journal of Consulting and Clinical Psychology,* **78**, 298–311.

Tyrer, P., Crawford, M., Mulder, R., Blashfield, R., Farnam, A., Fossati, A., . . . Reed, G. M. (2011). The rationale for the reclassification of personality disorder in the 11th revision of the International Classification of Diseases (ICD-11). *Personality and Mental Health,* **5**, 246–259.

Tyrer, P., Reed, G. M., & Crawford, M. J. (2015). Classification, assessment, prevalence, and effect of personality disorder. *Lancet*, **385**, 717–726.

Zanarini, M. C. (2004). Update on pharmacotherapy of borderline personality disorder. *Current Psychiatry Reports*, **6**, 66–70.

Zanarini, M. C., Frankenburg, F. R., Hennen, J., Reich, D. B., & Silk, K. R. (2005). Psychosocial functioning of borderline patients and Axis II comparison subjects followed prospectively for six years. *Journal of Personality Disorders*, **19**, 19–29.

Zanarini, M. C., Frankenburg, F. R., Hennen, J., & Silk, K. R. (2003). The longitudinal course of borderline psychopathology: 6-year prospective follow-up of the phenomenology of borderline personality disorder. *American Journal of Psychiatry*, **160**, 274–283.

Zanarini, M. C., Frankenburg, F. R., Reich, D. B., & Fitzmaurice, G. (2012). Attainment and stability of sustained symptomatic remission and recovery among patients with borderline personality disorder and Axis II comparison subjects: A 16-year prospective follow-up study. *American Journal of Psychiatry*, **169**, 476–483.

Chapter 6

Clinician stance

Introduction

Mentalizing in psychotherapy is a process of joint attention in which the patient's mental states are the object of scrutiny. The mentalizing clinician continually constructs and reconstructs an image of the patient in his/her mind to help the patient apprehend what he feels and why he experiences what he does. The patient has to find himself in the mind of the clinician and, equally, the clinician has to understand him/herself in the mind of the patient if the two together are to develop a mentalizing process. Both have to experience a mind being changed by a mind.

While this process sounds rarefied, in practice it is not. The clinician must ensure that his/her primary concern is the patient's state of mind and not his behavior. The clinician's principal interest is in what is happening in the patient's mind *now*, even if it is focusing on a past event; his/her curiosity is about what the patient is experiencing while talking about the events. In effect, the clinician moves from an interest in the events themselves, to the patient's experience of the events at the time, to his/her reflection about the events, to his/her current feelings about talking about the events (see Figure 6.1).

If the dialogue is about an experience in therapy itself, the clinician needs to recognize that neither he/she nor the patient experiences interactions other than impressionistically. This requires the clinician to monitor his/her own mind as much as that of the patient's and to keep an eye on any occasional enactments, however small. Despite our contention that individuals with borderline personality disorder (BPD) have a reduced capacity to monitor the mind states of others accurately, their abilities to use an external mentalizing focus to inform themselves about others' motives and affects are well honed. They may pick up, with remarkable and sometimes uncomfortable accuracy, your errors, your personal weaknesses, and your underlying feelings. So, as we will see, appropriate humility and capacity on the clinician's part to learn about him/herself from the patient is an important part of treatment.

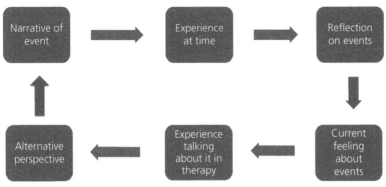

Fig. 6.1 Mentalizing process—trajectory.

Some general considerations

The clinician's mentalizing therapeutic stance (Box 6.1) includes:

- Humility deriving from a sense of "not-knowing"
- Patience in taking time to identify differences in perspectives
- Legitimizing and accepting different perspectives
- Actively questioning the patient about his/her experience—asking for detailed descriptions of experience ("what" questions) rather than explanations ("why" questions)
- Careful eschewing of the need to understand what makes no sense (i.e., saying explicitly that something is unclear).

Box 6.1 Mentalizing stance

- Mentalizing in psychotherapy is a process of joint attention in which the patient's mental states are the object of attention
- The clinician continually constructs and reconstructs an image of the patient, to help the patient to apprehend what he/she feels
- Neither clinician nor patient experiences interactions other than impressionistically
- Differences are identified
- Acceptance of different perspectives
- Active questioning.

An important component of this stance is monitoring and acknowledging one's own errors as a clinician—getting things wrong and owning up to these mistakes. This not only models honesty and courage, and tends to lower the patient's arousal through the clinician taking responsibility for interactional difficulties, but also offers invaluable opportunities to explore how interpersonal problems can arise out of mistaken assumptions about opaque mental states and how misunderstanding is a significant aversive experience. In this context, it is important to be aware that the clinician is constantly at risk of losing his/her capacity to mentalize when faced with a nonmentalizing patient. The primary task of the clinician at this moment is to regain his/her own mentalizing. Consequently, we consider clinicians' occasional nonmentalizing errors as an acceptable concomitant of the therapeutic alliance, something that simply has to be owned up to. As with other instances of breaks in mentalizing, such incidents require that the process is "rewound" and the incident "explored." Hence, in a collaborative, mentalizing relationship, the patient and clinician have a joint responsibility to understand what goes on between them.

We have often said that clinicians do not need to be overly worried about the primary task of MBT, that is, stimulating mentalizing when it is lost, since they are probably already doing it without being aware of it. Any technique that promotes mentalizing is valid. Rather than beginning afresh, our model requires the clinician to re-examine his/her current practice from the perspective of whether his/her interventions stimulate mentalizing or actually inhibit it. To this extent, the clinician should differentiate between a stance that primarily focuses on descriptive narrative and one that requires attention to mental states. MBT clinicians need the facts, and should not avoid eliciting the facts about important events. Indeed, these are necessary before mentalizing work is done about such events.

CLINICIAN: Tell me what happened? [This is a question eliciting facts.]
PATIENT: I walked into the house and found my boyfriend with another woman. They were in the living room and had obviously been fondling each other. I shouted at them and she told me to get out.
CLINICIAN: What did you do then? [A further question likely to elicit a story.]

This is a dialogue that elicits facts about events. Once enough detail has been obtained, the clinician returns to the events and begins exploration around the mental states associated with the events.

CLINICIAN: What sort of frame of mind were you in on your way home?
PATIENT: I felt quite good. I was looking forward to seeing my boyfriend. We had had a nice evening the day before.
CLINICIAN: So what was your general feeling about your relationship with him before this?

This is the beginning of a mentalizing dialogue moving slowly toward understanding the internal states the patient was experiencing in reaction to the events. In principle, MBT clinicians elicit the facts of the events and then rewind to establish the internal experience of the events.

In addition, the clinician needs to be aware of his/her own state of mentalizing. As we have put it before, "Ironically, when you become aware of your non-mentalizing interventions (or excrementalizing!), you are mentalizing. A further irony: when you start obsessing about mentalizing in the middle of a session, you have lost mentalizing, because you are no longer paying attention to your patient" (Allen, Fonagy, & Bateman, 2008, p. 163). Paying attention to your patient's mind is at the heart of mentalizing. Paradoxically, it is the clever or highly trained clinician who is more likely to turn off a patient's mentalizing by taking an expert role. Once he finds himself knowing why something is wrong with the patient and how it can be corrected, that is, he takes over the patient's mentalizing, he is not mentalizing. A general reluctance to admit to himself that he does not know what is happening in therapy sessions compounds the problem!

Knowing takes many forms: we profess a deep understanding of unconscious process, we are sure about good and bad thought processes, we empathically tell patients what they are feeling—all of which are nonmentalizing stances. The MBT clinician needs to stimulate a joint consideration of underlying processes rather than claiming to understand them, to explore different components of thought processes rather than Socratically demonstrating their inaccuracy, and to help the patient attend to his feelings rather than methodically naming them for him. The clinician focuses on the process rather than the content of the patient's thoughts and feelings, and in doing so he/she asks the patient to attend consciously to the processes within both his own and others' minds and to maintain this attention as his feelings fluctuate. To develop this process the clinician uses a range of interventions, which share the primary aims of maintaining mentalizing and reinstating it when lost.

Clinician attitude

The attitude of the clinician is crucial. The clinician will stimulate in the patient a recognition of mentalizing as a core process of successful interaction with others, in part through a process of modeling and identification. The clinician's ability to use his/her own mind and to demonstrate delight in changing his/her mind when presented with alternative views will be internalized by the patient, who will gradually become more curious about his own and others' minds and better able to reappraise himself and his understanding of others. This continual re-working of perspectives exemplified by the curious attitude of the clinician, along with consideration of alternatives within the therapeutic relationship, is key to a change process, as is the focus of the work on current rather than past experience.

In an attempt to capture this clinician stance, which gives the best chance of achieving mentalizing goals, we have defined a mentalizing or "not-knowing" stance.

Mentalizing or not-knowing stance

The mentalizing or not-knowing stance is *not* synonymous with having no knowledge. The term is an attempt to capture a sense that mental states are opaque, and that the clinician can have no more idea of what is in the patient's mind than the patient himself and, in fact, probably will have a lot less. Your position is one in which you attempt to demonstrate a willingness to find out about your patient's mind, what makes him "tick," how he feels, and the reasons for his underlying problems. Your initial task is to see things the way your patient sees them, taking the patient's perspective. To do this you need to become an active questioning clinician (see Box 6.2), discouraging excessive free association by the patient in favor of detailed monitoring and understanding of interpersonal processes and how they relate to the patient's mental states.

Your aim is to get the patient to monitor his own mind states in real time. If you take a different perspective from the patient this should be verbalized and explored in relation to the patient's alternative perspective, with no assumption being made about whose viewpoint has greater validity (see Box 6.3).

The task is to determine the mental processes that have led to alternative viewpoints and to consider each perspective in relation to the other, accepting that divergent outlooks may be acceptable. Where differences are clear and cannot initially be resolved they should be identified, stated, and accepted until resolution seems possible.

Box 6.2 Examples of active questioning

- Describe how you understood what he said.
- I wonder if that was related to the group yesterday?
- Perhaps you felt that I was judging you?
- What do you make of her suicidal feeling [in the group]?
- What made him behave toward you as he did?
- What do you make of what has happened?

Box 6.3 Highlighting alternative perspectives

- ◆ I saw it as a way to control yourself rather than to attack me [patient explanation]; can you think about that for a moment?
- ◆ You seem to think that I don't like you and yet I am not sure what makes you think that.
- ◆ Help me see it like that. I am not aware that you did not do well. It seems that it was a success to me.

The activity of the questioning clinician is illustrated in the following vignette.

The disappointed patient

PATIENT [Talking about her follow-up meeting with her former psychologist]: I don't think he bothered about what I was saying at all.

CLINICIAN: What makes you say that?

PATIENT: I had to repeat myself and he still didn't say anything except to ask me the same question that I had just answered [possible nonmentalized statement].

CLINICIAN: I can see how you get to that [validation without agreement that the psychologist was or was not bothered]. What effect did it have on you? [A question eliciting mental state rather than narrative.]

PATIENT: It made me upset that I had been seeing someone all that time who always seemed to want to listen to me but was actually a fake.

CLINICIAN: It is difficult, isn't it, when someone seems to have changed so quickly, but what about this sense that he didn't listen?

PATIENT: He was seeing me and so was supposed to be listening to me whatever else he was doing. He just didn't say much [explains how she has come to her conclusion]. I was not wanted there.

CLINICIAN: That's right, and I can see that it made you feel not wanted, but how did that compare with your feelings for him before? [Affectively based intervention and suggests contrast of her different experiences of him.]

PATIENT: I used to think that he always listened to me and was interested in what was going on in my life, but this . . . I won't be going again.

CLINICIAN: It is really upsetting, isn't it, when someone doesn't seem to be how they usually are? Maybe you were influenced by that awful feeling of disappointment that you were not going to see him again [links finality of decision to stop seeing her psychologist with the problematic feeling that was evoked. This goes further than the not-knowing stance, as the clinician suggests that another mental state might be important, but it is a mental state that he has suggested. Technically, this is not fully on the model. It would be better for the clinician to ask if there were other feelings about seeing her psychologist for follow-up].

PATIENT: Maybe, but when I was there it felt like hard work. But you are right, that was not how he usually was. But it was hurtful. He didn't seem to mind that he was not going to see me again.

CLINICIAN: Hmm. Let's consider how that left you feeling and how you are managing it [now moving the therapy on to consider what effect it will have that she will not see the psychologist again].

The doing clinician

Early in therapy, patients may experience clinicians as understanding their needs only if they provide them with explicit and concrete evidence that this is the case. Pressure for the clinician to do something is high because the teleological psychological function often apparent in people with BPD (see Chapter 1) means that their understanding of the world is dependent on what happens in the physical world—outcomes in the "real" world define meaning. Clinicians will, at times, demonstrate their understanding through appropriate action within the boundaries of therapy—a supportive letter for housing may be necessary, a telephone call to the patient to help him explore the precipitants of an interpersonal crisis and to monitor what is happening in his mind, or even a home visit with a colleague between sessions in an emergency. Many of these acts can become integral to therapy.

Any letter or report written on the patient's behalf should be shared with him before it is sent off, and rewritten if necessary, as part of the joint attention given to the patient's needs. The first draft by the clinician gives his/her perspective, while modification in discussion with the patient demonstrates a process of change and the influence of a mind on a mind. If joint agreement cannot be reached about an aspect of the letter, the clinician must decide whether to remove or retain the opinion. Whichever course of action is taken, the reasons for the decision should be explained to the patient. Of course, some reports are supportive of the patient while other reports, for example, those to probation, courts, or child protection teams, might raise complex issues for therapy.

> A clinician wrote a report about a patient for the child protection team. He gave the initial draft of the report to the patient to read. She corrected a number of minor factual errors but was most concerned about his view that her emotional volatility meant that her ability to focus on the needs of her baby was compromised. The clinician discussed

how he had come to that opinion. She disagreed. Some work was done defining the "elephant in the room" (affect focus; see Chapters 7 and 9) and repairing the therapeutic alliance by accepting the difference in opinion—for her part, the patient was concerned that the clinician would never change his mind and she would not be able to demonstrate her stability; for his part, the clinician was concerned that the patient would cover up her problems and so ensure that treatment was a sham, appearing to be effective while in reality being ineffective. Both agreed that they would openly talk about this when either of them thought it was interfering with therapy.

The aim of this openness about reports or other actions taken on behalf of the patient is to maintain mentalizing around the content of the report or action, which, after all, is about the patient. It is not to take over responsibility from the patient, and work may need to be done in helping them be more effective, for example, in dealing with housing or other organizations. Any major actions taken on behalf of the patient should be carefully considered—preferably with another team member—before they are undertaken, and certainly discussed with the team if they have already taken place within a session. This protects against inappropriate enactments.

The monitoring clinician

Being human, you will inevitably make errors in therapy, some more serious than others. Here we are not talking about structural blunders, for example, forgetting sessions or failing to organize appointments with due care. Gross structural errors require apology, acceptance on your part for your failure, and later demonstration within the therapy process that you are aware of the effects of the event on your patient. We are talking about a requirement to own up to your own mentalizing errors, that is, those that undermine mentalizing rather than promote it; for example, telling the patient how she feels, insisting that your perspective is right, arguing with psychic equivalence. You must not to attempt to cover up your errors or to deny them when confronted. Mistakes are treated as opportunities to revisit what happened and to learn more about contexts, feelings, and experiences—"How was it that I did that at that time?" (see Box 6.4). It is not enough to recognize silently within yourself that you have made an error and change your interventions accordingly. You need to articulate what has happened, not only to model honesty and courage, but above all to demonstrate that you are continually reflecting on what goes on in your mind and on what you do in relation to the patient. This is a central component of mentalizing itself.

Authenticity

This brings us to a controversial aspect of MBT—the clinician's mental processes must be available to the patient. Mental processes are opaque. This opacity, combined with the person with BPD's characteristic vulnerability to loss of

---

Box 6.4 Indicators of clinician self-reflection

- Is there something I have said or done that might have made you feel like that?
- I am not sure what made me say that. I will have to think about it.
- I believe that I was wrong. What I can't understand is how I came to say it. Can you help me go back to what was happening here before things went wrong?
- Have I missed something that is obvious?

---

mentalizing within relationships, sensitivity to external cues such as facial expressions (Lynch et al., 2006), and assumptions about internal mind states, means that the mentalizing clinician needs to make his/her mental processes transparent to the patient; as he/she tries to understand the patient, he/she openly deliberates while "marking" his/her statements carefully. This requires a directness, honesty, authenticity, and personal ownership of what the clinician feels and thinks, which is problematic partly because of the dangers of boundary violations in the treatment of people with BPD. Our emphasis on the need for authenticity is *not* a license to overstep the boundaries of therapy or to develop a "real" relationship; we are merely stressing that the clinician needs to make him/herself mentally available to the patient and must demonstrate an ability to balance uncertainty and doubt with opinion and professional perspective. This becomes particularly important when patients correctly identify feelings and thoughts experienced by the clinician. The clinician needs to be prepared for questions and assertions that put him/her on the defensive—"You're bored with me," "You are fed up with me," "You don't like me much either, do you?" and so on. Such challenges to the clinician can arise suddenly and without warning, and the clinician needs to be able to answer with authenticity. If he/she does not do so, the patient will become more insistent and even evoke the very experience in the clinician he/she is pointing out (if, indeed, the clinician was not already feeling it at the time!). Worse still, the clinician invalidates the patient's correct perception because he/she is embarrassed and uncomfortable. Commonly this is done by the clinician reflecting the question, which is a frequent mentalizing error.

A patient's accurate perception of what is in the clinician's mind needs validation:

You are bored with seeing me, aren't you?

This is likely to be asked from a position of psychic equivalence, in which the patient's internal thoughts and experience are assumed to be the same as outside experience. Within psychic equivalence, the patient cannot distinguish self and other easily, and so he operates from a perspective that others have the same experience as him.

If the clinician is indeed feeling bored, it is important that he/she says so in a way that stimulates exploration of what within the patient–clinician interaction is boring. An MBT clinician will take equal responsibility for creating boring therapy and move to making this a focus of therapy for that moment:

> Now you mention it, I was feeling a bit bored and I am unsure where that is coming from. Is it related to what you are talking about or how you are talking about it, or is it more me at the moment? You know, I am really not sure.

Alternatively, if the clinician is in fact not bored, then he/she needs to find a way to express this that opens up the possibility of exploring what stimulated the patient's question. To do this the clinician first needs to be open about his/her current feeling, rather than attempting to stimulate the patient's fantasies about what he/she, the clinician, is feeling. This follows a basic MBT principle—*DO NOT make interventions that assume mentalizing when a patient is not mentalizing*. To ask a patient to imagine what the clinician's experience is, and for that image to be given meaning, it has to be represented in the patient's mind and contrasted with his own experience. This process requires a reasonable mentalizing capacity. Asking a question like "What makes you think I am bored?" to the nonmentalizing patient, without clarifying first whether or not his perception is accurate, is likely to induce pretend mode or, alternatively, simply lead to the development of psychic equivalent fantasy. It is better for the clinician to tell the patient what he/she is experiencing within the therapy at that moment:

> As far as I am aware, I was not bored. In fact, I was trying to grasp what you were saying. I felt muddled. But now I am intrigued that you and I were having such a different experience of this at the moment [marked alternative perspective].

The aim here is for the clinician to stimulate exploration of alternative perspectives. If this is to occur, the different perspectives have to be clear. Here, the patient has a specific perspective. Now the clinician has placed an alternative viewpoint but emphasized that it is his/her own state of mind that he/she is reflecting on (marking) and not that of the patient. In doing so he/she is not stating that the patient's state of mind is wrong, but setting up a platform from which to explore alternatives.

Counter-relationship or feelings engendered in the clinician and marking mental states

In the past, we have blithely used the term "countertransference" to describe the feelings of the clinician occurring in treatment sessions. Correctly, concerns have been expressed about our use of the term. Indeed, our use of the term has been somewhat loose and lacked psychological precision in relation to the complex definitions found in the psychoanalytic literature. The meaning of the word has a long and illustrious history and its sense has changed over time. Yet, whatever definition is used, a core persists, namely, that "countertransference" refers to feelings in the clinician and links to his/her self-awareness, which in turn relies on his/her affective pole of mentalizing. This is the focus in MBT, and so we often talk about the "feelings in the clinician in relation to the patient" rather than using the term "countertransference" because this has implications for the source of the feelings, which are usually considered to be arising from the patient. Some clinicians tend to default to a state of self-reference in which they consider most of what they experience in therapy as being projected by the patient and technically part of countertransference. This default mode needs to be resisted. As clinicians, we need to be mindful of the fact that our mental states might unduly color our understanding of the patient's mental states and that we tend to equate our own mental states with those of the patient without adequate foundation. The clinician has to "quarantine" his/her feelings. These feelings are defined as those experiences, both affective and cognitive, that the clinician has in sessions and which he/she thinks might help to further develop an understanding of mental processes relevant to the problems of the patient or those in treatment itself. How the clinician "quarantines" his/her counter-relationship feelings informs his/her technical approach to feelings engendered in him/her during treatment.

We frame our technical work with feelings within the clinician (broadly, countertransference) with an exhortation for the clinician to be "ordinary." Inexperienced clinicians frequently have ideas about how a clinician should behave and act in therapy that lead them to become wooden, unresponsive, and dedicated to technical application. We suggest that being ordinarily human is a better way forward when working with counter-relationship feelings. We do not license clinicians to behave in any way they please or to say whatever they like—any more than they would do in a respectful relationship with a friend. Rather, we recommend that the clinician openly works on his/her state of mind in therapy in a way that moves the joint purpose of the patient–clinician relationship forward, keeping mentalizing on-line. To do this the clinician will often need to speak openly from his/her own perspective (this is termed "marking") rather than from his/her understanding of the patient's experience. The key word here is "openly." Counter-relationship experience expressed verbally by the clinician is an important aspect of therapy, but when it is being expressed it must be marked as an aspect of the clinician's state of mind. It should not be attributed to the patient, even though it may be a reaction to the patient. In essence, marking implicitly or explicitly speaks to the question about whose mind we are talking about: is it mine, is it my representation of your mind state, or is it a combination of both?

Counter-relationship experience can be powerful in the treatment of BPD, with clinicians struggling with feelings of rage, hatred, hurt, rejection, care, and anxiety. Patients seem able to hit our sensitive spots and sometimes will even focus on them as they try to control the emotional processes in a session. The task of the clinician is to help the patient recognize that what he/she does and says evokes a state of mind in the clinician, just as what the clinician does and says stimulates mental processes in the patient. The patient needs to consider the effects he/she has on others within his/her own mind, rather than to ignore them or maintain that they are of no consequence.

A patient with antisocial personality disorder (ASPD) had a threatening and menacing demeanor. He sat forward in sessions glowering at the clinician. Unsurprisingly, the clinician was fearful. So the clinician decided to try to talk about the problem he was having with offering treatment while feeling scared.

CLINICIAN: I think I need to bring up one aspect of our sessions, which I don't want you to take as a criticism [anticipating patient reaction prior to expressing the clinician's feelings]. But as you sit forward in the way you are now and raise your voice as you talk to me it makes me feel nervous. I can't think properly when I am nervous, so it prevents me listening carefully to what you are saying. Could you sit back and lower your voice a little?

PATIENT: You don't need to be. I am not threatening you [common ASPD dismissal of others' mental state].

CLINICIAN: I appreciate that, but nevertheless it is the effect that it has on me.

In this example, the clinician has managed to maintain his own mentalizing by expressing his own state of mind, namely, the emotion that is reducing his capacity to mentalize in the current session. This is in line with one of the primary principles of MBT—the clinician ensures that he maintains his own mentalizing. The response from the patient suggests that he has no concern about the effect that he is having on the clinician. This is a characteristic mentalizing problem found in people with ASPD and has to be addressed in MBT-ASPD (see Chapter 13).

In summary, the mentalizing clinician is not neutral but engaged in a process of reflective engagement (see Box 6.5), making it essential for him/her to monitor his/her responses more openly than in many other therapies; his/her role is potentially iatrogenic in terms of the interpersonal process. The question for the clinician is what aspect of him/her contributed to what happened and what element of the patient stimulated that involvement, or what aspect of him/her provoked it and what did it stimulate in the patient. His/her reflection about these processes needs to be open and genuinely thoughtful rather than closed and introspective.

This sort of exploration of shared experience requires an open-minded clinician, safe in his/her own failings and appropriately doubtful about his/her viewpoints, so that the patient can manage to open his own mind and begin to question his own rigidly operating schemas about himself and others in the same way that the clinician does. A detached, aloof, refined, defended clinician is unlikely to form a relationship with a patient that helps the patient find himself in the mind of the clinician in an accessible and meaningful way. Patients with BPD have a reduced capacity for understanding the subjective mental states of others; they cannot fathom the inscrutability of a remote mind, and such a clinician stance is most likely to stimulate uncontrolled paranoid reactions. But, equally, they cannot tolerate a clinician who bubbles with emotion, fails to differentiate different perspectives, and exposes them to excessive feelings in others, which might take them over. The clinician needs to become what the patient needs them to be, to feel what the patient wants them to feel, but at the same time to be themselves, while able to preserve a part of their mind that accurately mirrors the patient's internal state.

Box 6.5 Reflective engagement

- Clinician's occasional enactment is an acceptable concomitant of the therapeutic alliance
- Own up to enactment and rewind and explore
- Check out understanding
- Joint responsibility to understand over-determined enactments
- Monitor your own mistakes
- Model honesty and courage via acknowledgement of your own mistakes—past, current, and future
- Suggest that mistakes offer opportunities to revisit to learn more about contexts, experiences, and feelings.

It is important to emphasize that this "mentalizing the counter-relationship or feelings in the clinician" is not a process of reversal in which the patient is giving the clinician some therapy or the clinician is exploring his/her own pathology in front of the patient or engaging in self-disclosure—all of which are likely to burden the patient rather than help him understand himself. Reflection on interactions is by necessity focused on the patient–clinician relationship, with both parties being considered responsible for looking at all the elements that potentially contributed to the exchange. This might include the patient's provocative goading and projective processes on the one hand or the clinician's sensitivities and unresolved conflicts on the other. This can be discovered only by understanding the mental processes contributing to the problem. So, a "Stop, Rewind, Explore" (described later in this chapter) is necessary, taking the session back before moving it forward again "frame by frame" or "mental state by mental state." Just as the patient's behaviors cannot be understood in isolation from the mental processes that have led to them, so interventions by the clinician cannot become meaningful unless their contributing determinants are identified.

Emotional closeness in therapy sessions

Once the clinician has adopted the mentalizing stance and stimulated a mentalizing process, his/her task is to maintain mentalizing within him/herself and the patient while at the same time recognizing that therapy will potentially destabilize mentalizing by stimulating the attachment system (see Chapter 1 for a discussion of this phenomenon). Mentalizing will be threatened simply because the clinician probes, stimulates feelings, and asks questions, all of which are likely to make the patient anxious. Alert to this, the clinician moves emotionally closer to the patient during a session only to the point at which he/she judges the patient is on the verge of losing mentalizing. At this moment he/she moves back, distancing him/herself from the patient, to reduce the level of emotional arousal. Here we encounter a clinically significant paradox—just when the clinician would naturally move emotionally closer to the patient, we ask that he/she moves away. Any person talking with someone who is becoming increasingly disturbed or upset will naturally become more sympathetic and caring. At such times the clinician is likely to become gentler in his/her demeanor, speak more quietly, and try to demonstrate an ever more profound understanding of the patient's emotional state. Yet this will stimulate the patient's attachment system, leading to further impairment of his/her mentalizing capacity; this is particularly the case in patients with BPD because of the hypersensitivity of their attachment system.

For this reason, we ask the clinician to curb his/her natural tendency to become increasingly sympathetic when the patient becomes emotional, and to distance him/herself emotionally by becoming less expressive and perhaps more cognitive, even if only momentarily. Once mentalizing is regained, he/she can recapture emotional involvement and begin again to probe, empathize, and focus on the patient–clinician relationship. However, he/she should not be surprised to find that this rekindles the patient's attachment system. He/she needs to monitor sensitively for further losses of mentalizing and to step back rapidly when necessary. This recommendation of becoming more cognitive does not amount to a recommendation that a caring clinician becomes uncaring. However, caring that manifests itself as sweetness, concern, and sympathy at this moment will only add fuel to the fire, inflaming attachment needs and stimulating further mental deterioration in the patient just at the moment when it is crucial to find a way of stimulating more robust mental processes.

> A patient became distressed when talking about her boyfriend being sexually unfaithful. She talked about leaving him, but said that she loved him and so she could not do so. The clinician made many sympathetic noises during this story, and made increasingly supportive statements about the problem for the patient in coping with her conflicting experience. The patient became more and more distressed, becoming inconsolable for most of the rest of the session. This evoked a feeling in the clinician that she should offer an additional session. This immediately intensified the patient's needs; she then asked if the current session could go on for longer, saying that she thought she could not leave the room.
>
> Inadvertently, the clinician had aroused the patient's dependency and made her even more vulnerable by becoming more sympathetic and offering additional sessions to the patient at a time when she needed to step back from the patient.

Stepping back in the face of distress requires conscious effort on the clinician's part if it is to be done sensitively. It is counterintuitive. Not only does it go against instincts and natural tendencies, but it also defies all that was learned in training. Clinicians tend to lower their voices, speak softly, and express apprehension in their facial expressions as they become increasingly concerned and sympathetic. In order to reduce the power of the emotional interaction, the clinician needs initially to respond in a somewhat matter-of-fact manner or move the patient away from his/her current focus, rather than continuing to focus on either affect or the interaction between patient and clinician, both of which will continue to stimulate the patient's attachment needs. In the earlier example, the clinician would have done better to move the patient away from an internal focus on her affect and to de-emphasize the patient–clinician relationship (a counterbalance). One way of doing this might have been to focus the session more on practical aspects of how she might manage living on her own, for example. Thus, the clinician moves to a more cognitively dominated discussion.

This is an example of a *contrary move*: the more the patient is dominated by affect, the more the clinician becomes focused on cognitions. The clinician should aim to help the patient maintain some elements of mentalizing, in this case cognitive processing, when other aspects are overwhelmed, in this case the capacity for affective reflection about the self. Insistence on further exploration of internal states at times of emotional arousal will only overburden the patient; we suggest the use of contrary moves at these times.

Contrary moves

This movement of stepping back from excess emotional stimulation is part of a general technique to rebalance mentalizing that becomes fixed at one end of one of the four dimensions of mentalizing (see Chapter 1, where we discuss the dimensions of mentalizing in detail). In clinical practice, we recommend that you consider moving patients along or rebalancing the dimensions when they become fixed at one end, for example, excessive cognitive rationalization without affect, or persistent focus on self rather than consideration of the experience of others (see Table 6.1).

The clinician technically attempts to refocus the patient outwards when he/she is self-focused, or toward him/herself when he/she is excessively externalizing or is other-focused. This is also represented in the clinician–patient interaction, with the clinician moving him/herself toward the patient—that is, making the dialogue more emotionally personal—when the patient moves away, and moving away when the patient becomes emotionally fixed on the clinician.

We envision a "balancing act," maintaining flexibility of mentalizing around the four dimensions. This advances the scope for reflection and dialogue. In terms of the interpersonal interaction, we anticipate that you and the patient will oscillate back and forth as you titrate the intensity of the attachment relationship. In addition, within him/herself, the person with BPD may at some

Table 6.1 Contrary moves

Patient/clinician	Clinician/patient
External focus	Internal focus
Self-reflection	Other reflection
Emotional distance	Emotional closeness
Cognitive	Affective
Implicit	Explicit
Certainty	Doubt

moments be self-focused, and this is often to be commended; however, this self-reflection may begin to take on a ruminative quality, or the patient may get stuck in a rigidly negative, shameful, self-condemning mode. At such times, taking into account his/her current mentalizing capacity (see later for a caution), you will try to move the patient out of his/her mind and into another person's mind: "How do you think that affects her?"; "What was going on for him that led him to do that?" You should not be deflected from this task once you have decided that it is an appropriate move in treatment. Many patients respond by saying they don't know, and quickly return to their ruminative concern with their own state of mind. You may therefore need to be more insistent: "Bear with me a bit—I was wondering what you made of what was happening for him that made him respond like that?"

There will also be times when you will need to make the converse move. Patients who are preoccupied with understanding others and what they are like may need pushing to reflect on their own state of mind: "What did you feel about that?"; "How do you understand your reaction?" This is feasible even when the patient is in psychic equivalence.

There is one caution for the clinician when working with contrary moves, particularly when exploring events about problems in a relationship. In this context the clinician may be tempted to ask the patient about the motives of the other while at the same time exploring the motives and experience of the patient. If the patient is currently in psychic equivalence mode, asking him/her to consider the mind states of an "other" is to suggest an impossible task. At this point the patient's experience of the other's mind state is dictated by his/her own psychic equivalence experience.

PATIENT: My probation officer is trying to trick me so that she can send me back to prison [unelaborated statement stating other's motive, suggesting that it is held in nonmentalizing mode].

CLINICIAN: What makes you say that? [Attempt to stimulate the patient to think about the other person's motive.]

PATIENT: She asked me why I did not attend the police station yesterday and she already knew where I was.

CLINICIAN: Really?

PATIENT: She does not like me. She knew that I was at the anger management meeting and that is why she arranged for me to be at the police station at that time.

CLINICIAN: Do you think there is any other reason that she could have done that?

PATIENT: [Thinks for a moment.] She is a cow?

CLINICIAN: Oh! Any other reasons? I was thinking more that she might not have known about the conflict of appointments [asking to explore other possible motives of the probation officer].

PATIENT: [Thinks again.] Well if it is not because she is a cow. Maybe she is just a shit.

In this verbatim transcript the clinician has not appreciated that the patient is holding her experience of the meeting with the probation officer in psychic equivalence mode. Asking her about possible alternative motives of the probation officer merely stimulates different ways of saying the same thing. The patient is not in a position mentally to be reflective because of psychic equivalence, in which the patient's mental reality is experienced as being external reality. The clinician will have to stimulate the patient's mentalizing in the session before returning to this interaction with the probation officer to explore whether the patient can work on how she manages her relationship with the probation officer.

Contrary moves along the dimensions of mentalizing aim to embed increasing flexibility in mentalizing. The patient who is affectively overwhelmed needs to have some cognitive processes brought to bear on the problem—so the clinician tries to stimulate this in the patient by becoming more rational in his/her responses. The patient who is overly intellectual and rational needs to harness some affective experience related to the problem—and so the clinician tries to trigger some affective response to the problem. To this extent there is a constant reciprocal flow of dialogue between patient and clinician along the dimensions of mentalizing and an attempt to instill flexibility in the internal mentalizing process of the patient irrespective of the context.

Labeling with qualification ("I wonder if . . ." statements)

Labeling with qualification, or "wondering" statements, can sound woolly and be received as irritatingly uncertain ("How should I know? You are supposed to be the therapist"), but when used appropriately can propel a session forward and achieve further discussion and revelation. The mentalizing stance of "not-knowing" implies that the clinician will "wonder" more often than he/she "knows," but it is important that if he/she "knows" he/she does not "wonder." Hence, the not-knowing stance is not a continuous "wondering" stance. In our experience, a clinician who "wonders" too much is in danger of not sharing his/her perspective with a patient; for example, he/she wonders when in fact he/she has a viewpoint. This creates a false interaction—the patient may well understand the clinician's underlying subjective state of mind even if it is not openly expressed and reacts to it unconsciously, constructing a "pretend" interaction in which both patient and clinician are tentative while both are certain.

"I wonder if . . . " statements may be useful to ensure that the patient discovers what he/she is feeling. The patient should not be told what he/she is feeling because this takes over his/her mentalizing. The manifest feeling may be labeled without qualification, but the clinician's task is to identify the consequential experience related to that feeling. This is where labeling with qualification is important: "Although you are obviously dismissive of them, I wonder if that leaves you feeling a bit left out?"

The process clinician

Finally, it is important that the clinician concentrates on developing a mentalizing therapeutic process (see Box 6.6). More attention needs to be devoted to this than to detailed understanding of content. An implicit mentalizing process is a major goal of treatment, and this will develop only if the patient can be freed from rigid views held firmly within a schematic belief system. To achieve this shift, the clinician should focus on the relationship between patient and clinician, as it exemplifies different perspectives and offers opportunities for alternative understanding.

Overt schematic delineation of beliefs will generate explicit mentalizing, and this forms the basis of many cognitive interventions for BPD. This in itself may be helpful, but your goal is the development of an implicit mentalizing process within the therapeutic relationship. Explication of affective states embedded within the current relationship is therefore emphasized more than cognitive exposition in order to generate an experience of "feeling felt" in which the patient feels affirmed, validated, and not alone, and remains in the feeling while being aware of the feeling. Our emphasis on process is in line with other dynamic therapies for BPD, and clinicians who have been trained in the conversational model or cognitive analytic therapy will have little difficulty in recognizing the importance of "listening" to the process rather than paying too much attention to the exact content (see, for example, Meares, 2000; Meares & Hobson, 1977; Ryle, 2004).

Box 6.6 Mentalizing process

- Not directly concerned with content but with helping the patient
- Generate multiple perspectives in the patient ➜ to free him/herself from being stuck in the "reality" of one view (primary representations and psychic equivalence) ➜ to experience an array of mental states (secondary representations) and ➜ to recognize them as such (meta-representations).

Aspects of process that need special attention are the negotiation of a negative therapeutic reaction, a sudden rupture in the alliance, or rapid emotional dysregulation in the patient; all may leave the clinician perplexed and uncertain about how to react. Ruptures frequently result from the conjunction of relationship patterns in the patient and clinician (Aveline, 2005), thereby being the product of both rather than one alone; clinicians must be skilled in repairing them (Meares, 2000). In our experience, the explicitly reflective clinician, who retrieves his/her own mentalizing ability quickly following a collapse in the relationship, is the most likely to negotiate severe ruptures in the alliance successfully, and this capacity may be a key factor in maintaining people with BPD in treatment. Here again is the principle underpinning MBT—the clinician needs to maintain his/her own mentalizing and to work to recover it before he/she can help the patient further.

Ruptures represent a failure of mentalizing. The clinician's initial response should be open consideration of their part in the rupture—"What have I said or what is it you feel I have done to bring about this sudden change?"—as a demonstration of a continuing process of self-reflection. This allows the clinician to tease out the different contributions to events in therapy without apportioning blame and firmly embeds the dialogue within the immediacy of the patient–clinician relationship. The gravest danger at these times is increasing your use of the techniques that you believe are crucial to patient change, for example, transference interpretation, behavioral challenge, or delineation of cognitive distortions. First, the therapeutic alliance must be repaired by staying in the rupture and seeking a vantage point from which to view it. You and the patient need to move to a position betwixt and between the "heat" of the rupture. You both become detectives seeking clues about what has happened; this is best done by "stopping" and "rewinding" and then moving forward to the point of rupture. This brings us to the final topic of this chapter, which is to emphasize the importance of the clinician managing the process of each session.

The mentalizing focus—managing process

A number of basic mentalizing techniques are used to manage the mentalizing process in each session. We have previously emphasized that MBT is organized around various trajectories. First, there is the trajectory of treatment over 12–18 months, with different aims and processes at the beginning of treatment compared to the middle and end of treatment. Second, there is the trajectory through each group and individual session. There is the opening component of a session in which a focus is developed. This is followed by exploration of the focus from a range of perspectives, for example, the perspective apparent at the time when the problem occurred, the current perspective in the session, and the perspective on similar events in the future. Finally, there is the trajectory of intervention—often synchronized with the session trajectory—which moves from empathic validation at the beginning of a session, to affect exploration and focus, to mentalizing the relationship, and back to empathic validation and summary toward the end of the session. These trajectories need careful management by the clinician, and we have defined some techniques that can be used to manage the process. These are grouped together as "Stop, Listen, Look" and "Stop, Rewind, Explore." These aide-memoire "catchphrases" refer to the actions of the clinician as he/she tries to reinstate a mentalizing process in the session.

Technically, the clinician may Stop, Rewind, Explore the process in the session itself or Stop, Rewind, Explore the content of the narrative, asking for more detail. The minds of both patient and clinician need to stop and/or rewind together to understand the process in the session better or, alternatively, to identify important elements of the events at hand. The purpose of both strategies is to reinstate mentalizing when it has been lost or to promote its continuation in the furtherance of the overall goal of therapy, which is (to re-reiterate) to encourage the formation of a robust and flexible mentalizing capacity that is not prone to sudden collapse in the face of emotional stress. As a session moves forward it is sometimes necessary either to pause, to consider, and to explore the moment, or to move back to retrace the process or re-examine the content.

Exploration: Stop, Listen, Look

As an individual or group session unfolds, the clinician needs to listen constantly for nonmentalizing processes and interactions. Indicators of poor mentalizing such as failure to respond to feelings expressed by others, dismissive attitudes, trite explanations, or lack of continuity of dialogue suggest that the clinician needs to Stop, Listen, Look (see Box 6.7). To do so, he/she holds the group or individual session in a suspended state while investigating the detail of what is happening by highlighting who feels what about whom, and what each member of the group understands about what is happening from their own perspective (see Box 6.8).

On the one hand, the clinician has to be active about this exploration of the current state of the group or individual session, but on the other hand, he/she must also listen to the responses carefully to piece together the complexity of the interactions and make sense of the affective process that is interfering with each person's capacity to think about themselves in relation to the others. Once the group has worked around the "stop" point it can move on.

It is only when mentalizing is seriously disrupted that a "Stop, Rewind, Explore" takes place.

Box 6.7 Process of exploration (1)

During a typical nonmentalizing interaction in a group or individual session:

- ◆ Stop and investigate
- ◆ Let the interaction slowly unfold—control it
- ◆ Highlight who feels what
- ◆ Identify how each aspect is understood from multiple perspectives
- ◆ Challenge reactive "fillers"
- ◆ Identify how messages feel and are understood, and what reactions occur.

Box 6.8 Process of exploration (2)

If the patient is NOT in psychic equivalence:

- • What do you think it feels like for X?
- • Can you explain why he did that?
- • Can you think of other ways you might be able to help her really understand what you feel like?
- • How do you explain her distress/overdose?
- ◆ If someone else was in that position, what would you tell them to do?

Stop, Rewind, Explore

Stop, Rewind, Explore is indicated when either the patient, the clinician, or the group has lost mentalizing. The clinician has to stop the group or individual session and insist that the session rewinds back to a point at which constructive interaction was taking place or he/she was able to think clearly and was maintaining his/her mentalizing stance. The clinician has to take control, rewind, and, with a steady resolve, explore while moving forward "frame by frame," diverting the path that led to the loss of mentalizing. To do this he/she must retrace the steps that led to the point of loss of mentalizing by reverting to the point at which the patient or patients were able to think about themselves and others constructively, albeit with some difficulty (see Box 6.9).

Stop, Rewind, Explore should be implemented as soon as the clinician thinks the group or individual session has become uncontrolled and/or is in danger of

---

Box 6.9 Process of rewind

Draw attention to disjunction in topic/dialogue/tone:

- ◆ Let's go back to see what happened just then.
- ◆ At first you seemed to understand what was going on, but then . . .
- ◆ Let's try to trace exactly how that came about.
- ◆ Hang on, before we move off, let's just rewind and see if we can understand something in all this.
- ◆ Oh, I thought we were talking about your child, and now you are suddenly on to the gearbox in your car? What happened there to make such a jump?

---

rapid self-destruction, for example, patients walking out or engaging in inappropriately aggressive discourse.

The suicidal patient

A patient talked in a group about how suicidal she felt and about her plans to take an overdose. The group, with the help of the clinician, worked hard with her to understand what had precipitated her negative and destructive state of mind in which she felt no one cared if she lived or died and she did not feel that she had anyone or anything to live for. Many attempts to help from other members of the group were rebuffed, and it was apparent that the frustration of the group was building up. Before the clinician could control this and highlight the underlying frustration, the following interaction took place:

PATIENT   [to the suicidal patient]: I am fed up with all this. Whatever we say it is no good. Why don't you put everyone out of your misery and just do it?

[Immediate silence in the group.]

CLINICIAN: That is a serious thing to say [stop] and I suspect that while you mean it at this moment it has come out of somewhere which we will all regret and so we had better go back [rewind] to see how we have reached this point in which one of us doesn't care if someone else lives or dies [explore].

PATIENT: So it will all be my fault I suppose now when she takes an overdose.

CLINICIAN: No [stand]. We are going to go back to see what has happened that has led you to be so frustrated that you don't care if she takes one or

> not [stop]. Actually, I don't think that it is like you, and so perhaps
> we can start with going back to the point at which you began to feel
> frustrated [rewind]. When did you first feel like that? [Explore.]

When implementing a "stop" the clinician may initially use exploratory probes in an attempt to help the patient reflect—"What happened there? We seem to have gone off topic."

In conclusion, the clinician stance is inquisitive, active, empathic, and at times challenging, but most importantly the clinician should refrain from becoming an expert who "knows." His/her mind is focused on the mind of the patient and he/she is intrigued, curious, questioning, and not-knowing. The clinician's primary aim is to stimulate a robust mentalizing process and to do so he/she needs to manage the process of sessions carefully. Sessions need to be focused and well paced, and this is the responsibility of the clinician. At times it is useful to effect closure of a session through a summary of the session, working with the patient to ensure that the summary reflects both the patient's and the clinician's perspectives. Many patients request a copy of each note made in their electronic record. The summary is a good way to ensure that this is accurate and meaningful.

References

Allen, J. G., Fonagy, P., & Bateman, A. (2008). *Mentalizing in clinical practice.* Washington, DC: American Psychiatric Press Inc.

Aveline, M. (2005). The person of the therapist. *Psychotherapy Research*, **15**, 155–164.

Lynch, T. R., Rosenthal, M. Z., Kosson, D. S., Cheavens, J. S., Lejuez, C. W., & Blair, R. J. (2006). Heightened sensitivity to facial expressions of emotion in borderline personality disorder. *Emotion*, **6**, 647–655.

Meares, R. (2000). *Intimacy and alienation: Memory, trauma and personal being.* London, UK: Routledge.

Meares, R., & Hobson, R. F. (1977). The persecutory therapist. *British Journal of Medical Psychology*, **50**, 349–359.

Ryle, A. (2004). The contribution of cognitive analytic therapy to the treatment of borderline personality disorder. *Journal of Personality Disorders*, **18**, 3–35.

Chapter 7

Principles for the mentalizing clinician

Introduction

In this chapter we discuss some general characteristics of interventions designed to promote mentalizing and some clinical principles to follow when deciding which intervention to give when. As we shall see, being an effective clinician is not simply a matter of giving the right intervention. It is only too easy for clinicians to make technically correct interventions in therapy, but to use them at the wrong moments and without compassion and humanity—that is, adherence to the model without competence—rendering therapy shallow and functional. In an attempt to overcome this problem we provide some guiding principles (see Box 7.1).

There will be many times when the principles are, and should be, broken; being intuitive is an important part of therapy. Here, we can only offer advice that we hope experienced clinicians will not find patronizing and condescending. Our training program is aimed at generic mental health professionals who gallantly implement our treatment without having had extensive therapy training but having had good general experience of risk management, emergency assessment, and crisis intervention. Paradoxically, this initial therapeutic naivety of practitioners might be an important part of successful treatment, enabling them to follow basic principles without too much deviation. Experienced clinicians have, often necessarily, come to believe in their therapy, their methods, and their techniques, and may be in danger of becoming inflexible. Enthusiasts who are setting out on their therapeutic journey and have fewer preconceived ideas and hobby-horses to ride may stand a better chance of taking a mentalizing or "not-knowing" stance (see Chapter 6). But enough said before we are accused of forming straw men, stereotypes, and archetypes, all of which are examples of nonmentalizing phenomena!

Maintain or regain clinician mentalizing

The initial principle to follow is to maintain your own mentalizing, and if it is lost your first task is to regain it—"maintain or regain." Treatment is impossible if the clinician is not able to think or to reflect. The easiest way to maintain and regain is to halt the session by saying something like "Can we hold on for a minute?

Box 7.1 Guiding principles

- Maintain or regain mentalizing of clinician
- Monitor patient's mentalizing capacity
- Manage arousal levels
- Focus on patient's mind
- Address current events and immediate states of mind
- Stepwise intervention process starting with empathic validation.

I cannot quite follow what we are talking about." This helps the clinician to re-orient his/her mind; it is easier to get back on track from a stationary position. In addition, rather than flailing around in the dark or rushing headlong into danger, having managed to halt the flow of nonmentalizing dialogue, the clinician returns to a point at which they felt they could think and could follow what the patient was saying. In other words, whenever the clinician is in considerable doubt and uncertainty, he/she should stop digging a hole, return to the basic principles, and couple this with a "Stop, Rewind (to a point at which the dialogue was understandable) and Explore" (see Chapter 6) before moving forward again.

Clinicians inadvertently lose mentalizing frequently, for example, arguing with patients, trying to persuade them of a different point of view, presenting their own perspective as the correct one, telling the patient how he/she feels, or joining in with a reciprocal role. Remember that nonmentalizing begets nonmentalizing and clinicians can easily hold thoughts in psychic equivalence or begin to believe their own story in pretend mode. The key issue in this situation is for the clinician to be monitoring him/herself carefully and, to some extent, openly. If the ability of the clinician to think clearly is compromised, this is stated, as long as he/she simultaneously engages in a process to regain mental clarity; if the clinician feels unable to identify how he/she feels, he/she must begin a process of elaborating the difficulty in treatment with the patient, as long as it is in the service of moving forward constructively to address the patient's target problems better.

Identify and consider patient mentalizing capacity

The MBT clinician listens for nonmentalizing modes and mentalizing dimension imbalance. Is the patient currently working mentally in psychic equivalence, pretend mode, or understanding him/herself and others through teleological process? Is the mental processing a mix of these? The reason for monitoring and identifying the nonmentalizing modes throughout a session is that the clinician should avoid inadvertently creating situations where the patient is forced into talking about mental states that they cannot immediately link to subjectively felt reality. A number of simple but hard-to-observe implications follow from this general principle. First, a focus far removed from the patient's conscious awareness creates an opportunity for pseudomentalizing. It is far less risky to stick to conscious or near-conscious content available in working memory than it is to aim to reveal unconscious meaning. The clinician's aim is enhancing mentalizing rather than engendering insight. The former is in many ways commensurate with the latter. It has been argued that therapeutic progress in all therapies is based on achieving representational coherence and integration. Our point here is that while this is arguably best achieved by enhancing insight in less severely disturbed patients, at the more severely impaired end of the spectrum of interpersonal functioning a challenge to the patient of a complex mentalizing account of what is going on, somewhat removed from what is consciously accessible to the patient, can inadvertently generate disintegration and incoherence of the representational world. This is a simple point, but an all-important one. If a person is struggling with maintaining a grip over the massive distortions of their subjective experience, an expert who describes complex mental states of conflict, ambivalence, or nonconscious motives is more likely to generate turmoil than bring about integration. Probably similar turmoil is created in patients with less severe disturbance too, when the complexity of their mental functioning is brought to the foreground of consciousness by the clinician's intervention. In this context, however, against a background of competence in dealing with subjective experience, such turmoil can be the catalyst for reorganization. The higher-functioning patient tolerates the confusion to understand better their internal state. In contrast, in borderline patients sensitized to the possibility of confusion, it undermines rather than enhances a fledgling capacity for finding real meaning behind behavior.

Thus, the clinician is less concerned with the use of metaphor, analogies, puns, and symbolism extracted from the content, and more focused on developing an increasingly robust mentalizing process. Metaphors, analogies, puns, and symbolism require a high level of mentalizing and are likely to be beneficial in furthering understanding only at those moments when the person with BPD is able to balance internal emotional states with inner reflection. At other times such interventions will be met with either incomprehension, envious admiration, dismissal, or development of pretend mode (see Chapter 1).

The clever clinician

A patient complained that her housing association had done nothing about the leak in the roof of her flat. She had reported it a number of times but workmen had still not visited to repair the roof. She believed that her flat would flood if it rained too hard and this would ruin her furniture.

CLINICIAN: Perhaps you feel that I am doing nothing to repair the leak that has opened up in your mind and if I don't do something quickly your feelings will get out of control and ruin everything.

PATIENT: They should come round and repair it. I got angry with them again and soon I will go around and "start" on them if they don't come.

CLINICIAN: So then your feelings really are going to leak badly at that point.

PATIENT: What are you talking about? Stop going on about my feelings, will you. You would be frustrated if people didn't turn up to repair things, wouldn't you? So stop making out that what I am feeling is a problem. It is only a problem because they haven't done what they are supposed to do.

The session continued in this way until the clinician stopped trying to link the practical problem to what was happening in the therapy. It is not so much that the clinician is wrong here but that the timing is off-beat and the patient cannot increase her self-reflection when trapped in her mind about a very practical issue. Her current mental reality is fixed within teleological mode at this point, and so drawing analogous links is relatively meaningless to her.

Similar errors may occur when clinicians ask a patient to consider other people's motives. This is a superficially tempting intervention, and indeed it might stimulate mentalizing about others' motives. But, as we have discussed in earlier chapters and reiterate here, it becomes ineffective when a patient is not mentalizing, for example, when they are holding thoughts in psychic equivalence, and serves only to trigger confusion in this context (see the clinical example of the probation officer in Chapter 6, in the section on "Contrary moves"). If psychic equivalence is firmly rooted, the patient does not, at that moment, have the capacity to consider others' mental states and motives. Asking a question such as "What made your boyfriend say that?" or "Why do you think he did that?" is likely to either elicit a robust response of "I don't know, why don't you ask him?", "He is a shit," or stimulate pretend mode, in which you and the patient elaborate a fantasy about the boyfriend's motive. The patient cannot easily differentiate self from other when in nonmentalizing modes and so cannot consider the other person's state of mind as separate from their own. So, this commonly used MBT intervention of actively exploring self-understanding of others and contrasting mental states comes with a caution—it is recommended primarily when the patient shows some mentalizing capacities. When beliefs are held in psychic equivalence, the clinician is better off empathizing with the patient rather than immediately trying to challenge the patient's belief. Tables 7.1, 7.2, and 7.3 summarize some of the core clinical responses to psychic equivalence, pretend mode, and teleological process.

Table 7.1 Modes of nonmentalizing: psychic equivalence

Clinical form	Certainty/suspension of doubt Absolute Reality is defined by self-experience Finality—"It just is" Internal = external
Therapist experience	Puzzled Wish to refute Statement appears logical but obviously overgeneralized Not sure what to say Angry or fed up and hopeless
Intervention	Empathic validation with subjective experience Curious—"How did you reach that conclusion?" Presentation of clinician puzzlement (marked) Linked topic (diversion) to trigger mentalizing then return to psychic equivalent area
Iatrogenic	Argue with patient Excessive focus on content Cognitive challenge

Table 7.2 Modes of nonmentalizing: pretend mode

Clinical form	Inconsequential talk/groundless inferences about mental states Lack of affect. Absence of pleasure Circularity without conclusion—"spinning in sand" (hypermentalizing) No change Dissociation—self-harm to avoid meaninglessness Body and mind decoupled
Therapist experience	Boredom Detachment Patient agrees with your concepts and ideas Identification with your model Feels progress is made in therapy
Intervention	Probe extent Counterintuitive Challenge
Iatrogenic	Nonrecognition Joining in with acceptance as real Insight-oriented/skill acquisition intervention

Table 7.3 Modes of nonmentalizing: teleological mode

Clinical form	Expectation of things being "done" Outcomes in physical world determine understanding of inner state—"I took an overdose; I must have been suicidal" Motives of others are based on what actually happens Only actions can change mental process "What you do and not what you say"
Therapist experience	Uncertainty and anxiety Wish to do something—medication review, letter, telephone call, extend session
Intervention	Empathic validation of need Do or don't do according to exploration of need Affect focus of dilemma of doing
Iatrogenic	Excessive "doing" Prove you care in the belief it will induce positive change Elasticity (extending what you do, e.g., extra sessions, only to rebound with extra constraints) rather than flexibility

Meeting nonmentalizing in the patient with mentalizing in the clinician

In Chapter 4, in the section on enactment, we gave a clinical example illustrating the problem of meeting nonmentalizing in the patient with a mentalizing response from the clinician. Clearly, as outlined earlier, MBT requires the clinician to maintain his/her mentalizing as best as possible throughout a session. However, there is often the temptation for the clinician to seek appropriate solutions and to act "for" the patient, using his/her own mentalizing, and this is especially acute when the patient is in the teleological mode. The clinician is able to work out an appropriate solution or suggest a constructive response to the patient's problems and gives it to the patient. While the patient is likely to—rightly—feel grateful, no mentalizing in the patient has been stimulated by this action. This process of meeting the patient's nonmentalizing with a mentalized response from the clinician takes more subtle forms—a patient who cannot name feelings is given the name for the feeling; a patient who cannot express something clearly is told what they are saying; the clinician's understanding of projective systems is used to identify emotion. In all cases, the clinician's mentalizing takes over mentalizing for the patient. Overall, we ask that clinicians are aware of this and are cautious when they find themselves engaged in this process, for the simple reason that the patient's actual need remains unaddressed.

Management of arousal

The MBT clinician monitors the level of patient arousal throughout every session.

Absence of arousal prevents the development of attachment-based affect, which is the area of sensitivity in interpersonal interactions for people with BPD. Treatment becomes cognitively organized and the patient is detached from relational process. Pretend mode is often associated with absence of affect and may become persistent. Working on areas of interpersonal sensitivity that lead to loss of mentalizing becomes impossible because interpersonal meaning is absent. The avoidant strategies used by the patient may need to be challenged if some anxiety is to be stimulated.

Excessive arousal undermines mentalizing to the extent that no constructive work can be done. The clinician needs to reduce arousal to create circumstances in which mentalizing can flourish. Only then can therapeutic work begin.

It is the clinician's job to ensure that arousal is maintained within a range that is neither too low nor too high. As the patient's arousal increases, the clinician rebalances the interaction if necessary with cognitive process; as the arousal decreases excessively, the clinician rebalances with injection of affect. As a principle, any increase in arousal in the patient during a session has been created by the clinician until proven otherwise. The clinician takes responsibility for the affect change, asking him/herself and the patient what he/she may have done to create the distress and dysregulation apparent in the session. Table 7.4 gives a summary of MBT techniques to manage arousal.

Initially, de-escalating techniques may be necessary to reduce arousal. All clinicians working with people with BPD need to be conversant with interventions that are likely to reduce high arousal.

Table 7.4 Balancing in-session arousal

	High arousal	**Low arousal**
Dimension	Affective → cognitive	Cognitive → affective
Focus	Redirect	Emphasize
Patient experience	Validate	Challenge
Responsibility	Clinician accepts	Patient explores
Process	Go with the flow	Resist/challenge
Interpersonal interaction	Decrease	Increase

General characteristics of interventions

Interventions need to be within the mentalizing capacities of the patient and are therefore likely to be straightforward, short, and simple rather than long and complex (see Box 7.2). In addition, interventions promoting mentalizing show a number of other general characteristics: they are affect focused rather than concerned with behavior; they target the patient's subjective state of mind in addition to specific aspects of mental activity such as cognition; they relate to present events or current interpersonal interactions, that is, they are in proximal reality rather than distal reality and more often in current mental reality; they emphasize near-conscious or conscious content, that is, working memory rather than unconscious concerns; and they are concerned with maintaining process rather than interpreting content.

Straightforward and short

Keeping things straightforward and short is easier said than done but is necessary in the service of the key principle of ensuring that your interventions are in keeping with the patient's mentalizing capacity. The longer and more complex interventions become, the less likely they are to be within the patient's mentalizing ability, particularly if he/she is emotionally aroused at the time. The greater the use of "psychobabble" and jargon, the more likely it is that pretend mode will be stimulated. It is best to use an ordinary conversational style and everyday language.

The mentalizing capacity of patients with BPD fluctuates according to the level of stimulation of the attachment system. Thus, at one moment a patient may be able to understand and react to a complex intervention and yet at another he/she may be unable to comprehend or even listen to something straightforward. The more the clinician stimulates the emotional state of the

---

Box 7.2 General characteristics of interventions

- In keeping with patient's mentalizing capacity
- Affect focused (love, desire, hurt, catastrophe, excitement)
- Explicitly interpersonal and affective
- Relate to current event or activity—mental reality (evidence-based or in working memory)
- De-emphasize unconscious concerns in favor of near-conscious or conscious content.

patient and increases the arousal of the attachment system, the more fragile the patient's mentalizing capacity becomes, and so the clinician must tread more carefully in his/her interventions.

In the example given earlier, the patient is emotionally frustrated about the lack of response from the housing association and its failure to effect repairs to her flat. A straightforward intervention targeting the patient's emotional state would have been more appropriate, increased the therapeutic alliance, and allowed the patient to explore her current state and how this interfered with finding an effective way to manage the problem:

The clever clinician (continued)
A patient complained that her housing association had done nothing about the leak in the roof of her flat. She had reported it a number of times but workmen had still not visited to repair the roof. She believed that her flat would flood if it rained too hard and this would ruin her furniture.

CLINICIAN: Awful. That is frustrating for anyone [normalizing to some extent].
PATIENT: They should come round and repair it. I got angry with them again and soon I will go around and "start" on them if they don't come [indicator of feelings potentially getting out of control].
CLINICIAN: It can feel like that, can't it. How are you managing that feeling? [Tentative exploration of emotion and impulsivity.]

These interventions are experience near and very straightforward. The aim is to encourage the patient to focus on her mind state, to balance the emotion with consideration of a solution, and to help her reflect on herself without collapsing into her frustration.

Affect focused—"the elephant in the room"

All therapies for BPD are concerned with emotional states. Working with affect is discussed in more detail in Chapter 9. In MBT, the focus on affect has two components. The first component is helping the patient understand and label feelings associated with events and exploring any consequential feelings. This is a focus on affect. The reasons for actively identifying emotions and labeling them in this way are introduced through the psychoeducational session on emotions in MBT-I (see Chapter 11). The patient may feel angry in the context of an argument (the feeling associated with an event) and this results in feelings of shame or being unlovable (the consequential feeling). This exploration and labeling of affect often takes the form of discussing past events in the present sessions, and to this extent it is "there and then." But it can take place within the context of the patient's current state in the session—the "here and now"—because they still have the feeling associated with the events. In general terms, the exploration of affect around a past event is experience far, while that of current states is experience near.

The clinician needs to be sensitive to the ever-present danger that the patient will begin describing events and in doing so will re-experience the emotions associated with the events. This is likely to stimulate psychic equivalent feeling, which is to be avoided; to do so, the clinician needs to balance the affect with a more cognitive exploration of the events until the patient calms. This dialectic of balancing the dimensions of mentalizing using contrary moves is discussed in Chapter 6. Conversely, the discussion and labeling of affect can become an intellectual exercise with little meaning, raising the danger of inducing pretend mode. To avoid this, the clinician needs to balance distant affect with closer scrutiny of current affect states. This requires him/her to consider the second aspect of the affect focus.

The second component of the emphasis on affect is identifying the emotional interaction between the patient and the clinician. This is the *affect focus* or, better, the *interpersonal affect focus*. It overlaps with the "interpersonal affective focus" described in brief dynamic interpersonal therapy (Lemma, Target, & Fonagy, 2011) but differs to some extent in that it focuses more on the current interpersonal dynamic in the treatment session. We discuss this in more detail in Chapter 9, but in essence it means grasping the affect shared between the clinician and the patient in the moment, not so much in its relation to the content of the session or a past event but primarily as it relates to what is currently happening between them. This has become known as "the elephant in the room" because it makes something that is implicit within the session explicit. In effect this is a further dialectic of balancing implicit mentalizing with explicit mentalizing. A brief intervention identifying the current but unnamed feeling between patient and clinician is likely to propel a session forward within the interpersonal interaction more effectively than focusing on the detail of the content of a narrative.

> A patient had had her three children temporarily taken into care shortly before she started treatment. Once she was in treatment, there had been requests from the child protection services for reports about her ability to parent the children. In MBT, any report is always discussed in detail with the patient and agreed both in content and in opinion. Nevertheless, the patient constantly reassured the clinician that her visits to her children were going well. It seemed to the clinician that the patient may naturally be reluctant to talk openly about her feelings and what happened at visits because of the clinician's role in the child protection proceedings. Yet she was concerned to assess how the patient was managing with her children when she visited them and to explore her feelings about them. From the patient's perspective, she was concerned to make sure that she was seen to be managing. So the clinician identified the tension between them as part of the ongoing affect focus—"I listen carefully to how you are managing with the

children and I thought that you might be concerned to make sure that I appreciate how well you are doing. But in doing so I suppose that there is a tension about whether we can talk safely about any worries about how you parent them and whether you feel that you can talk to me openly."

Here the clinician is trying to identify an affectively infused relational factor that is interfering with treatment. This is done though explicit identification of the "elephant in the room."

Focus on the patient's mind, not on behavior

In working with challenging patients who have the propensity to act rather than think, to behave rather than feel, the temptation is always to engage with them at the level at which they are expressing themselves. This means, first of all, that the clinician is always tempted to respond to action with action. The patient challenges the clinician's mental equilibrium through acts of self-harm or aggression; the clinician feels compelled to "do" something and reacts by insisting on hospital admission without adequate assessment of risk or by asking the emergency psychiatrist to undertake a medication review. Alternatively, the patient is irritable and uncommunicative in a session; the clinician reacts to this behavior by providing excessively complex explanations, over-talking, or pressing the patient to respond.

The withdrawn patient

A patient attended her session wearing a baseball cap pulled down over her face. She sat with a downward gaze, unable to make eye contact with the clinician, exposing bandages on her arms. Initially, the clinician asked the patient if she wanted to talk about "what was going on." But her enquiries elicited no response. Gradually the clinician realized that she was becoming increasingly reactive to the patient's withdrawal, communicated through body language and silence, by not only asking more and more questions but also leaning forward in her chair, trying to force the patient to talk. Yet all she elicited was a grunt. The clinician eventually showed some frustration—"Is there any point in me keeping asking you questions?"

We must remember that talking is action and a verbal response may be a behavioral reaction to the patient's apparent retreat. A clinician's excessive verbalization following a piece of challenging behavior from the patient may be experienced by the patient as "punishment," in part because it is, whatever the motive of the clinician. The clinician ends up trying to force the patient to do something she cannot do—in this case, talk about herself. So what can the clinician do in these circumstances?

1 First, focus on the patient's state of mind—be empathic about her difficulty in expressing what is happening in her mind.

2 Establish the affect focus—identify the current interactive process.

As we mentioned at the beginning of this chapter, the principle to follow is that the clinician needs to go back to the point at which she was mentalizing. This was at the beginning of the session. From there she can focus on the patient's mind state, initially by empathizing with the predicament of being in the session and not being able to say anything.

Instead of this straightforward maneuver, the clinician reacted by attempting to force the patient to talk about her silent presentation and explore the meaning behind her presentation. While this appears to be focusing on the mind, it is in fact well outside the probable mentalizing capacity of the patient and is tantamount to guessing. Had the clinician been mentalizing herself, she would have realized that the patient is incapable of giving a reason for how she is at this moment. Coercing the patient to talk about her withdrawal is a nonmentalizing and unnecessarily confrontational, shaming, and undermining act that at best is likely to induce pseudomentalizing but is more likely to reinforce withdrawal.

The clinician initially needs to be able to set aside the behavior and its effect on her, not in the sense of pretending it is not happening but in the sense of playing Sherlock Holmes in relation to it, and get on with her task of focusing on the patient's mind. A starting point following the empathic statement may be asking about the impact that the behavior has on the patient herself.

CLINICIAN: Can you describe to me what it is like not being able to say anything or look at me? I don't want to make you feel uncomfortable.

PATIENT: [Grunts.]

The next step is to define an affect focus if it has become impossible to help the patient elaborate her current state of mind. This is essential if the clinician has been drawn into an overactive response.

CLINICIAN [after a silence]: I am not sure whether it helps for me to keep asking questions or if that makes you feel uncomfortable. It makes me uncertain about whether I should push you further or perhaps leave you alone [beginning of an affect focus to make the current interactive problem more explicit. A full affect focus would try to add the patient's component in this dynamic, affective interaction].

The attempt by the clinician to establish an affect focus is to create a shared platform from which she and the patient can develop the session. The clinician uses the current behavior as an indicator that feelings or thoughts must have arisen in, or at least are now being played out within, a relational context that creates a high level of arousal, intensifies the activation of the attachment system, or reinforces a tendency toward phobic avoidance and causes a general collapse of mentalizing. The clinician thus focuses the patient's mind, as she struggles with mental experiences within an interpersonal context, on some of the sensitivities that lie behind the withdrawal.

Overall, focusing on the mind rather than behaviors requires the clinician to distinguish between descriptive narrative and mental states by asking questions such as "What were you feeling at that point?" or "What was that experience like?" rather than asking "What did you do?", and "What are you feeling now?" rather than "What do you think you should do?" This is a false dichotomy of course, but the emphasis of the dialogue should be on the affect and not the behavior, even when exploring suicidal and self-destructive behavior.

Relate to current event or activity

The contemporary trend within psychotherapies is to focus on current external events or internal states. Schema-focused therapy and cognitive behavioral interventions define thoughts and schemas from the past that are operating in the present; transference-focused therapy uses "here and now" rather than "there and then" interpretive work; and behavioral treatments emphasize diary cards about immediate events. Reaching into the past, working with memories of childhood experience, forging causal links between current behavior and past events and the subjective experiences these *might have generated* is less apparent than a decade ago. MBT has never been focused in the past or been insight oriented, although it is respectful of past experience and how it affects the present. It is our view that explaining a person's current wish to please in terms of a continuing wish to satisfy a demanding image of a parent is a descriptor masquerading as an explanation. Furthermore, it potentially has the harmful side effect of stimulating pretend mode while avoiding the current interpersonal problem of the patient's overarching desire to please the clinician (for whatever reason). It sabotages more genuine interaction. Reaching into the past can be more comfortable for both patient and clinician but is far less real, thus encouraging pseudomentalizing between patient and clinician about what the patient might or might not have felt as a child or what the motive of his/her parents might or might not have been all those years ago.

The best way of circumventing this potential difficulty is by selectively focusing on recent experiences in the patient's world or on the immediacy of the situation in the room. The latter is not quite the same as the psychoanalytic focus often characterized ironically as "you mean me" interpretations. That kind of work also leads to pseudomentalizing in patients with BPD. The general principle is to focus on emotionally salient but perhaps apparently trivial events around which the thoughts and feelings of the protagonists may be productively elaborated. The task of the clinician is to wrap mentalizing around the events.

In general, the clinician aims to work with whatever is current in the patient's mind, in other words, in working memory. It is important that the experience should have mental reality for the patient, that it should feel like a real experience when talked about. At times, experiences from long ago can have this level of emotional saliency. The clinician must be careful, however, that the mental reality associated with past experience has "real depth" rather than being a stereotypic repetitive reproduction, a kind of mantra where it is the experience of recall that is real rather than the reality of the experience.

Clinical pathway for interventions

There are four main principles to follow in MBT when considering the clinical process and interventions (see Box 7.3).

1 In Chapter 6, we discussed the movement of the mentalizing process along a pathway from narrative to alternative perspective (see Figure 6.1). The overall aim in moving along the pathway is to stimulate a natural therapeutic process, with the emphasis being less on content and more on process as both clinician and patient move flexibly around the anchor points, identified in Box 7.3. The schematic stepwise movement is a principle and not a rule, and there will be many times when it is necessary to skip a step.

2 Intertwined with this gradual shift of focus in a session are interventions that help stimulate or maintain mentalizing. These are organized according to their propensity to trigger interpersonal anxiety, with the least stimulating being empathic validation. Following the pathway will move the patient from the least intensely felt introspection to the most intense if the clinician remains focused on affects and the interpersonal domain. For this reason, the clinician most often starts at the empathic validation end of the intervention spectrum. Only once the patient and clinician experience a shared affective platform developed through empathic validation can the clinician

Box 7.3 Clinical process

* Narrative to alternative perspective
* Intervention spectrum from "surface" to "depth"
* Intervention choice determined by arousal level
* External events to current treatment process to patient–clinician interaction.

move to exploration. Clearly, there are exceptions to this generalization, and at times focusing on the emotional interaction between patient and clinician, most commonly the most concentrated emotional area, may be rendered cold and intellectual and represent a move away from the "heat" of an external or treatment context—an example of adherence to treatment without competence.

3 The clinician's assessment of the patient's level of arousal, and to some extent the mode of nonmentalizing, determines where to start on the intervention spectrum. If the patient has high arousal, the clinician is recommended to start at the empathic position. If the patient shows low arousal, it may be more appropriate to focus more on the affective processes and the therapy relationship to see whether this will shift the downregulated state.

4 Finally, there is a fourth principle to follow to ensure safe delivery of treatment without overstimulating attachment processes. In any given session, the patient is encouraged initially to talk about outside events. Important aspects of this narrative, once mentalized, can be linked carefully to treatment itself, and then to the patient–clinician relationship. There is then a movement from a focus on external events to processes in treatment and vice versa, with each bringing an understanding of the other.

Appraisal of outside interpersonal interactions is immediately meaningful to patients with BPD and, when discussed "after the event," is less likely to induce the powerful emotions evoked at the time of the interaction. So, making time for retrospective reflection allows the patient and clinician to "strike while the iron is cold" or better still "while it is cooling down"—mentalizing interpersonal events without too much danger of mental collapse or loss of attention. Similar work can be done within, for example, an individual therapy session about a patient's interactions within an earlier group session, reflecting on what *was* rather than what *is*. While this is no substitute for a patient addressing their feelings in the heat of the moment, in our experience the ability to reflect and to act constructively while emotionally aroused gradually develops only as the person is able to consider their own and others' states of mind retrospectively. We all reflect with greater honesty with hindsight than we do within the hurly-burly of an emotional interaction itself. But, in the end, our lives are led and possibly determined within the subjective immediacy of interactions; patients with BPD need to learn to use these moments constructively.

We are not recommending downgrading therapeutic work within the immediacy of the patient–clinician relationship; in fact, quite the opposite. However, it is important to move toward working in this way with sensitivity, without overwhelming the patient with emotional states that they cannot understand or address. Moving too quickly and without adequate preparation will stimulate a gradual failure in mentalizing, which if uncontrolled may lead to a crisis in the session and become iatrogenic, provoking the very behaviors you seek to address.

Which intervention when?

Here we discuss further the rationale to follow to help in deciding which interventions to use at any given moment, following the four principles identified earlier. We have arranged the spectrum of interventions in order of complexity, depth, and interpersonal emotional intensity, with empathy and support being the simplest, the most superficial, and the least intensive, and mentalizing the relationship/transference being the most complex and, for the most part, the most emotionally intensive (see Box 7.4). Commonly, the decision about which intervention to use when will be taken outside consciousness, and be all the better for it, but we believe that there are some general principles to follow. These are summarized in Box 7.5.

The basis for our recommendations is simply that, in general, mentalizing capacity in patients with BPD is inversely related to stimulation of the attachment system. As the attachment system is activated, so the capacity to mentalize is inhibited, emotions become bewildering, the self fractures, and actions to restore precarious safety and a sense of self become inevitable. Remember that the attachment system is stimulated by fear of any kind. A patient could have a frightening thought, which triggers the attachment system, so he/she is motivated to seek proximity to someone for safety. This process causes the well-described volatile pattern of relationships of intimacy and distance found in patients with BPD who try to maintain their mind when it becomes overwhelmed. It results in the appearance of characteristic schemas that can stabilize confusion, for example, experiencing oneself as the victim of a victimizer. It is senseless to reproduce this pattern of wildly fluctuating affects or fixed

---

Box 7.4 Spectrum of interventions

- Empathic validation—including reassurance, support, and empathy
- Basic mentalizing—clarification, exploration, and challenge
- Basic mentalizing—affect identification and affect focus
- Mentalizing the relationship.

Box 7.5 Which intervention to use when?

- If in doubt, start at the surface—empathic validation
- Move to "deeper" levels only after you have performed earlier steps
- If emotions are in danger of becoming overwhelming, take a step toward the surface
- Type of intervention is inversely related to emotional intensity: empathic validation when the patient is overwhelmed with emotion; mentalizing relationship when the patient can continue mentalizing while "holding" the emotion
- Intervention must be in keeping with the patient's mentalizing capacity. There is danger in assuming that people with BPD have a greater capacity to mentalize than they actually have when they are struggling with feelings.

schemas in an uncontrolled manner early in therapy by overstimulating the patient, focusing on complex mental states, and provoking intense emotions. Balancing stimulation of the attachment system with capacity to mentalize places the clinician in the delicate position of having to mobilize affect while controlling its flow and intensity. Without emotion there can be no meaningful subjective experience, but with excess emotion there can be no understanding of the subjective experience.

As we have argued before, one of the gravest dangers for clinicians treating borderline patients is iatrogenic harm by using well-meaning but mistimed and misguided interventions that diminish rather than increase mentalizing capacity through excessive activation of the attachment system. Therefore, the overarching principle to be followed when selecting interventions is to minimize iatrogenic effects by balancing emotional intensity with the patient's continuing capacity to subjectively monitor his/her own mind and that of another.

At the surface level, sensitively given support and empathy are unlikely to provoke complex mental states in borderline patients who, feeling that someone else is showing interest and is attempting to understand their emotional state from their point of view, will feel safe enough to explain their feelings and give their perspective about what has happened or is happening to them. The patient's mind is not threatened. Hence, these types of interventions, along with motivational interviewing, problem-solving, psychoeducation, and other behavioral techniques, are useful early in therapy and indeed at the beginning of a session. So, when a patient's emotions are high, it is best to be empathic rather than to ask them to do complex psychological work. On the other hand, when a patient is stuck at the affective pole of mentalizing, rebalancing is also necessary. Becoming increasingly sympathetic will potentially make the patient worse by stimulating his/her attachment processes more and increasing regression. Consequently, the clinician is empathic, seeing the patient's experience, but rebalances by working cognitively on the effect the emotion has on the patient.

At the intermediate level of intervention, clarification, exploration, and challenge create more difficulty because they force self-scrutiny and imply that another mind might have a different perspective, which has to be considered and integrated. If the intervention incorporates interpersonal content and current affect rather than being intellectual, it forms part of basic mentalizing because the relational world is invoked, which heightens the emotional intensity. If the intervention is then linked to "you and me" and underlying motivations are brought into play, the danger of overwhelming the patient's mentalizing capacity increases considerably, as does that of inducing action: for example, the patient walks out of a session or cuts him/herself to restore his/her mind. This cascade of psychological disaster can be avoided if clinicians move slowly down the levels of intervention, only reaching the greatest depth having worked on the surface levels first. You should move down a level only when you judge that the patient's degree of anxiety, and therefore mentalizing capacity, allows them to consider your perspective further, or they are willing to elaborate more about themselves. If in doubt, your interventions should be tentative at first; inject more pressure into the dialogue only when the therapeutic relationship is robust.

It is not our intention to suggest that clinicians must adhere rigidly to the principles outlined here. But if clinicians follow our clinical pathway and sensibly implement our recommendations about the timing of interventions, we believe they will be less at risk of causing harm and will have the greatest chance of stimulating a positive therapeutic relationship within which mentalizing can flourish.

Basic principles—a clinical example

We are commonly asked how to deal with many of the critical issues that beset borderline patients and their clinicians. It is impossible to outline how to manage every situation, and so we urge clinicians to follow the basic principles that we have set out in this chapter. The most difficult behaviors for clinicians to face are suicide attempts and self-harm. Here we outline the principles once again in relation to these behaviors.

Suicide attempts and self-harm

To reiterate some of the principles, interventions should be straightforward and short, aim to manage arousal, be affect focused, refer to the current/immediate context, focus on mental states rather than behavior, and initially address conscious or near-conscious content. The pathway for interventions moves from empathic validation, that is, a contingent response, to affect identification in relation to external events and interactions, to exploration of those events, through to context and meaning within the current interpersonal interaction. Intervention therefore moves from surface to depth only when the patient's emotional state allows reflective mentalizing. Finally, it is important to adopt a nonjudgmental attitude to all behaviors, including suicide attempts and self-harm or other destructive activities, and to refrain from assuming that any action is aimed at the treatment itself or even to attack the clinician.

The clinician should not assume responsibility for the patient's actions. A comment early in treatment defining the extent of his/her responsibility is necessary, for example:

> I can't stop you harming yourself or even killing yourself, but I might be able to help you understand what makes you try to do it and to find other ways of managing things.

The agreement of joint goals early in treatment will have specified self-harm and suicide attempts and other destructive behaviors as a clear focus for the initial sessions.

The MBT clinician works therapeutically from the perspective that the primary purpose of self-harm and other actions is, from a mentalizing perspective, to maintain self-structure following sudden destabilization. The action is not carried out to express aggression or to attack someone else: it is to manage an attachment loss. While motivations are complex, we suggest that self-harm and suicide attempts occur when mental existence is in doubt following an attachment loss, and personal integrity can only be re-established through the body with blood, for example, supporting existence within the teleological understanding of the patient at that moment. Collapse with emptiness and absence become partially filled by action. More simply, the patient has to be in a non-mentalizing mode to self-harm (see Box 7.6). In pretend mode, the patient can experience emptiness and loss of existence; self-harm becomes a way of managing the extreme pain and experiencing being alive once again. Psychic equivalence thoughts and feelings are overwhelmingly real; self-harm distracts and places physical pain where there was emotional pain. Teleological processing shows the patient what they were feeling in a context of inchoate emotion—"I took an overdose so I must have been suicidal."

Box 7.6 Understanding suicide and self-harm in terms of the temporary loss of mentalizing

- ◆ Loss →
  - Increases attachment needs → triggering of attachment system →
- ◆ Failure of mentalizing →
  - Psychic equivalence → intensification of unbearable experience
  - Pretend mode → hypermentalizing, meaninglessness, dissociation
  - Teleological solutions to crisis of agentive self → suicide attempts, self-cutting.

Intervention

Start at the beginning of the pathway. Use supportive and empathic interventions and establish the events of the self-harm, including any interpersonal context (see Box 7.7). It is essential here that the initial response is contingent to the patient's current state of mind.

> So things had become impossible at that point. You mustn't have known what else to do.
> It must have been really bad for you to end up harming yourself.

This is, to some degree, validating the patient's struggle at the time but does not address the current state of mind. This still needs to be discovered.

> Tell me where it all started to go wrong.

First, ask the patient to give you the outline of the story leading to the self-harm or suicide attempt. This is narrative. It is necessary so that the clinician

---

Box 7.7 Stepwise intervention

- ◆ Contingent response = empathic validation with current state
- ◆ Establish joint reflection on suicide/self-harm/violence
- ◆ Affect focus if no joint reflection—presentation of shared dilemma
- ◆ Identify moment of "loss," attachment trigger and context
- ◆ Work toward recognition/awareness of vulnerability points and context representation.

can start to assess risk from the perspective of the context: for example, was the action impulsive or planned, was a note left, was someone contacted after the overdose? Do not confuse this with exploration of the affective and cognitive processes leading up to the action. Define the interpersonal context whenever you can. Gently explore who the patient was with or who he/she was thinking about before the event happened.

Once the story of the self-destructive act has been told in adequate detail, find out when the feelings leading to the act began, by taking the patient back to a point when they were clear that they did not feel like harming themselves in any compulsive way—a Rewind and Explore (see Chapter 6). The most common error is for clinicians not to rewind far enough. Do not be put off by a patient who says "I am always thinking of self-harm." Many patients treasure self-harm in the back of their mind as a way of managing feeling states but this is not the same as the compulsive urge that builds up into a self-harm state, which is what the clinician is trying to identify here. Ask the patient when their thoughts seemed to change or what they were like a few days ago. Insist that they contrast their states of mind over time. This has become known as a *mentalizing functional analysis* (see later) (Bateman & Fonagy, 2012) and may kick-start a mentalizing process.

Do not be put off by the patient's wish not to talk about the event of self-harm. If this occurs, empathic validation should be used to establish a shared sense of how difficult it is to talk about painful topics and how it creates an immediate sense of anxiety that things will be made worse. This will maintain a lower level of arousal in the session and, indeed, the session may focus on how talking about things can make them worse. People with BPD commonly begin to experience events in psychic equivalence as they talk about them. Thus, the clinician focuses on how the narrative of the self-harm is held, rather than on the thoughts associated with the action itself. Following empathic validation of this process, the clinician may be able to move on to the mentalizing functional analysis if anxiety is reduced. In summary, there are many occasions when patients will not want to talk about self-destructive acts. In this case the clinician can do a number of things (see Figure 7.1 for a decision algorithm):

1 He/she can reconsider the contract made at the beginning of treatment, in which addressing self-harm will have been agreed if it was part of the symptoms and behaviors associated with BPD. The contract needs to be re-discussed.

2 He/she can gently insist by talking around the topic about the difficulty of talking about such actions, recognizing that by talking the patient feels shame and might even begin to relive the events in psychic equivalence. The clinician then needs to manage anxiety levels carefully.

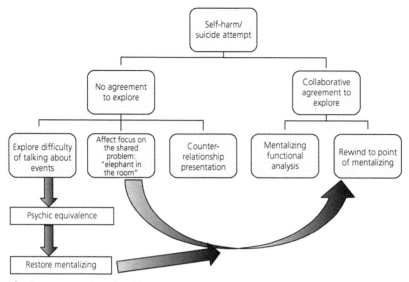

Fig. 7.1 Intervention algorithm.

3 He/she can use an affect focus, identifying the difficulty being manifested between patient and clinician in not talking about the action. This leaves the clinician worrying about the patient's level of risk and unable to concentrate on the topics the patient talks about. In contrast, the patient is sensitized to the clinician raising the question of self-harm, and this will distort the interaction between them. This "elephant in the room" can be explored. In doing so, the immediate toxicity of talking about the act of self-harm may be reduced.

Mentalizing functional analysis

In a mentalizing functional analysis, the first step for the clinician is to help the patient explore the content of the self-damaging event. The clinician must focus on the event even if the patient does not want to talk about it. Of course, if focusing causes too much anxiety for the patient, the clinician needs to allow the patient to talk about other things and then sensitively return to the topic when the patient is more able to talk about it. Second, the clinician must probe by asking what was going on in the patient's mind before the event took place. This is as important as finding out about the external context. The mentalizing functional analysis is concerned with the patient's changing state of mind and its interdependent interaction with external circumstances. Often the patient is not able to remember what triggered the reaction—after all, the main function of the reaction is to elude the precipitating event and the emotions that it creates. The clinician's task is therefore to go back to "neutral territory," through a Stop, Rewind, Explore, and then begin to progress in time. Alternatively, the clinician can ask the patient when he/she first began to realize that he/she might self-harm. Having found this point, the clinician can rewind further. Using this method, the triggering process is explicated and can be further explored in relational terms when appropriate (see Boxes 7.8–7.10).

Box 7.8 Mentalizing functional analysis (1)

- Seek point of vulnerability
- Stop and Rewind to point before mentalizing was lost
- Stop and Explore a point when mentalizing was taking place
- "Micro-slice" mental states toward the self-destructive act
- Continually move around self and other mental states
- Place responsibility for keeping mind "on-line" back with the patient
- Ask patient to identify when he/she could have possibly re-established self-control.

Box 7.9 Mentalizing functional analysis (2)

- Empathic validation and support → collaborative stance:
  - "You must not have known what to do?"
- Define interpersonal context:
  - Detailed account of days or hours leading up to self-harm with emphasis on mental/feeling states
  - Moment-to-moment exploration of actual episode
  - Explore communication problems
  - Identify misunderstandings or oversensitivity
- Identify affect:
  - Explore the affective changes since the previous individual session, linking them with events within treatment
  - Review any acts thoroughly in a number of contexts, including individual and group therapy.

Box 7.10 Mentalizing functional analysis (3)

- Explore conscious motive:
  - "How do you understand what happened?"
  - "Who was there at the time" or "Who were you thinking about?"
  - "What did you make of what they said?"
  - Challenge the perspective that the patient provides if therapeutic alliance is robust
- *Do not*:
  - Mentalize the relationship in the immediacy of a suicide attempt or self-harm
  - Interpret the patient's actions in terms of their personal history, the putative unconscious motivations or their current possible manipulative intent in the "heat" of the moment. It will alienate the patient.

The aim is to identify the "point of vulnerability"—the point at which the patient is on an unstoppable downward spiral—and then to start working on earlier warning signs that self-destructive behavior is inevitable. Only if the patient can intercept a collapse of mentalizing early is there a chance of maintaining stability and a coherent sense of agency. Once the point of sensitivity is reached, the patient has little chance of diverting the destructive trajectory.

Throughout the process, the clinician and patient focus on the period prior to the breakdown in mentalizing while identifying the build-up to nonmentalizing modes. Exploring and understanding the emotions that gradually stimulate psychic equivalence, teleological thinking, and possibly pretend mode form the core of the mentalizing functional analysis.

Once this process is complete, the clinician and patient may explore the consequences of the action and question the effectiveness of the behavior even if the outcome was apparently positive in terms of the "real" world, for example, the boyfriend apologizing and trying to repair the relationship. Self-destructive behavior is an ineffective way to manage emotional distress within an interpersonal context.

> The boyfriend of a patient with BPD announced that he and his friends were heading off to a football match. This was despite their agreement that she and her boyfriend were going to visit friends. This event eventually led her to cut herself. Her experience of being alone produced an unbearable stress that in turn produced a breakdown in mentalizing. The initial announcement by the boyfriend is an attachment loss—a loss

of anticipated physical and emotional "togetherness." Initially she felt that his choice of going to the football match rather than joining her meant that he did not love her. While this is understandable, the problem was not the thought but the fact that the thought began to take on all the characteristics of psychic equivalence. Her thought became a fact with certainty and his absence was additional proof that he did not love her. Further development of this idea led her to more rigid schematic thinking in which she "knew" he was really out on a date with somebody else. This inevitably produced more intolerable feelings, which the patient could not manage. Her only option, or rather the only possibility she could think of, was to cut herself. This self-destructive act made her relax, but unfortunately it also produced shame. When her boyfriend returned he became angry on noticing her bandaged wrist. This perpetuated her cycle of self-criticism.

By working through these patterns of rapidly changing mental states in a wide range of circumstances, the patient gradually learns that feelings are not something that spontaneously arise. Rather, they are created by interactions with others and interpretations of those interactions. Understanding and representing the process as it is happening allows mentalizing to be maintained.

The emphasis needs to be on feeling states as part of an overall mental state and not solely on cognitive states or antecedent triggers. So, the mentalizing functional analysis is more about how the context interacts with the feelings and mental state of the patient—"What was going on in your mind at the time?" In particular, look out for communication difficulties and oversensitivity, which lead to difficulties in managing feelings of rejection, abandonment, and humiliation or, conversely, powerful feelings of love, desire, and need that lead to a flood of affect overwhelming the mind and destabilizing the self. Remember that, within the context of a collapse of the mind, patients with BPD experience feelings at the level of psychic equivalence. Thus, "feeling bad" becomes "I am bad." Your interventions must reflect a sense that you understand this and are not underestimating the power of their experience.

It is the conscious determinants of the self-harm that should be explored without trying to second-guess more complex psychological reasons. During this exploration the patient's explanation should be questioned if it is schematic and formulaic because these are nonmentalizing phenomena and will prevent the development of a more robust mental buffer to future emotional experiences that might result in self-harm. The patient's action of self-harm or suicide attempt should not be interpreted in terms of their personal history, the putative unconscious motivations, or their current possible manipulative intent in the "heat" of the moment. This will alienate the patient. Only later will you be able to build up evidence for underlying vulnerabilities and sensitivities of which they are only vaguely aware, whether these be unconscious determinants or current events to which they are sensitized by their past.

Illustrative clinical example: "The abandoned cutter"
A patient talked about her self-laceration the previous day, glossing over what had happened and insisting that it was unimportant.

CLINICIAN: Tell me a bit more about what happened?

PATIENT: There is nothing more to say really. I cut myself with the cup I broke when I threw it against the wall after I got home.

CLINICIAN: Let's go back and tell me when you first began to feel something was wrong. [A rewind of the content.]

PATIENT: I don't know really.

CLINICIAN: Bear with me; can you remember what you felt, for example, yesterday or even before then? [Trying to identity a context or a time when the patient was aware of feeling OK.]

PATIENT: No. I was OK yesterday and I think it was when I got home early in the evening. I arranged to see two of my friends and we went for a drink as I said, and it was only when I got home after that I began to feel miserable.

CLINICIAN: So you were aware that you were miserable at that point. It sounds like something might have occurred during the evening. Tell me about the evening, starting with how you felt before you went out.

The session continued in this way, with the clinician insisting on exploring the detail of the miserable affect along with the positive enjoyment of being with her friends. It turned out that the patient had felt abandoned (an earlier feeling than the misery) by her two friends when they had gone off to the toilet together and left her alone for what she felt was an excessive length of time.

PATIENT: I felt so hurt [a further affect complicating the internal state of the patient at that time] that I nearly cut myself then with my knife but I scratched myself with my fingernails to get a bit of blood out instead. Then I got the idea that I should just get up and go so that when they came back they would not know where I was [motive of revenge appears to have been stimulated by the severe scratching; only with a mentalizing mind can the patient have revenge feelings, which require self and other representation, and hence her revenge fantasy occurs after she has scratched herself]. But just as I was about to go they came back.

CLINICIAN: And?

PATIENT: I didn't say anything at all. What's the point? They had already spent ages together.

CLINICIAN: Drawing blood is a strong reaction to them being in the toilet for a long time. What were you thinking and what was the hurt about? [Trying to focus on the strength of the reaction—the problem is less the feeling of being left alone when they went to the toilet but more the reaction to the feeling, which is excessive and inappropriate and probably based on a psychic equivalent experience.]

PATIENT: They always exclude me. [Use of words like "always" that have a totality and absolute component commonly imply nonmentalizing.]

CLINICIAN: So you felt excluded and hurt and didn't know what to do about how you felt [empathic and validating statement]. Scratching yourself made you a bit clearer and I can understand how you could become momentarily revengeful to get back at them although you then became miserable later. I guess that you felt that cutting was the only way you could make things feel better at that point.

The clinician is focusing on affective relief from cutting and also hinting at a stabilizing effect of the action—it brings back the patient's mind at the point at which it is lost. Cutting and other actions are ways of reinstating a mentalizing mind. However, there is a danger here of the clinician overstating his own understanding and going beyond the patient's mentalizing capacity.

PATIENT: It always clears how I feel and then I can get on with things again. I was OK with them until we left the pub and I was able to watch TV for a time.

CLINICIAN: But you cut yourself again.

PATIENT: Soon after I got home I felt awful again and so really wanted to do it that time.

CLINICIAN: Can you say what was going on then?

PATIENT: Don't know.

Here the patient is struggling to reflect more on what led her to self-harm. The clinician can empathize with this at that point.

CLINICIAN: It's difficult to grasp what it was like then, especially if things are OK now [empathic statement].

PATIENT: I cannot remember. I was just alone. I went to bed after that.

CLINICIAN: Tell me more about the awful feeling before you broke the cup.

PATIENT: I just felt that the evening had been ruined and that every time I try to enjoy myself something goes wrong. I was then on my own again.

CLINICIAN: In this case what has gone wrong is that you felt excited about seeing your friends and then were more sensitive to being left out. This

PATIENT: seems to have returned when you were alone at home and you did not know how to manage it. We need to go back to consider how you manage your feelings of being left out.

PATIENT: Hmm.

At this point the clinician decides that the patient does not feel able to reflect more on what has been happening and so the conversation moves on to other topics. However, later in the session the clinician assesses the patient as mentalizing more robustly at a time when she is talking about sensitivity to being let down. So he brings the patient back to the experiences that led to self-harm, bringing her attention to the need to be alert to such experiences so that she can begin to manage the emotions either by redirecting them or by using interpersonal interaction more constructively to reduce her urges to self-harm.

References

Bateman, A., & Fonagy, P. (2012). *Handbook of mentalizing in mental health practice.* Washington, DC: American Psychiatric Press Inc.

Lemma, A., Target, M., & Fonagy, P. (2011). *Brief dynamic interpersonal therapy: A clinician's guide.* Oxford, UK: Oxford University Press.

Chapter 8

The mentalizing focus: support, empathy, and validation

Introduction

In MBT, the primary goal is to help the patient be alert to his/her own mental process and focus more on how he/she and others think and feel at any given moment. To this end, the clinician needs to learn more about how the patient thinks and experiences him/herself in the world. This requires the clinician to constantly explore the current state of mind of the patient while putting forward his/her own understanding of the patient's state of mind. The task is to develop a joint process of contrasting states of mind, taking interest in detail, puzzling over difference and nuance, and thereby maintaining the mentalizing focus throughout treatment. This ability to attend to mental states "on the fly," as they occur, needs to become increasingly automatic for the patient. Uncertainty about mental states—whether they are one's own or those of others—needs to become explicit. It is better to feel confident about saying "I am not sure what I think" than it is to make up an opinion; it is more appropriate to say "I am not sure what you mean" than to make an assumption.

In furtherance of understanding mental states and making them explicit, the clinician's mind is "open" to the patient in MBT. For instance, when the patient questions your view you should give a clear explanation of how you have come to your opinion and express any uncertainties you have about your perspective. As the interaction develops you may change your mind about your understanding of the patient's experience, and you will need to demonstrate this to the patient if further mentalizing is to be stimulated. A statement from a clinician such as "I understand now what you are saying. That means that what I said is not quite right. Perhaps it is more like . . ." is a valuable way to stimulate mentalizing in the patient and to demonstrate interpersonal respect. This "models" reflectiveness and allows the patient to recognize that having one's mind changed by another mind is not humiliating but constructive and developmental in a relationship.

There are a number of techniques that are likely to promote mentalizing. Many of these are well known to clinicians. We hope you will begin to feel, as you read this section, that you are already doing much of what is described here. It is very likely that you are. Our aim is not to teach new techniques, but to recommend that you focus your therapy differently by placing greater emphasis on some aspects of treatment while reducing emphasis on others.

Motivation

Motivation to change and enthusiasm for treatment are highly variable in people with BPD. As a clinician you must be constantly alert to decreases in motivation and alter your interaction with the patient accordingly. As a generalization, the patient's level of motivation is inversely proportional to his/her degree of agitation and emotional distress. The patient will not be able to maintain a state of reflective thoughtfulness about treatment when his/her arousal overwhelms his/her ability to process feelings and experiences.

A great deal has been written about maintaining motivation, and much of this information has been incorporated into good therapeutic technique for many years. Even if you have not been trained in the specific techniques there are a number of principles that will help you maintain a patient's motivation for treatment and which are in line with a focus on mentalizing. Motivational interviewing is fully consistent with an overall mentalizing approach. In sum, the main point of contact between motivational interviewing and a mentalizing-focused approach is the collaborative endeavor to promote treatment engagement by maintaining a spirit of curiosity and inquisitiveness.

Some motivational techniques are summarized in Box 8.1.

Box 8.1 Maintaining motivation

- Demonstrate support, reassurance, and empathy as you explore the patient's mind
- Model reflectivity
- Identify the discrepancy between the experience of the self and the ideal self—"How you are compared with how you would like to be?"
- "Go with the flow" or "roll with the resistance"
- Re-appraise gains and identify areas of continuing problems
- Highlight competencies in mentalizing and listen for mentalizing strengths.

It is natural that the patient will not immediately seek change at the beginning of treatment. This is a problem for the clinician and not a problem for the patient. The clinician needs to gradually bring the patient toward a process of change. However, the change cannot be one suggested by the clinician; it has to be change agreed between the patient and clinician. The patient will have spent many years adapting to their circumstances and will have found the best adaptation to meet daily challenges, even though, to an observer, the adaptation seems ineffective and manifestly counterproductive. An early challenge to the patient's ways of adjusting to life stresses is likely to increase opposition rather than create a change process. We all naturally defend our position when we feel threatened and this will rigidify mentalizing rather than loosen it. So, as we have repeatedly emphasized, first it is necessary to go alongside the patient to see things from their perspective. This is primarily done through reflection on the patient's position and, later, a full empathic response to their problems. Initially, though, this might take the form of a level of agreement with their perspective. This is not a trick or false agreement, and nor does it mean that the clinician must agree with something that is manifestly distorted or ineffective. The clinician needs to find an area of agreement. This is the skill of *validation*. Only when authentic validation occurs will the patient feel that the clinician understands; it is from here that the patient and clinician can diverge and start considering different perspectives.

PATIENT: I don't think this therapy is going to be any use.

CLINICIAN: It might not be. It is difficult to know, isn't it? You are right to question it.

PATIENT: I don't like groups either.

CLINICIAN: Yes, that adds to the difficulties for you. I can see that. Maybe we need to consider how you can decide if you want treatment.

PATIENT: It will take too long and I haven't got the time. I have waited ages to come here and now I don't think it will be of any use and I feel exhausted.

CLINICIAN: It is tiring trying to manage things, and almost certainly the effort for treatment is high and going to be more exhausting.

The clinician is continuing to go alongside the patient's anxiety and concerns about treatment. He/she is not arguing that treatment will be effective or trying to persuade the patient to come into treatment. The clinician stays alongside the patient, who needs to consider the effort required to engage with treatment and to make a decision based on an assessment of the advantages and disadvantages to him/herself of change.

The development of a shared focus is essential at the beginning of treatment (see Chapter 5). Equally essential is a regular review of joint goals during treatment. Goals are defined jointly by the patient and clinician on a 3-monthly basis. The patient needs to experience treatment as being relevant to his/her needs and feel that the clinician is paying attention to the his/her concerns. There are a number of motivational elements to this process:

- The generation of joint goals is itself motivational.
- Identifying the pros and cons of goals implies that change is important.
- Each short-term goal is considered in relation to a longer-term goal, providing a coherent strategy for treatment.
- The process of joint review and the recognition that some goals have been achieved is motivating for the patient.

It must be the patient who recognizes the progress, and not the clinician. If the patient does not feel that they have made any positive steps in reaching goals, do not try to persuade them that they are mistaken and have not yet recognized their achievements. Empathically validate the patient's experience of lack of progress. Revisiting the goals to consider why there is no change may increase motivation—mentalizing about the lack of progress details the "failure," making it less absolute, and may bring a more nuanced perspective. The patient and clinician together explore the goal and consider why they have been ineffective in making change. Responsibility for lack of progress is shared between patient and clinician, with the clinician taking the lion's share of the blame without becoming self-deprecating.

PATIENT: I don't think this therapy is working.

CLINICIAN: Tell me in what way you mean that.

PATIENT: I don't think that I am any better.

CLINICIAN: Hmmm. That's not good. Shall we have a look at the initial goals that we agreed?

PATIENT: Can't remember what they are.

CLINICIAN: Goodness me! Let's go over them. My memory says that we agreed on two main initial goals, which were reducing how often you isolated yourself from family and friends and also increasing your ability to stand up for yourself.

The clinician has initially asked an open question to promote elaboration of the patient's statement that therapy is not working. In answer, the patient repeats the same statement, albeit in a slightly different form. On this occasion the clinician decides to revisit the goals rather than explore the patient's experience of not being any better. Either response is a reasonable maneuver in MBT.

The clinician also correctly expresses a little surprise about the patient's lack of memory about the goals, and re-states them.

CLINICIAN: Now that I mention them, does that chime with your memory?
PATIENT: Now you say them, yes.
CLINICIAN: Let's consider each of them. Do you have any preference which one we start on?
PATIENT: No.
CLINICIAN: Let's start on the standing up for yourself.
PATIENT: Well I don't do that.
CLINICIAN: What makes you say that?

Gradually, the clinician now asks the patient to explore what makes him say that he does not stand up for himself, and the patient gives a number of examples. The clinician then asks the patient to contrast the current situation with his examples, and to identify differences.

CLINICIAN: I can see that in those examples people did what they wanted and you couldn't do anything about it or find a way of saying what you wanted or what you thought about it. How does that contrast with now? You have been able to say exactly what is on your mind so that we can consider it. What is the difference here?

Now the clinician is asking the patient to contrast his current ability in the session, which seems to meet the goal of standing up for himself, with an outside situation in which he was unable to do so. This continued exploration of the goal led to the patient being less catastrophic about his lack of change and more thoughtful about progress.

Reassurance and support

Reassurance and support are necessary components of all therapies, and the therapeutic skills of reflective listening and accurate empathy are fundamental aspects of MBT (see Box 8.2). These are not the same as agreeing with everything the patient says and, as we shall see, challenge is an equally important aspect of therapy. They are more synonymous with listening nonjudgmentally, refraining from criticism, and abstaining from guessing about how a patient feels, while maintaining a positive, hopeful attitude, a "can-do" approach to problems, and an active determination to make progress.

Open questions are the road to reassurance—"Tell me a bit more about the problem." As the patient explores in detail how he/she feels about something, a quiet nod of encouragement from the clinician may be all that is

Box 8.2 Supportive attitude

- Respectful of patient's narrative and expression
- Positive/hopeful attitude but questioning
- Demonstrate a desire to understand
- Authentic curiosity
- Constantly "check out" your understanding
- Spell out emotional impact of narrative based on common-sense psychology and personal experience
- For the patient but not *acting* for them—to retain patient's responsibility.

required. Positive and hopeful questioning provides some reassurance for the patient and demonstrates your desire to know and to understand his/her problems. You will have to constantly "check out" your understanding—"As I have understood it, what you have been saying is . . ."; "Does that sound right?"

Inexperienced practitioners often confuse having theoretical knowledge with knowing the answers, and may believe that giving advice is in itself supportive. This is more consistent with an "expert role" that is recommended in some therapies. But using your theoretical knowledge without teasing out the patient's perspective is likely to lead to gross assumptions on your part, diminish the individuality of the patient's problems, and gradually move the patient–clinician relationship toward one in which the patient passively looks to the clinician for answers and the clinician unwittingly gives suggestions or uses problem-solving techniques excessively. This not only deviates from the not-knowing stance of MBT but also, to some extent, goes against the principle that MBT sessions are an "advice-free zone" (see Chapter 13); advice may be given, but only after the patient has worked out a solution. The aim in MBT is to generate with the patient a process that leads to the identification of a solution; the patient finds the solution through serendipity, recognizes it as their own, and works out how to put it into practice. He/she does this through the interactive mentalizing process with the clinician. The aim in MBT is not to act for the patient but to remain alongside him/her, helping him/her to explore areas of uncertainty and to develop meaning. The clinician needs to keep an image in their mind of two people looking at a map and trying to decide which way to go; although they may have agreed on the final destination, neither party knows the route, and indeed there may be many ways to reach the destination.

Empathy and empathic validation

Using empathic statements is a way to deepen the rapport between patient and clinician. Our clinical approach to empathy as a psychotherapeutic intervention follows on from our understanding of the neurobiology of mentalizing and contingency. The therapeutic relationship is an emotionally invested relationship in which the representation of the other person's mental state is closely linked to the representation of the self. This does not mean that the thoughts and feelings of self and other are identical, but rather that they are highly contingent on each other. A change in the mental state of one is highly likely to be associated with a change in the mental state of the other. When two minds are experienced as having overlapping thoughts and feelings and influencing each other, empathy is taking place. When two minds are experienced as having exactly the same thoughts and feelings, for example, if both are in panic, self and other are unconsciously assumed to merge (identity diffusion). This is not empathy, and in the context of the therapeutic relationship is likely to be experienced as intrusive and destabilizing.

The construct of empathy accounts for an experience of similarity between feelings of self and other. This is a two-way process and moves between self and other and other and self, with both remaining distinct agents. It is a process in which the emotional experience is more congruent with the other person's situation and state than one's own. The other person's mind is the focus and he/she experiences the interaction as such; the clinician demonstrates that he/she is "in the mental shoes" of the patient and is able to understand the patient's feelings and emotions without being taken over by them. This is important as, if the clinician experiences too high a level of personal distress linked to the emotions of the patient, he/she is likely to become partially self-oriented and so lack the ability to communicate full attention to the other's experience. Overall, the person being empathized with experiences a compassion, understanding, care, and tenderness from the other person; there is a feeling of not being alone. It is a uniquely human experience and is more than sympathy. Sympathy is an expression of concern for the other through the expression of comprehension of their plight or emotional state. The MBT clinician shows sympathy too, but is mostly concerned with empathic validation of the patient's experience.

From the point of view of developing a treatment strategy in a session starting with a focus on empathy, the clinician needs to come to a conclusion about the overall shape of the current relationship from the perspective of the patient. Broadly, there are two possibilities:

- A current relationship in which the patient conceives the clinician as having a mental state highly contingent on that of the self (i.e., the patient)—this is an empathic and validating relationship

- An interaction whose relationship representations suggest little contingency between the thoughts and feelings of the patient and the clinician—this is an unempathic and invalidating relationship.

If the first possibility is uppermost in a session, the clinician is in a position to develop a shared platform to explore problems. If the second possibility is apparent, the clinician must actively work to establish an empathic and validating position before he/she can do anything else.

Accurately reflecting underlying emotional states can be problematic in the treatment of patients with BPD. These patients often cannot readily discern their own subjective state, and this difficulty tends to trigger in the clinician a need to tell them how they feel. Yet, patients cannot benefit from being told how they feel. This is the most common error when clinicians are trying to be empathic. You should refrain from telling the patient what they are saying or what they are "really feeling." Some examples of proscribed statements in MBT are given in Box 8.3.

The problem is compounded if the clinician persists in telling the patient what his/her underlying feeling is or what he/she is really saying, and for good measure gives him/her the underlying reasons as well. This will not make the patient feel that the clinician is empathic, standing in his/her mental shoes, or that he/she is the focus of compassionate concern. It is more likely to result in one of three possible negative responses. First, it may lead to passive acquiescence and acceptance that the clinician "knows" things about the patient that the patient doesn't know him/herself; second, it may result in inappropriate

---

Box 8.3 Proscribed statements

- "What you really feel is . . ."
- "I think what you are really telling me is . . ."
- "It strikes me that what you are really saying is . . ."
- "I think your expectations of this situation are distorted"
- "What you meant is . . ."

bickering about who is right; third, it may lead to pretend mode. In essence, the clinician stance has moved away from the mentalizing or "not-knowing" stance to one of knowing the internal states of others. Such a stance is likely to lead to interactions between patient and clinician that create problems within the therapy. These problems are a product of the therapy itself, rather than specific to the patient. It is better to ask the patient to describe the feeling to you—"Can you describe what you feel or where you feel it?" This is useful when the patient cannot name his/her feelings. Working with identifying affect is discussed in Chapter 9. Here we are concerned with using empathy. When a patient has difficulties in naming how he/she feels, the empathic position is expressing to the patient that you are aware of the shame or embarrassment that is being triggered by asking him/her to do something that she cannot easily do.

Components of empathy

There are a number of components to empathy. Basic elements include interest, reflection, summarizing the dialogue, normalizing statements in the context of past and present experience, and respect. These are all inherent to the not-knowing mentalizing stance. But in MBT we ask the clinician to consider two major components of empathy, which coalesce around affective mental states within the interpersonal context.

The first is his/her identification with the feeling of the patient. The clinician recognizes the feeling, manages it in him/herself, and is not taken over by it. In other words, he/she becomes momentarily sad, for example, but his/her mental process is not substantially affected by the feeling. For an empathic intervention to be effective in strengthening the therapeutic alliance, the patient needs to experience the clinician as recognizing his/her emotional state and yet not being disturbed by it. Demonstrating this identification to the patient in a manner that shows you have grasped the form and strength of his/her feeling so that he/she "feels felt" is the difficult part. To do this, we suggest that you first engage in the process of "being ordinary" that we have already mentioned (see Chapter 6, section on the counter-relationship). If in doubt, say to the patient what you would say to a good friend if he/she was telling you the same story while sitting in a café and you wanted to transmit a sense that you were "getting" their emotional state (the café is important here because there is a social constraint, to some degree, on what you can say and how you can behave in that context!). Your friend's outrage, say at her boyfriend's betrayal, has to be mirrored without you being equally disabled by the outrage. Yet you cannot be wooden in your response; to be so lacks the common humanity required to be supportive and empathic. Initially, a normalizing and validating response said with some feeling will suffice—"Anyone would feel like that under these circumstances. What on earth is he up to?"

The second part of empathy considered by the MBT clinician is this: if the patient feels like this, what are the consequences to her of that feeling? For example, if you are asking the patient to name a feeling she cannot name, this has an effect on her. Here, to be empathic it is necessary to identify her shame or annoyance, for example, and how this leaves her feeling inadequate, which in turn has the effect of making her feel inferior to you. Or, if the patient describes events that suggest to her that her boyfriend does not love her, this leaves her struggling with the *effect* of her *affect* that is she is an unlovable person.

At the age of 10 years a patient had wanted to see her 12-year-old brother when he was ill in hospital. She was not allowed to by the nurses and her parents on the basis that her brother was too ill. She protested strongly but with no effect. She did not see him for 2 months. When he returned home he looked different because he had lost a considerable amount of weight, lost his hair, and was taking medication. She was upset that she had not been able to visit him, and protested to her parents. They were unsympathetic. On describing all this during a session, she was upset and a little bitter. Having identified this feeling, the clinician identified the effect that it had on her:

CLINICIAN: It is awful being a child in those situations [noting the affect], at the mercy of other people and so helpless [attempting to identify the effect that the affect and context had on her].
PATIENT: I never wanted people to have control over me ever again. I felt that they did not understand.
CLINICIAN: They probably didn't—or at least they had no idea how powerless they were making you.

In this brief vignette the clinician is identifying the effect that the upset had on the patient, which in this case was crucial for treatment. The patient was a person who insisted on autonomy from others but did so by making sure that she had no need of others.

So, in MBT the clinician identifies the emotional state (*affect*) of the patient and recognizes the *effect* it has. This takes the empathic interaction beyond simple identification of the feeling. Returning to the example of talking with a friend in a café, you might say something like, "Feeling betrayed as you do, how is that affecting you in the relationship now? Can you manage that?" This moves the conversation on toward how your friend is managing her feelings and the effect it is having on her and on the relationship. This can then become the focus of therapeutic work.

Clinical example: "The bastard boyfriend"
PATIENT: That bastard has done it again.

CLINICIAN: Which bastard, and what has he done?

PATIENT: My boyfriend didn't turn up last night until after midnight and said that he had been at work. I know he wasn't because I rang there and they said he had left at 7 pm.

The clinician does not question the patient's assertion at this point. He has no idea whether it is likely to be accurate or not, and the first step is to empathize with the patient's current predicament. It is not to question the accuracy of her perceptions and explanations. Doing so will alienate a person with BPD, who will naturally feel that you are not understanding them. Elaboration of how the patient has come to her conclusion can wait until you think the patient has a capacity to mentalize around the events.

CLINICIAN: I imagine waiting for him all that time without knowing where he was caused some trouble.

Here the clinician states that he is using his mind to imagine the patient's state, while not saying that this is how the patient feels.

PATIENT: I couldn't sit still and when he came in I attacked him.

CLINICIAN: Tell me a bit about what was going on in your mind all that time.

PATIENT: I felt that he didn't care about me. Anyone who cared would have called to let me know where they were. Don't you think that would have been the normal thing to do?

CLINICIAN: Certainly. I can see how him not phoning would lead to you to feel he didn't care about you and that he didn't think about you enough to bother to let you know [normalizing her feeling to some degree].

PATIENT: When he eventually arrived home I felt furious that he could do that to me, but it seemed typical that I would be treated like that.

CLINICIAN: Doesn't make you feel good about yourself.

The MBT clinician is now trying to get at the effect that the emotional states have had on the patient, with one feeling state cascading into other feeling states. Eventually, the clinician will try to elaborate the knock-on effect of each emotional state. The aim here is for the patient to capture emotional states of mind early, identify them, and disrupt the inevitability of moving into more dangerous states of mind.

PATIENT: I felt like a piece of shit that people just tread on and then try to wipe off.

CLINICIAN: Anyone might feel uncared for and unimportant if someone does not let them know they are very late. You would be anxious about what had happened to him. This seems to have led to you experiencing yourself as a total piece of shit though. Maybe it is that bit that started the real trouble.

Now the clinician is asking the patient to consider how her feeling uncared for leads to a crushing feeling of being a piece of shit.

Identifying and exploring positive mentalizing

Positive attitudes in the clinician instill hope in the patient; appropriate use of praise creates a reassuring atmosphere within therapy. But clinicians are naturally more sensitive to negative reactions to events in patients' lives. Consequently, constructive responses by the patient to difficult situations are not given adequate recognition. So the MBT clinician is alert to examples of the patient managing his/her emotions constructively, expressing them appropriately and effectively, and when he/she has been able to negotiate a complex interpersonal problem. The question is when to use praise for maximum benefit. We do not suggest that the clinician is unwaveringly positive and encouraging, but that he/she expressly recognizes when a patient has used mentalizing with positive results (see Box 8.4).

The clinician does not become a "cheerleader" supporting the patient from the touchline but stands alongside the patient, provoking curiosity about motivations and exploring how understanding oneself and others improves emotional satisfaction and control of mood states (see Box 8.5).

Box 8.4 Supportive and empathic approach (1)

- Identifying and exploring positive mentalizing:
  - Use judicious praise—"You have really managed to understand what went on between you. Did it make a difference?"
  - Examine how it feels to others when such mentalizing occurs—"How do you think they felt about it when you explained it to them?"
  - Explore how it feels to the self when an emotional situation is mentalized—"How did working that out make you feel?"
- Identifying nonmentalizing fillers:
  - Fillers are typical nonmentalizing thinking or speaking, or trite explanations
  - Highlight these and explore the lack of practical success associated with them.

Box 8.5 Supportive and empathic approach (2)

- ◆ Provoke curiosity about motivations:
  - Highlight own interest in mental states
  - Qualify own understanding and inferences—"I can't be sure but . . .";
    "Maybe you . . ."; "I guess that you . . ."
  - Guide patient's focus toward experience and away from "factual
    fillers"
- ◆ Demonstrate how subjective information could help to make sense of
  things.

The principle to follow is: *Use praise judiciously to highlight positive mental-izing and to explore its beneficial effects.*

The clinician alights on how a patient has understood a complex interpersonal situation, for example, and examines how this may have helped him/her not only to understand how he/she felt but also to recognize the other person's feelings.

PATIENT: My mother phoned me and asked me to come to help her pack before she went on holiday. I told her I wasn't going to do that. She said that I had always been a selfish girl given all that she did for me, which of course upset me and made me feel like a little girl.

CLINICIAN: Of course, given that you have worked so hard to have a different relationship with her [work done in therapy earlier] and here she is treating you like you are a child, telling you what to do. Like your efforts have not yet had an effect [empathic statement indicating affect and the effect on her].

PATIENT: This time, though, I didn't put the phone down but told her that I couldn't help her pack because I had to go to work. She made me feel guilty about that but I said that it was too late for me to ask for time off. In the end I was able to say that I would also miss her because of all she did for me.

CLINICIAN: You sound like really managed to explain something to her this time. How did that make you feel?

PATIENT: I felt so much better that I had not given into her demands. I think that she just wanted to know that I still love her and that I would miss her when she was away. I sort of will.

Later, the clinician explored how the patient thought her mother felt about the whole conversation. The patient and her mother had managed to say goodbye to each other in a constructive way, which seemed to leave them both feeling satisfied at the end of the phone call.

The clinician praised the patient's ability to manage her own emotions and the way that she had addressed her mother's state of mind. In effect, the patient had made a counterintuitive response to her mother's criticism or perhaps naturally used opposite action as a response. She had said that she would miss her mother rather than demonstrating how upset she was. This was helpful in calming them both down, which allowed the patient to express other feelings that she had for her mother.

Nonmentalizing fillers

Judicious praise of mentalizing strengths is balanced by identification of non-mentalizing "fillers." Trite explanations, dismissive statements, assumptions, absolutes, rationalizations, etc., should all be identified and tackled as they arise. Most nonmentalizing fillers do not help to develop constructive, satisfying relationships or increase understanding of situations or oneself. These negative effects need to be highlighted.

The use of nonmentalizing fillers enables the patient to avoid problems and even ensures that quasi-explanations and understanding become acceptable and not subject to review. The clinician first makes sure that the patient recognizes the fillers, primarily through the not-knowing stance, and second, seeks to bring the patient back to question his/her current state of mind.

CLINICIAN: What makes your boyfriend like that?
PATIENT: I think that he is irritable with me because he does not know how to show any of his feelings. He had a difficult time with his father and so he can't express any of his feelings. So he spends all his time doing things and doesn't talk to me much. When I talk to him it is an irritation. Mostly I see this as him trying to have a relationship with me without really having one. But he wants one.
CLINICIAN: I am not sure where his father comes into this?
PATIENT: Well his father was an awful man who never cared about him.

At this point the patient engaged in a long description about her boyfriend's father. While this may have been important as an understanding of her boyfriend's character, the clinician decided that the excessive detail of the description and the complex reasoning behind the patient's understanding of the boyfriend was hypermentalizing, an overattribution of motives and mental states.

CLINICIAN: So you think that there are reasons fueling his irritability. But what is it in your relationship that he is struggling with, and how does it affect you? [Attempting to get the patient to focus on her current state of mind in relation to the boyfriend.]

PATIENT: Oh! I feel sorry for him.

CLINICIAN: In feeling sorry for him, how does that influence you in your relationship? [Trying to explore the effect of the affect to promote some empathy.]

The brevity of this chapter should not give the impression that delivering supportive and empathic interventions validating the patient's experience is cursory in treatment. Nothing could be further from the truth. Unless this level of intervention is skillfully implemented, the therapeutic alliance will be poor and other interventions will never be optimal in their effect. The first aim of the clinician in any MBT session is to establish a shared affective platform from which to explore the patient's problems further. This can be achieved only through appropriate validation of the patient's experience.

Chapter 9

The mentalizing focus: clarification, affect elaboration, affect focus, and challenge

Clarification

Clarification is self-explanatory. It is the "tidying up," making meaning of and giving context to behavior that has resulted from a failure of mentalizing (see Box 9.1). Clarification extends what the patient is talking about, minimizes obfuscation, and reduces ambiguity and misunderstanding. To a large extent the clinician seeks to stimulate the patient to clarify, rather than to show that he/she, the clinician, is clear. Unwary clinicians tend to misconstrue some interventions as clarifications. Clarification is not simply repeating or reflecting what the patient has said; this is low-level validation. It is not the re-stating of facts; this confirms a shared narrative.

In order to "tidy up," important facts have to be established and their relationship to underlying feelings identified. Initially, it is necessary to establish the facts of events. Do not mistake this for mentalizing, which is the process of reflecting on the story. Establishing facts is essential if the patient has engaged in any destructive behavior or if the clinician needs information, for example, for an official report. Some patients spend considerable time elaborating the facts associated with a story, and on occasion it is appropriate to ask for an edited version if the patient is talking around the event particularly long-windedly. Actions should always be traced to feelings whenever possible by "rewinding" the events and establishing the moment-by-moment mental process that led to an action. Within this process the clinician should be alert to any possible failures of communication that indicate a problem in understanding others. When this problem is apparent in the story, the clinician questions it and seeks an alternative perspective. Asking open questions and the process of focusing on moment-to-moment events are common clarification techniques.

A 22-year-old patient reported that he had left his university course. He had failed to attend lectures and seminars for a few weeks, preferring to stay at home and smoke cannabis. The first time he re-attended, his tutor asked him where he had been. Taking offence, he told the tutor "Stick your course up your arse," and then walked out. He had

> ## Box 9.1 Clarification
>
> - Clarification is the "tidying up" of behavior that has resulted from a failure of mentalizing
> - Establish the important "facts" from the patient's perspective
> - Reconstruct the events
> - Make behavior explicit—extensive detail of actions
> - Avoid mentalizing the behaviors at this point—begin promoting mentalizing only once the facts are available
> - Trace action to feeling
> - Seek indicators of lack of reading of minds.

not returned after that. The clinician asked the patient to go back to the point at which he had stopped attending the lectures, and traced the events leading up to his absence. Having spent considerable time looking at preceding events and tracing the pathway to the patient's eventual return to university, the clinician alighted on the obvious failure of mentalizing when the student shouted at his tutor and walked out. While this was an appropriate focus, the failure in mentalizing had started earlier. The patient had attended the meeting in a sensitive state of mind, feeling that he was going to be reprimanded and thrown off the course. In the transcription of the tape of the session, the clinician makes many comments such as "Take me through what happened"; "Not so quickly. Can you go slowly there and tell me what was in your mind at the time"; "Just to be clear—you felt that your tutor was criticizing you and sneering about your lack of attendance"; "Looking back, do you think that what he said could have been meant any other way?"; "Have there been other times when you have felt he didn't like you?" These are all attempts to clarify the pathway leading up to the failure of mentalizing while linking it to what was going on in the patient's mind at the time.

It transpired that the patient's understanding of his tutor's mind was that his tutor was being censorious, when an alternative understanding was that his tutor was in fact expressing concern for him and showing that he had missed him. In an attempt to link the patient's experience of the motive behind his tutor's question to his action, the clinician asked what the tutor would have had to say, and perhaps have thought about, for the patient to feel differently and not to have acted so precipitously.

Affect elaboration

Affect elaboration requires the clinician to explore empathically the feeling states of the patient (see Box 9.2). Before this can be done as an integral part of the process of therapy, it is necessary to be sure that the patient has understood the importance of feelings as sources of information and comprehends their

Box 9.2 Affect elaboration

- Normalize when possible—"Given your experience, it is not surprising that you feel..."
- Identify, name, and give context to emotion—that is, use labeling
- Explore absence of motivating emotions—relentless negativity is wearing to others
- Identify mixed emotional states.

close interaction with mentalizing. This is covered in MBT-I (see Chapter 11) but the individual clinician may need to revisit some of this information. The patient has to recognize that emotions are important sources of information and often act as an early warning sign of developing problems. Emotions are to be welcomed and not avoided. In MBT, the basic emotions—those that are necessary for survival—are emphasized (see Chapter 11). Of these, one of the most important, but often neglected, is curiosity. The patient needs help to be curious about his/her own internal states as well as those of others. Without curiosity, no constructive social and intimate relationships can take place. If necessary, restate the principle of curiosity and genuine interest. This may be especially important in the MBT group when patients ask questions of each other but are not interested in the answers.

Normalizing emotions

Emotions are normal. Humans need emotions and the clinician can readily affirm emotions that are a normal reaction to an everyday situation—such as feeling hurt when someone is insulting, or feeling happy when a close friend shows he/she cares. Normalizing feelings whenever possible means patients begin to consider themselves less as "odd" or even "freaks" and more as sensitive people who have normal feelings but experience them too strongly. Do not normalize over-reaction, but normalize the feeling itself: "Anyone would feel anxious waiting for exam results"; "It is natural to feel jealous when you see your former boyfriend with another young woman."

Question the certainty of feelings when held in psychic equivalence by working in the not-knowing stance. This reminds the patient that feelings are not facts, but they are useful experiences; just because you *feel* that someone thinks something does not mean that they actually do. Exhort the patient to check it out whenever possible:

PATIENT: He was seen near the cinema and he was with a girl. My friend saw him. Of course I was jealous. So I said to him, "What were you doing having sex with that girl you were with at the cinema?"

CLINICIAN: Help me see how you get from him being seen near the cinema to them having sex.

PATIENT: His mother lives round the corner from there.

CLINICIAN: I can see that him being seen with a girl would make you jealous, especially as you haven't trusted him for some time [normalizing]. But what makes you so sure that he had sex with her?

PATIENT: Because I know, and his mother would let him use her house.

CLINICIAN: It is really difficult to know how to cope with jealousy when it jumps straight to infidelity, isn't it? [Trying to identify the effect of the initial emotion.] Let's look at how it jumped so far so quickly.

The problem in this clinical example is that the patient's feeling is held in psychic equivalence. Checking out her belief by asking her partner if he has had sex with another woman at his mother's house will be ineffective, as she will not believe his response if he denies it. It is better to ask the patient to question her assumptions and to look more carefully about how she collapses into psychic equivalence, rather than arguing with the belief. If this fails, then consider moving to an allied topic, work to turn on a general reflective process and then—and only then—revisit the question of the boyfriend's infidelity (see Table 7.1 in Chapter 7 for a summary of this process in psychic equivalence).

Identifying emotions

Many patients with BPD have difficulties naming emotions. Their lack of descriptors to communicate their emotional states limits interaction, reduces their ability to be soothed by someone else who understands how they feel, and militates against their developing contextual meta-representations of their inner state. For soothing to take place, the other person has to be able to respond in a contingent manner; this is difficult if the individual cannot accurately and efficiently describe how they feel. To address this immediate problem for patients of describing their current internal states, MBT focuses in detail on experiences in the session itself as well as on feelings the patient has felt in different contexts at different times. Both of these discussions are encouraged. At times it may be necessary for the clinician to "label" the emotion for the patient—"If that was me I would feel disappointment"; "When I have that increase in tension in my body I start to think it means I am frustrated." It is apparent that "giving" the patient his/her feeling breaks one of the principles of MBT—do not take over the patient's mentalizing—but there are always exceptions to principles, and this is one of them. Any patient who has not developed a capacity to differentiate feelings and give emotional expression to them will need help to translate bodily feeling into mental emotion. This is the core psychological process used to help patients who are alexithymic.

The clinician should keep in mind that the focus on affect in MBT is primarily on the dominant feeling in the moment of the session as manifested between patient and clinician—that is, the here-and-now rather than the there-and-then. Nevertheless, it is important to elicit feelings experienced during events in the there-and-then, if only to illustrate the principle that strong feelings disrupt mentalizing. Furthermore, talking about recent but past events may trigger less arousal.

In exploring feelings, the patient can become increasingly aware that he/she is bewildered about feelings and even begin to experience them in psychic equivalence. As a result his/her mental agitation will increase, quickly overwhelming his/her capacity to be reflective. In effect, the clinician is asking the patient to undertake a task that creates stress. Rather than elaborating feeling states, feelings become dangerous reality for the patient; physical agitation, panic, and defensive maneuvers result. If this occurs in a session, the clinician can focus on the importance of the bodily experience and note that these experiences indicate a need to find ways of expressing the feeling more effectively. Identifying feelings and their bodily precursors, then placing them in context, helps to reduce the patient's perplexity and reduces the likelihood that his/her feelings have to be managed through action.

Absence of motivating emotions

Many patients exhibit emotions that are unlikely to induce sympathy in others. Relentless pessimism and hopelessness is wearing to others. The absence of pleasure and joy that characterizes many of the relationships of people with BPD is exhausting—not just to the patient but also to people they are with. It is possible that the persistent absence of happiness in a relationship is worse for constructive interaction than the presence of distress. The absence of such feelings should become a focus of therapy. Working toward enjoyment of things in life is as important as working to reduce emotional turmoil.

Clinicians may become exhausted by the relentless hopelessness experienced by the patient and the lack of progress over time. In MBT, there are two possible interventions in this situation. First, the clinician can "affect focus" the problem (see below); second, the clinician can challenge the fixed position of the affective pole of the affective–cognitive mentalizing dimension.

A patient who felt that she was useless, that nothing ever worked for her, and that no one could help was unable to see any different perspective on her problems. So the clinician started to work specifically on the shared affect focus.

CLINICIAN: What is it like for you to feel that everything you try or touch always fails? [Not-knowing exploration.]

PATIENT: I just get more hopeless and tired.

CLINICIAN: It must be exhausting to try to harness some energy only to find it is wasted [initial empathy].

PATIENT: Yes.

CLINICIAN: So it occurs to me that you are sitting here wondering what else can be done, feeling you have tried everything and are now exhausted. For my part I am also sitting here wondering what else we can try. I am not sure either.

PATIENT: Well, if you are not sure that makes things worse.

CLINICIAN: I can see that, but it is not quite what I meant. I thought that perhaps you were tired of trying all the time and I was thinking that I am tired, which usually means we need to find another way around the brick wall we keep banging our heads against.

The clinician is trying to address the current interactive process shared between him and the patient that is interfering with progress of treatment. From here, a challenge may be necessary to twist the process or to stimulate the patient to consider another perspective.

Mixed emotional states

Finally, the clinician needs to be sensitive to overtly expressed emotions covering another feeling. The danger is focusing only on the manifest feeling and not recognizing the underlying struggle.

A patient spent considerable time in the group standing up, talking with a raised voice. The clinician remarked on how angry he was. This upset him and he reacted strongly, saying that he was not angry.

PATIENT: Why do people say I am angry all the time? I am not.

CLINICIAN: Well, I thought that you were as you are standing up, you raise your voice, and you are gesticulating with your arms [describing the external focus of his mentalizing]. You come across as angry to me [presentation of clinician's experience of patient's state]. If you are not angry, can you say how you do feel [suggesting identifying feeling state] so that I can understand it better?

PATIENT: Not angry.

CLINICIAN: I accept that. So, can you describe what you do feel at the moment? Start by saying what your body feels like, if that helps. [Seeking to get the patient to focus on his internal state initially; later, the clinician will ask the patient to translate this into a mental state.]

PATIENT: I feel tense, which is why I am standing up. Actually, I am frustrated as I don't think people ever really listen to me.

CLINICIAN: What would tell you that we were listening?

PATIENT: [A bit more hesitant.] Not sure.

This patient is now able to reflect a little more, so he is more able to feel that people are listening.

PATIENT: I don't really think that you all see me as important.

Now the patient has uncovered another feeling, which was masked by his agitation and apparent anger. This allows the clinician to be much more empathic about the patient's plight.

CLINICIAN: That is really helpful. So when I see you as angry and agitated, I really need to consider if you are feeling unimportant, which I can easily miss. Is there something at the moment that we are doing that makes you feel unimportant? [Empathic statement rooted in the interpersonal relationship.]

The elaboration of the manifest feeling, which reveals an underlying state, is more likely to provoke a caring or concerned response. A common example of this process is the use of anger and hostility to cover more problematic feelings such as closeness and intimacy. Here, the clinician should make careful use of the counter-relationship; this may be the first indication of the patient's underlying state.

Affect focus

This topic was introduced in Chapter 7. The affect focus refers to the "atmosphere" or "shared affect" between patient and clinician which is present in a session. It is the "elephant in the room," that is, something that is apparent in the interpersonal/relational domain but is unexpressed (see Box 9.3). It is an aspect of implicit mentalizing that is influencing the interaction but is hidden and unstated. Both patient and clinician may be skirting around the "elephant," even pretending it is not there, anxious about identifying it for fear that it will trigger an emotional storm or stimulate an interaction that cannot be negotiated constructively. The unstated processes are not necessarily unpleasant or painful, and the most problematic and uncomfortable affect focus can be identifying a warmer and more supportive affective interaction.

Box 9.3 Affect focus

- The "elephant in the room"
- Define the current affective state *shared* between patient and clinician
- Do this tentatively, from your own perspective
- *Do not* attribute it to the patient's experience
- Link the current affective state to therapeutic work within the session itself
- Moves implicit process to explicit mentalizing
- Defines explicitly any interaction interfering with the process of therapy.

The intervention of defining the affect focus in the patient–clinician relationship is to make implicit mentalizing explicit. It is a dialectic move to rebalance the relationship along the implicit–explicit dimension of mentalizing. The aim is to increase the complexity, depth, and intimacy of the relationship while managing the associated interpersonal affect and while maintaining mentalizing. It is the beginning of identifying some of the core difficulty of people with BPD whose mentalizing is vulnerable to being lost in the context of close emotional interpersonal interactions. To this extent, identifying the affect focus may destabilize the current interaction in a session by increasing anxiety unless it is done sensitively and skillfully. On the other hand, when it is done well, the relationship will be enhanced and mentalizing will be increased despite some change in anxiety. In this case the clinician can use the affect focus as a stepping stone toward mentalizing the relationship.

The affect focus indicates that the unspoken can be spoken, that it is safe to share emotional aspects of relationships and check out personal understanding of an element of the relationship. Openness in relationships increases trust and stimulates a more secure attachment, establishing doubt in the natural wariness about learning from relationships that is often experienced by people with BPD. Epistemic trust is rekindled. For this to be effective, the affect focus is defined as an "elephant" that both patient and clinician are contributing to; it is not something that is solely created and formed by the patient.

The avoidant patient

A patient showed avoidant attachment strategies in his life. These were evident in sessions by the patient's avoidance of eye contact and turning away from the clinician to look out of the window. These avoidant behaviors indicated underlying anxiety, which, at times, had led the patient to leave the session. Indeed, the clinician was also anxious—about addressing topics in more detail when it triggered immediate avoidant behaviors, and fearful that it could make the patient leave the session.

CLINICIAN: When we talk about this you start avoiding eye contact and keep looking away. Can you say why?
PATIENT: I don't know. My mind goes a bit blank.
CLINICIAN: Can you describe it?
PATIENT: I feel anxious and I am nervous about talking about it.
CLINICIAN: Perhaps that is something that we share—at the moment I am a bit anxious that if I keep asking about things it will make you more anxious and make you avoid things more. So perhaps both of us are uncertain whether to avoid or not.

The clinician is trying to identify the implicit avoidance in the session that permeates the relationship. He verbalizes the dilemma as something that is currently shared between them. He does not focus on the patient's anxiety and its underlying cause. This might promote self-exploration and may be a reasonable intervention. However, the clinician is trying to make the process increasingly relational, so starts to identify the dynamic affect focus shared between him and the patient.

Challenge

Challenge (see Box 9.4) is an underrated and underused intervention. The clinician has one primary aim when using challenge—to reinstate mentalizing

---

Box 9.4 Challenge

- Aim is to bring nonmentalizing to an abrupt halt, even if only momentarily
- Surprise the patient's mind; trip his/her mind back to a more reflective process
- Grasp the moment—Stop and Stand—if the patient seems to respond. Use steady resolve
- Intervention should be outside the expected frame
- Use humor when possible.

when no other intervention has succeeded. It rebalances mentalizing that has become stuck at one end of one or more of the dimensions: it triggers affective response in the context of excessive rationality; it forces scrutiny of internal states if external mentalizing is leading to rapid assumptions; it shifts the patient's attention from ruminative self-scrutiny to the mind of the clinician.

Our descriptor "Stop and Stand" is a reminder that if the nonmentalizing comes to a halt as a result of the intervention, the clinician is asked to hold the session almost in freeze-frame, otherwise the nonmentalizing will soon resume. Challenge, when effective, provides both a breathing space and a pivotal moment for exploration and clarification to become more focused. It generates an alternative perspective around an apparently insoluble problem.

Indicators

The primary indicator for challenge as an intervention is any persistent non-mentalizing (see Box 9.5). But the more specific indicator is the presence of pretend mode. Pretend mode is pernicious and is one of the main causes of ineffective treatment. It can be difficult to recognize initially, but the clinician should be alert to pretend mode if the patient seems to be doing well in treatment itself but there is no change in his/her outside life or the sessions seem to be going nowhere despite efforts and apparent clinician and patient understanding about problems.

Persistent nonmentalizing leads to action, and so challenge needs to be considered in situations in which the patient is at risk of action or treatment is in danger of ending. Hence, challenge may be necessary when a patient is actively suicidal, thinking of leaving treatment, or engaged in self-destructive activities, such as alcohol or drug use, which interfere with treatment. Once the clinician fails to trigger doubt in the patient's perspective about his/her need to kill him/herself, for example, and becomes increasingly concerned that the extent of the patient's nonmentalizing may lead to action, challenge becomes imperative. To some extent this will feel counterintuitive to the clinician, who is more likely to

---

Box 9.5 Challenge—indicators

- Persistent nonmentalizing, especially in high-risk contexts
- Pretend mode
- Fixed position in one or more dimensions of mentalizing
- Inadequate progress in treatment.

become increasingly protective of a patient in these circumstances and actively avoid doing anything that might cause further upset. But in such a situation there is urgency and things cannot be left alone. Challenge cuts through the "bullshit" and is often used in these high-risk situations.

Characteristics

Challenge has to be infused with compassion, otherwise it may be inappropriately used against the patient rather than for them. It is most effective when it comes as a great surprise to the patient, when it is unheralded, when humor is used, when it confronts severe nonmentalizing with an alternative perspective, and when the maneuver "trips up" the patient's mental processes and halts them abruptly. It comes from left-field and is outside the normal patient–clinician dialogue. To this end, a challenge has certain characteristics, which are summarized in Box 9.6.

Saying something infused with some or all of these characteristics to the patient tends to "trip up" their mind, startle, stop the diatribe, or at least create hesitation. The clinician calls a halt, as it were, without alienating the patient, and seeks to stimulate reflection.

Challenge should always be accompanied by exploration of the patient's underlying feeling state; it is not a cognitive analysis of the logic of the conversation. The feeling state needs to be validated within the challenge process, even if only at the level of reflection about their struggle.

Humor is a key feature of effective challenge. Using humor may immediately reduce tension in a session but, most of all, it brings attention to the absurdities of life and adds an alternative perspective, thereby lessening mental pain. One patient who complained that her sessions with one of the authors (AB) were only 40 minutes long whereas patients seeing other therapists all had 50-minute sessions was answered with "Forty minutes of me is worth 50 minutes of everyone else." The arrogance of the statement was followed by an explanation of the reason for the shorter sessions.

Box 9.6 Challenge—characteristics

- Infused with compassion
- Nonjudgmental
- Unheralded, left-field, surprise
- Outside the normal therapy dialogue
- Targets affect using empathic validation more often than cognition.

Of course, it is necessary to gauge the sense of humor of the patient; turning something into a "joke" can undermine an alliance, leaving the patient feeling he/she is not being taken seriously. To this extent, using humor in challenge is a high-risk intervention, potentially giving high gain but equally risking a breakdown in the therapeutic alliance if it goes wrong. Timing is the key.

A female patient was "ranting" about services and complaining about the way the emergency services were organized. There was no progression in the session and the clinician was unable to interrupt the flow of her diatribe. At one point the clinician looked out of the window, thinking about how to challenge this uninterruptible flow of words.

PATIENT: Don't you look out of the window! You listen to me.

CLINICIAN: I can look [pointing at his eyes] and listen [pointing at his ears] all at the same time. I can multitask.

The patient stopped talking at this point, uncertain what to say.

CLINICIAN: And do you know why I can multitask? Because I am a man.

At this point the patient appeared to be about to react.

CLINICIAN: [Stopping and standing.] Don't carry on now that I have a chance to say something. I can only multitask for a short time, being a man!

The patient was momentarily uncertain whether to laugh or react with anger. Having caught the patient's attention, the clinician was able to hold the session for a moment to try to refocus and, in doing so, trigger a more constructive mentalizing process.

CLINICIAN: Look, I can see and hear that the emergency services have not reacted in a way that was useful, and the effect this seems to have is for you to be angry about them, but I also have the sense that you are frightened about how you will manage if they respond in the same way again when you are so vulnerable [empathic statement about her current state (affect) and the underlying concern (effect)].

Given the arousal level in the session, the clinician has correctly returned to the level of empathic intervention rather than moving to a relational level.

The complaining patient

A patient complained throughout the session that no one understood his problems. He had made a number of written complaints about the ill-treatment that he had received from mental health professionals whom he felt had never believed his reports of neglect as a child and so had not taken his problems seriously. Because he could function to some extent and was gainfully employed, they had told him that he was all right and didn't need further help. As he talked about this he continually pointed out to the clinician that she didn't understand, and treatment with her was going to be useless.

CLINICIAN: So I suppose that if I don't understand it will make it difficult for you to come to see me, especially if it means to you that I am not going to take your problems seriously [a basic supportive, empathic mentalizing intervention linking the theme to the clinician–patient relationship and the consequential anxiety].

PATIENT [challenging tone and dismissive attitude]: You can't understand because you have never experienced what I have. I think I will have to go to one of those user groups where everyone has had the same experience. At least they might know how I feel.

CLINICIAN: Is there anything else that you would like to tell me about my childhood while we are talking about it? [Challenge—it is unexpected and direct.]

PATIENT: [Looks confused momentarily.] What?

CLINICIAN: You were telling me about my childhood and that I had never experienced neglect as a child?

The patient's nonmentalizing process has now been disrupted and the patient is having to focus in the moment. For her part, the clinician is now in a precarious position. The patient may ask if she was neglected and, if so, in what way. The clinician needs to be ready for this.

PATIENT: Well you didn't.

CLINICIAN: But what makes you say that?

[Silence.]

PATIENT: Well did you?

CLINICIAN: I can see that that is a reasonable question given my provocative statement. But it wasn't really my point. You feel very strongly that all these mental health professionals should not have made assumptions about you being OK and not needing help. But when it comes to you making assumptions about me and basing your attitude to me on those assumptions, it is somehow OK [attempt to bring attention to nonmentalizing]. I am someone who can be dismissed as just another person who will not be able to understand because you assume that I have not experienced neglect.

PATIENT: That's different.

CLINICIAN: In what way is it different?

PATIENT: It is.

CLINICIAN: Is it? How come you make a formal complaint to the hospital board because other people have made assumptions about your difficulties and then acted on them? You seem to be doing the same thing to me.

The reader may feel that the clinician was becoming a little too challenging in this session, but the clinician felt strongly that this was a core element of the patient's difficulties, to the extent that as soon as he found his underlying feelings problematic he became dismissive of others without reflection, lost the ability to mentalize others momentarily, inflated his focus on himself, and as result left therapeutic relationships with his feelings unaddressed and holding a grudge that no one understood him. The session continued to focus on this area. The challenge had reinstated some reflection on the part of the patient, whose mostly preconscious assumption about the clinician was now conscious and "on the table" for discussion as something that might stimulate feelings that would lead him inexorably toward leaving therapy and repeating his previous interactions with clinicians, and possibly writing a further letter of complaint. The clinician moved on to identify the fears the patient had of never being understood and his current feeling that the clinician would never be able to comprehend authentically his wish to be understood as a person who has his own needs and desires, who requires support and emotional care, and who needs help.

Challenge is effective over the long term only when used prudently. Excessive challenge disrupts the flow of a session, and when employed too frequently is counterproductive. Clinicians must use their judgment about when a gross assumption has been made or pseudomentalizing is gaining hold and is likely to result in a serious distortion of the process of therapy or in further acting out by the patient. Challenges should not be made in an unpleasant manner or with anger, but they require the clinician to persist and to decline from being deflected from exploration: "Bear with me, I think we need to continue trying to understand what is going on." The clinician maintains a steady resolve to examine the problem: "I can understand that you want me to move off this discussion about what you are doing, but I don't think that would be right because . . ."

As previously stated, challenge may be necessary to reduce threats to the integrity of therapy, for example, when antisocial aspects of a patient's function predominate and justifications of dangerous or illegal actions mount one on top of the other, or the clinician becomes unclear about the veracity of a patient's story.

The well-dressed patient

A 26-year-old male patient on probation for fraud attended the session looking distinctly different in appearance. Instead of his usual slightly unkempt look he was wearing designer jeans and fashionable shoes.

PATIENT: How do you like my new look?

CLINICIAN: You do look very different, I must say. What has happened to change things?

PATIENT: I just decided to buy some new stuff and to make myself look good. My grandmother gave me some money [said hurriedly].

CLINICIAN: That was kind of her, and you decided to spend it on clothes. You do look good, but can you think about what made you begin to think about yourself a bit differently and want to present yourself to me and to others looking clean and well dressed?

PATIENT: I think that most of you just see me as a bad person, and I am more than that.

The session continued in this way, but gradually the clinician became preoccupied with two thoughts. First, she thought that the patient might have shoplifted the clothes and that his explanation of money from his grandmother was specious; second, that he had done it to present himself nicely to her. Eventually she brought her preoccupations into the session as sensitively as she could.

CLINICIAN: Going back to when you said that most people only see you as being bad, I wonder if one problem for you is that because people know you have been to prison for fraud you fear that everything you do makes them think that you might have committed further fraud. A bit like me thinking that you might have got your new clothes in that way, rather than from your grandmother [a tentative affect focus capturing potential worry of the patient mirrored by that of the clinician].

PATIENT: Do you?

CLINICIAN: It did occur to me that something like that might have happened, particularly if you wanted to look good to come here.

PATIENT: So you don't really trust me then do you. You think I stole them, don't you?

CLINICIAN: I don't know how you got them, but you have said very little about your grandmother since you started in therapy, so she has come "out of the blue" for me. Why don't you tell me more about her and what led her to give you some money?

PATIENT: You won't believe me anyway.

CLINICIAN: I think that we have to face the fact that you have committed fraud using credit cards and been to prison for it, and so if you suddenly appear with expensive things then people are going to be suspicious. That is something that you are going to have to live with for a time at least. But first, let's consider what you expected me to think, especially since you have never mentioned your grandmother before. To me she is a fictional person.

In this vignette the clinician is trying to balance honesty about her state of mind with reflection about how this affects her responses in therapy. She has been candid and expressed her own assumptions while stopping and standing to allow the patient to begin further exploration of what is in his mind and what he understands might be engendered in the mind of the other. In fact, in this case the patient's grandmother had visited from the North of England and given him some money, which he had spent on his appearance. The key area for further examination turned out not to be the patient's dishonesty but his attachment to the clinician and his wish to present attractively to her.

There are times when a patient is blatantly dishonest or attempts to gloss over obvious deceit, and at those times therapy itself is under threat. Initially, it is important to convert frank deceit into a clearly stated truth. Until this has been done it is impossible to continue therapy.

Deceit is interesting from the perspective of mentalizing. To deceive effectively, an individual must have a capacity to understand the mind of the other person and to be able to predict what he/she will and will not believe, and under what circumstances. To this extent the patient with antisocial personality disorder (ASPD) may have a highly tuned capacity for cognitive mentalizing, but it is our experience that this apparent ability is actually highly restricted and rarely generalizable to complex interpersonal situations. We discuss this in Chapter 13. ASPD patients are able to mentalize some specific mind states; for example, the exploitative patient easily picks up the subjective state of the dependent borderline patient and tunes in to her needs. Able to cognitively understand her underlying feelings, he exploits her for his own ends rather than affectively empathizing, initially stimulating an erroneous trust and misguided affection on her part. This is a misuse of mentalizing. An unequal relationship follows, which deteriorates at the point at which the borderline patient expresses more complex mental states and feelings that the ASPD patient fails to understand and cannot react to other than with violence or coercive action to bring his partner back to a position in the relationship that he does understand. These relationships are dangerous for the dependent borderline patient and will interfere with treatment if the relationship is between two patients who have met through group therapy. More sinister for treatment is the psychopathic patient who has the ability both to charm and to "read minds" effectively but misuses this with serious exploitative or even sadistic behavior. In common with other treatments, we have no answer to this problem, although we have discussed some of the underlying mind states leading to violence elsewhere (Bateman, Bolton, & Fonagy, 2013; Bateman & Fonagy, 2008).

Strategies

Challenge strategies are summarized in Box 9.7.

Counterintuitive statements

Responding counterintuitively ensures that the challenge comes as a surprise to the patient. A counterintuitive intervention—for example, at a simple level, a counterfactual question—goes against the grain, may reverse the understanding currently being generated, and reframes the perspective. The key element here is really the surprise. The patient has to think for a moment rather than assuming. It is not a "trick" in the sense of reverse psychology; the clinician is not saying one thing in the hope that the patient will naturally oppose the suggestion and move in the direction the clinician wants. He/she is saying it to stimulate mentalizing so that the patient can begin to reflect. For example, if the patient is saying "I am going to leave the session because it is meaningless," the clinician might say "I was just thinking how important this was." At this moment the clinician will "stop and stand" the statement and say what was important. The aim is to pull the patient's attention away from a fixed position of self-absorption to consideration of the other. The patient may still decide to leave the session, but has had to consider it from a different perspective, even if only momentarily. The "center of gravity" has changed.

There is considerable overlap with paradoxical interventions, and many clinicians, from Adler (1956) onwards, have recommended challenge interventions

---

Box 9.7 Challenge—strategies

- Counterintuitive statements
- Mischievous or "wacky" comments
- Clinician's emotional expression to rebalance patient's emotional expression
- Frank but fair.

based on counterintuitive statements, especially for oppositional patients (Beutler, Moleiro, & Talebi, 2002).

Mischievous or "wacky"

At times, making a mischievous or wacky comment can quickly "trip" nonmentalizing into a mentalizing frame. Mischievous statements are provocative and may be left-field; wacky statements are puzzling but definitely left-field and will make a patient turn, almost wondering whether they heard properly. It is akin to a doctor making conversation with a patient who is phobic of injections and giving them the injection when they are focused on the conversation, so that the injection is over by the time they notice. This comment could be in the form of a parallel dialogue, for example, the clinician talking about a different subject or suddenly changing the focus. It could be a peculiar statement with ambiguous meaning; an example of this type of comment was famously delivered by the footballer Eric Cantona who, when asked in a press conference about a community sentence he had recently received, answered with "When the seagulls follow the trawler, it is because they think that sardines will be thrown into the sea." This so perplexed the assembled press that it led to a frenzy of reflection about its meaning. This is the exact reaction that challenge seeks to stimulate in a session. The attention of both patient and clinician twists toward another area and becomes jointly focused.

Emotional expression

Patients rightly expect their clinicians to be measured in their emotional responses, and even nonreactive. For a clinician to make contrary moves in terms of emotional expression comes as a surprise and may make patients reconsider their experience as they are faced with unexpected incongruity. For example, their dismissal of the seriousness of a problem is met with earnestness and gravity, or their extreme anxiety is answered by minimizing the problem. This overlaps with our principle of managing arousal of a patient throughout a session. The clinician is always balancing the level of arousal through his/her interventions and expression, to ensure that the patient's attachment system is not over- or under-stimulated. To do so, he/she makes contrary moves. As a generality, the clinician is more likely to challenge under-arousal.

> A patient who minimized an episode of self-harm in which she had cut herself badly and then woken up to find blood on her bedroom walls, without any idea how it had got there, said this was "not a big deal." The clinician stated that he was horrified and that he thought they had to talk about it. This discussion moved around the importance of the event, with the clinician insisting that this was a horrific event—and indeed his voice confirmed this reaction. It was authentic in this situation and not made up. He was concerned that she could dismiss the event as a small aberration.

The opposite reaction to a problem may also challenge the mental processing of the patient. The clinician may fall silent at a particular point and become nonresponsive, and wait until there is noticeable change in the patient. Once the patient notices the change in behavior, it is likely to cause some change in their affect. The patient may ask why the clinician is not saying anything and the clinician might answer, "I am pleased that you noticed me. Thanks for asking. I seemed to be talking into space."

Of course, these interventions need to be centered within an empathic, validating stance in which the patient's struggle is seen as the core process for attention.

Frank but fair

In the example of the well-dressed patient and the question of deceit, the clinician is open and frank about her concerns. There is no cover-up and she tries to frame the challenge within an area of affect focus. Being frank but fair and resolutely pursuing an area of importance with an open mind may appear insensitive at times, but it has to be done without a judgmental attitude and without censure. The clinician knows why she is pursuing an avenue of enquiry and treats the topic like any other; the problem is a result of nonmentalizing and a collapse in ability to manage emotions and urges. It is not a moral issue. She is direct and resolute, confident and authoritative—all characteristics suggested to be essential in clinicians who treat people with BPD (Gunderson, 2008). Only once the situation is stable and a safe level of arousal has been established does the clinician become more doubtful and uncertain.

Frank and fair challenge is often necessary in high-risk situations. Patients may not want to talk about a suicide attempt. To do so triggers psychic equivalence experience and they naturally wish to avoid the pain. The clinician starts by empathically validating this problem but gradually marches on, insisting on exploring the suicide attempt while managing the level of arousal. It is the *attitude* that is important, rather than the *content* of the exploration.

Challenge as an intervention for boundary violation

An intimate relationship between two or more patients is very likely to create severe difficulties for clinicians and other patients. There is no single correct response that meets all situations, but this is a situation in which challenge has to be considered. It may occur in the context of group therapy. The open reporting of such events has to be encouraged if they are to be explored within treatment. Otherwise, if they occur, they are likely to be conducted in secret, which distorts the dynamics of group therapy even further. A "hidden" couple within a group acts like a foreign body, unknown and quiescent, but dangerously infective if left for too long without exposure and detoxification. Once a more intimate relationship between patients outside the group becomes apparent, the clinician allows the group to react and considers their responses, and addresses the effect that it has on them and the group. Thus, our first response to a relationship between two participants is to be frank and fair and ask them to discuss openly the development of their relationship and its effect on their involvement in treatment and their understanding of its effect on others. From a mentalizing perspective, the problem is that the formation of a pair rigidifies mentalizing across a whole group and may precipitate chronic pseudomentalizing—"I think that it is nice that they have met each other, so why do we need to worry about it," or even teleological thinking—"Good for them—at least they have got something really good from the group that they can take home!" In these circumstances, the clinician has to recruit other members of the group and force the group to move from a "dialogue of the deaf" to a mentalizing discussion.

Once all avenues have been explored and it becomes clear that the relationship is to continue, a challenge to the impasse should take place (see Box 9.8).

The boundaries of treatment are reiterated, along with an understanding of the patients' position toward these boundaries:

> You feel that your relationship has helped you, and I understand that it has made you feel happier. Our concern is that the special relationship that you have together will not only interfere with your ongoing treatment but also distort the treatment of the other patients in the group who are excluded from your special relationship. I realize that your view is that it may have little effect on what you decide to do, but our experience is that things can go wrong for everybody and so we will have to consider discharging one of you from treatment with the proviso that you may return to treatment if the relationship ends or if you want to reapply for treatment after 6 months, when we could consider you for different groups.

Box 9.8 Challenge in boundary violation

- Clarify your boundary—should be a repetition of the boundary agreed when treatment began
- When all avenues have been explored, state the impasse—"As far as I can tell we are going round in circles. When I say something you simply dismiss it as rubbish, and while I am willing to accept that it sometimes is, I cannot accept that it always is"
- State own position—"If we can't get around this I may have to say that treatment has failed and we should finish"
- Monitor feelings of clinician to ensure no impulsive action by clinician.

It is possible that the challenge could focus on the two patients deciding between them which of them is to leave treatment.

Challenge as an intervention to a patient who wants to change clinician

On occasion, a patient and clinician will decide that their relationship has reached an impasse and they cannot continue the treatment relationship. If this is the case, it should be discussed with the clinical team before a final decision is taken. Hopefully, there will have been considerable discussion earlier in the team about the problems in the treatment, so the discussion about finishing the treatment relationship will come as no surprise.

However, there are other occasions when a patient wishes to change clinician but the clinician is concerned that this is an inappropriate request. Initially, the clinician discusses this with the patient and attempts to listen with an open mind, putting aside any concerns about failure, reputation, or professional hurt. If an impasse is reached, then challenge may be an appropriate intervention.

> A patient had a history of many failed relationships and two failed therapies. So the clinician, having exhausted exploration, challenged the patient: "I tell you what. You go away and think about it for a couple of weeks and so will I. The question we need to answer is: if you change clinician, am I colluding with something you are actually coming to treatment to address? That is, when the going gets tough you change the relationship, and I accept that at the moment our relationship is tough. We need to know if that is going on or not."

This is a relatively modest "frank and fair" challenge and it places the reflection about the problem on both patient and clinician. It is not simply a request for the patient to do the thinking—this would be frank and *unfair* as the patient will have marked problems in stepping outside his/her need for a change of clinician to scrutinize his/her motives. The clinician needs to do it sincerely as part of the modeling process and demonstrate that he/she has done so at the next meeting, perhaps with teleological evidence in the form of some salient points written down.

References

Adler, A. (1956). *The individual psychology of Alfred Adler*. New York, NY: Basic Books.

Bateman, A., Bolton, R., & Fonagy, P. (2013). Antisocial personality disorder: A mentalizing framework. *Focus: The Journal of Lifelong Learning in Psychiatry*, **11**, 1–9.

Bateman, A., & Fonagy, P. (2008). Comorbid antisocial and borderline personality disorders: Mentalization-based treatment. *Journal of Clinical Psychology*, **64**, 181–194.

Beutler, L. E., Moleiro, C., & Talebi, H. (2002). Resistance in psychotherapy: What conclusions are supported by research. *Journal of Clinical Psychology*, **58**, 207–217.

Gunderson, J. G. (2008). *Borderline personality disorder: A clinical guide*. Washington, DC: American Psychiatric Publishing.

Chapter 10

Relational focus of mentalizing: transference tracers and mentalizing the relationship

Introduction

There are compelling reasons to use the patient–clinician relationship as a vehicle for careful scrutiny in the treatment of people with personality disorder. First, our main contention is that attachment and the interpersonal domain are at the root of personality functioning and its disorders—a view that we elaborated at the beginning of this book. Second, interpersonal avoidance as a strategy can become an answer to the pain of relationships experienced by people with BPD. This is recognized in long-term outcomes that suggest that people with BPD continue to have lives that they feel are "second best." Third, studies of the outcomes of all treatments show that intimate relationships remain a problem for people with BPD. Even though patients' interpersonal adaptation improves with MBT, there is evidence that more improvement could be achieved by better concentration on relationships. Finally, the clinical relationship itself and feelings in the clinician engendered in treatment are known to cause considerable problems for services and individuals both within and outside health services. The relationship cannot be ignored.

Transference tracers

"Transference tracers" are interventions that link the content, for example, patterns of behavior, and process of the session either to the patient–clinician relationship (an inward movement) or to the patient's life outside (an outward movement), but they do not have the depth and complexity of mentalizing the relationship. They are a significant and necessary aspect of mentalizing and point the way toward mentalizing the relationship. The aim of tracers is to move therapy toward the here-and-now aspect of interpersonal interactions, to identify attachment patterns and their consequences, and to focus attention on salient interpersonal interactions. Hence they may be used early in treatment and in the assessment phase. They are current; they do not link the past to the present or move therapy from the present to the past with its ever-ready danger of stimulating pretend mode, but link the present outside to the current process in treatment or, conversely, move the current emotion in the session to the outside life of the patient. Depending on the intensity of emotion within a session, "transference tracers" moving inward from the outside may link to the treatment facility (". . . like you feel about the department. . . "), the treatment itself (". . . just as you feel about the program"), the therapy (". . . I guess that mentalizing can become an equal pain"), the session, (". . . just as it is today. . . ") and sometimes the clinician him/herself ("maybe you feel the same when I. . . ").

As a general principle we assume that linking statements using a trajectory from the impersonal (e.g., departmental building) at one end to the personal (e.g., the clinician him/herself) at the other end represent an increase in interpersonal emotional intensity. The clinician has to choose the intensity of the link he/she makes at any given moment. This will depend on how much he/she wants to heighten the tension and the emotion of the session. The "hotter" the session, the more advisable it is to link to the lowest level of intensity for a few moments, to test whether the patient can easily tolerate greater intensity before moving toward the higher levels. Once direct links have been made to the clinician, you are in the realm of mentalizing the relationship.

A summary of typical aspects of "transference tracers" is provided in Box 10.1.

The involved patient
A patient talked extensively about her relationships with other women and bemoaned the fact that they always ended in acrimony after a few months. She

---

Box 10.1 Relational mentalizing

"Transference tracers"—*always* current:

- Linking statements and generalization—"That seems to be the same as before and it may be that . . ."; "So, often when something like this happens you begin to feel desperate and you feel that they don't like you"

- Identifying patterns—"It seems that whenever you feel hurt you hit out or shout at people and that gets you into trouble. Maybe we need to consider what happens"

- Making "transference" hints—"I can see that it might happen here if you feel that something I say is hurtful"

- Indicating relevance to therapy—"That might interfere with us working together."

felt that a pattern repeated itself, with her becoming more and more dependent until she felt trapped and compelled to escape, which usually occurred by her blaming her partner for problems.

PATIENT: I told her that she didn't care about me. She said that she did, but she doesn't. If she did she would have come after me. She never did, though, and nor did any of the others, even though I was upset and angry.

CLINICIAN: I was thinking that maybe this is something we need to remain aware of. It is possible you will feel very involved in treatment and it will make you feel trapped or that we aren't bothered about you. Then you will want to get out. I'll have to remember that we should come after you and contact you if that occurs if we are to help you come back. Maybe we could both look out for this and you could alert me to any sense you have of being trapped.

The clinician is now trying to share some responsibility for noting that this pattern may be activated in treatment.

PATIENT: Don't think it will happen here.

CLINICIAN: Hope not, but at least we know what to do if it does. You let me know if you see it coming and I will bring it up if I think it is happening.

PATIENT: Hmmm.

The intolerant patient

PATIENT: I don't like it if I don't know what people are thinking. I avoid them or ignore them by going quiet and keeping my own thoughts to myself. I don't share if someone else doesn't. It's dangerous.

CLINICIAN: So if you just go quiet and keep things to yourself, I will need to wonder if you are anxious about what I am thinking.

PATIENT: I won't talk about anything if I don't know what the other person is thinking.

CLINICIAN: Tell me a bit more about that. Will you be able to ask me what I am thinking or will you go quiet?

PATIENT: Might.

CLINICIAN: It would be good if you can. But I will try to remember that when you go quiet you might be worrying about what I am thinking. In general I will tell you what I am thinking, though. What happens to make you feel you don't know what the other person is thinking? Has there been a time today when you have felt like that?

Integrative mentalizing

We use the term *integrative* here rather than talking about interpretation. In the past we have talked about "interpretive mentalizing," but this became confused with interpretation as a technique used to engender insight in psychoanalysis and psychodynamic therapies. This is not what we are concerned with in mentalizing the relationship. Here, we are concerned with the piecing together of the patient's narrative beyond clarification. The basic structure of integrative mentalizing involves presenting a more detailed perspective on what the patient has said, placing it in a context of increasing complexity. Something becomes clearer having been mistaken for something else.

> In MBT-I, I use a "book" to illustrate the process. I show an object that to all intents and purposes looks like a book. When asked, the participants all say it is a book and when asked why they say it is a book, they point to the facts—it has a cover with a writing on it, a spine, pages. I suggest that we look at it in more detail, and turn it over. On the back it has further writing. So we are all convinced that it is a book. I suggest that we look at it in more detail, and open it up to see what the subject matter is. On opening the pages, it turns out to be a box of chocolates and not a book at all! Only by looking at increasing detail did we discover it was not what we thought it was but something else.

Normally, integrative mentalizing follows extensive elaboration of the experience the patient is describing. Elaboration, as we have already described in Chapter 9, involves the enriching of a description in collaboration with the patient. Thus, when the patient describes feeling angry about something, the elaborative work identifies connected emotions, perhaps of anxiety or shame, and links to a more complex and detailed depiction of the experience. For example, an initial statement about feeling "in a rage" with a manager becomes elaborated as having felt deeply anxious about being criticized and recognized as arising from the perceived facial expression and bodily posture of the manager, which was seen as threatening and undermining. While elaboration does not aim to mentalize the patient's reaction, in integrative mentalizing the clinician links the patient's reaction to a state of mind in a causal sequence involving cognition and affect. In the scenario just described, an integrative mentalizing statement might be to link the patient's rage reaction to the fear of criticism with a simple statement such as "Well, perhaps you felt frightened that you were going to be criticized and that made you just walk out in a rage." The aim is to elaborate the events in terms of mental process together with the patient and try to recruit the patient to take a joint look at how he and his manager were acting in the situation, using mental state language to make sense of their actions for both themselves and the clinician.

The steps in integrative mentalizing are:

1 Clarification and elaboration of both emotion and experience
2 Identifying the failure of mentalizing and encouraging active mentalizing around the same theme
3 Presenting an alternative view or perspective.

For example, a patient reports a painful argument with her partner in the context of an intense attack of possessiveness and jealousy on her part that ended in accusations of infidelity. In clarifying the experience, the clinician is able to elicit from the patient how her inability to understand the partner's behavior had totally persuaded her that he had cheated on her. The clinician recognizes this as psychic equivalence and an indication of failure of mentalizing the partner. While it is possible that the partner was unfaithful, this is by no means the only possibility. But first the clinician empathically validates the patient's experience, in keeping with his/her aim to rekindle mentalizing and to establish a shared platform to start further elaboration. So he/she validates the uncertainty the patient has, which has been engendered by her partner's secretiveness and his frequent late homecoming from work. This allows a shift from psychic equivalence on this occasion. In elaborating the patient's mental state from this point, it becomes clearer how the partner's lateness triggered a terror of abandonment, which in turn led to a sense of overwhelming jealousy and possessiveness. It also becomes apparent that the likely impact of this on the partner is not at all evident to the patient.

CLINICIAN: I've no way of knowing how John felt, but it sounds to me as though you just didn't know how to stop "going on at him," as you put it.

PATIENT: No, I just couldn't stop. There was nothing that he could say that would reassure me.

CLINICIAN: I wonder how someone might feel when nothing they could say could alter the situation?

PATIENT: I guess they would feel helpless, like I did.

CLINICIAN: Is that all that they would feel? [Trying to elaborate the feelings of the other.]

PATIENT: I don't know. I guess they would also feel very frustrated and angry.

CLINICIAN: Do you think John felt frustrated and angry?

PATIENT: He must have done; that's why he threatened me.

CLINICIAN: But I don't think that you were aware of that at the time. I don't think you knew what effect you were having on him [recognizing the nonmentalizing].

PATIENT: I didn't care, I just felt I had to go on and on, I had to get some reassurance, otherwise I was going to go mad.

CLINICIAN: It sounds to me as though you felt very desperate indeed, is that right?'[Elaboration of the feelings of the patient.]

PATIENT: Yes, I was totally desperate, I thought I was going to lose him and I'd be alone again.

CLINICIAN: In what way were you going to lose him? [Further elaboration.]

PATIENT: I wanted him there, so every time he walked away I followed him [description of teleological aspect of nonmentalizing at the time.]

CLINICIAN: So maybe you "wouldn't leave off," as you said, to make sure that you weren't left alone, and perhaps in that way even him threatening you was in a funny way reassuring for you? [Alluding to an alternative aspect in the interaction.]

PATIENT: I don't think we should go around threatening each other though. It is awful in the end.

The patient is now beginning to reflect more on her relationship and the understanding of the interaction has become less two-dimensional and more multifaceted.

Mentalizing the transference or mentalizing the relationship

We are often asked by both psychoanalytic and non-psychoanalytic colleagues whether MBT recommends "using the transference." Our standard reply is:

> It all depends what you mean by that phrase. If you mean do we focus on the clinician–patient relationship in the hope that discussion concerning this relationship will contribute to the patient's well-being, the answer is a most emphatic yes. If by "using the transference" you mean linking the current pattern of behavior in the treatment setting to patterns of relationships in childhood and current relationships outside the therapeutic setting, then the answer is an almost equally emphatic no.

While we might well point to similarities in patterns of relationships in the therapy and in childhood or currently outside the therapy, the aim of this is not to provide the patient with an explanation (insight) that they might be able to use to control their behavior pattern, but far more simply as just one other puzzling phenomenon that requires thought and contemplation, part of our general inquisitive stance aimed at facilitating the recovery of mentalizing.

Thus, when we talk about "mentalizing the transference," this is a shorthand term for encouraging patients to think about the relationship they are in at the current moment (see Box 10.2). One of the authors (AB) prefers to name this level of intervention "mentalizing the relationship," primarily because it reminds the clinician to focus on the relational aspect of the interaction in the moment and not worry about causality and insight. In addition, it moves away

> ### Box 10.2 Mentalizing the relationship
>
> Working with the relationship (*must* be a mentalizing process):
>
> - Emphasis on the current moment
> - Contrast patient's perception of the clinician to self-perception (or perception of others in the group)
> - Link to selected aspects of the treatment situation (to which they may have been sensitized by past experience) or to the clinician
> - Highlight underlying motivation as evidenced in therapy
> - Work toward alternative perspectives.

from academic discussion about what is and what is not "transference." As a result, we place "transference" in inverted commas throughout the rest of this section.

The aim of mentalizing the relationship is to create an alternative perspective by focusing the patient's attention on another mind, the mind of a clinician, and to assist the patient in the task of contrasting his/her own perception of herself with how he/she is perceived by another—by the clinician, or perhaps by other members of a therapeutic group. In addition, the patient may be sensitized through past experience to current situations, and so experience the clinician as having underlying motives which are not in reality there. The emphasis is on using the relationship pattern to show how behaviors and motives may be experienced differently by others. For example, an experience of the clinician as persecutory and demanding, destructive, and cruelly critical does not equate to their actual motive. It may be a valid perception given the patient's experience of the clinician's behavior, but there are likely to be alternative ways of seeing what lies behind the clinician's behavior. Once again, the aim is not to give insight to the patient as to why they are distorting their perception of the clinician (if they are) in a specific way, but rather to engender curiosity as to why, given the ambiguity of interpersonal situations, they choose to stick to a specific version. In focusing on why they might be doing this, we hope to help them recover the capacity to mentalize and in so doing give up the rigid, schematic psychic equivalent, teleological way of interpreting their subjectivity and others' behavior. Thus, while we look at the motivation the person might have for manifesting a particular type of "transference," the reason behind such exploration is, as always, the encouragement of a mentalizing process within the interpersonal interaction.

Indicators for mentalizing the relationship

There are a number of indicators that suggest the clinician should consider mentalizing the relationship (see Box 10.3). First, any break in the mentalizing process in a session may indicate that the patient and clinician should stop to think about what happened. Did the interaction suddenly jar? Was there a sudden change in topic? To start mentalizing the relationship in this context, the clinician may simply say, "Was there something in how I said that which made your mind go on to something else?" Second, the attachment strategies outlined in the formulation and agreed as being relevant to relationships may be apparent in the session or over a number of sessions. Commonly, mentalizing the relationship in this context will start with defining the affect focus. Third, the clinician may have a persistent counter-relationship feeling, for example, feeling stuck or useless. Again, this may begin with elaboration of an affect focus. Finally, the patient may be describing something of his/her current experience of the clinician. In this case, mentalizing the relationship is in the immediacy of the session.

Process of mentalizing the relationship

Perhaps the best way of explaining how MBT uses "transference" is to outline the six steps of mentalizing the relationship (see Box 10.4).

The first step is the validation of the "transference" feeling or the statement the patient has made about the clinician, in an attempt to move the patient out of psychic equivalence. This is the first task because unless the patient is able to develop a more robust mentalizing process, mentalizing the relationship is not possible. The danger of the classical approach to the "transference" is that it might implicitly invalidate the patient's experience. This alienates people with BPD. The individual who feels the clinician to be persecutory and who is functioning in a psychic equivalent mode is not helped by their experience being "interpreted away" as part of a distortion. In this situation, the patient will

---

Box 10.3 Indicators for mentalizing the relationship

- Sudden break in mentalizing process in the session
- Attachment strategies become apparent
- Persistent counter-relationship feeling
- Patient–clinician interaction stuck
- Patient describes immediate experience of clinician.

Box 10.4 Steps of mentalizing the relationship

- ◆ Validation of experience
- ◆ Exploration in the current relationship
- ◆ Accepting and exploring enactment (clinician's contribution, clinician's own distortions)
- ◆ Collaboration in arriving at an understanding
- ◆ Present an alternative/additional perspective
- ◆ Monitor and explore the patient's reaction to the new understanding.

---

experience the clinician as failing to understand his/her experience. In psychic equivalence, the internal is "equivalent" to the external, so the patient in this mode *is* being persecuted; reference to a victim–victimizer type of dyadic relationship based in past relationships will not generate reflection.

Thus, the first step of mentalizing the relationship is ensuring that the patient feels that their experience is being taken seriously and that it is real and legitimate, in the sense that there must be good reasons, which are normally to be found in the actions of the clinician, why they are experiencing the clinician in a specific way.

PATIENT: You are too modest. I thought that before and last night it annoyed me.

CLINICIAN: I'm not sure what I have done to make you think I am too modest. I am not sure that I quite see myself like that. Can you say where it has come from?

PATIENT: I was watching a YouTube video of you at a conference and one of the other people on the panel was rude to you. He criticized some of your work and you just accepted it. [The patient went on to explain this in more detail.]

CLINICIAN: You may be right. I can see that you thought I was not standing up for myself. In what way is that linked to being overly modest?

The clinician is trying to understand her own contribution to the experience the patient has of her being modest when she does not stand up for herself following criticism. From here, she needs to understand what has brought it to the patient's mind at this point in the session.

CLINICIAN: What made it come to your mind now?

PATIENT: I am not sure. I suddenly thought that you were hesitating in what you were saying.

The second step is exploration in the current relationship. The events in the session that generate the "transference" feelings must be identified. Similarly, the facts from the patient's perspective must be clarified. The techniques of elaboration and exploration discussed in Chapter 9 apply to "transference" feelings too. It is important to explore the complexity of the reported feelings. Taking another example, if the patient reports feeling angry or frustrated, what other feelings accompany or underlie these feelings? Is it disappointment in the clinician or a sense of humiliation at being stuck with someone who appears unable to help? Or perhaps even pleasure at defeating the clinician? The behaviors that the thoughts or feelings trigger need to be made explicit, sometimes in painful detail. The clinician must be cautious not to pseudomentalize the behaviors at this point, that is, explain them or link them to subjective experience too quickly. This can inadvertently have the effect of invalidating the patient's experience. It is more important to trace actions to feelings in the sense of exploring the emotional impact of what the clinician or the patient did, rather than the putative reasons behind them.

The third step is accepting enactment. Most experiences of the patient about the clinician are based on reality, even if on a partial connection to it or an exaggerated component. This may mean that the clinician has been drawn into the "transference" and acted in some way consistent with the patient's perception of him/her. It may be easy to attribute this to the patient's "manipulativeness"; however, to do this would be completely unhelpful if not harmful, suggesting, as it does, a conscious action on the part of the patient and no contribution from the clinician. On the contrary, the clinician should explicitly acknowledge even partial enactments of the "transference" as inexplicable involuntary actions that he/she accepts agency for. He/she "owns" them and does not attribute them to the patient. It is equally possible that the clinician has acted according to his/her own patterns. Drawing attention to such actions may be particularly significant in modeling to the patient that one can accept agency for involuntary acts and that such acts do not invalidate the general attitude that the clinician tries to convey. This may be essential in overcoming the patient's teleological stance whereby only actions are felt to be meaningful.

In the above sequence, the clinician identified with the patient that at times she was not only hesitant, which had stimulated this particular statement at that moment in the session, but that, at times, she underplayed herself whenever the patient talked about something that she admired about the clinician.

CLINICIAN: So when I am uncertain it makes you feel annoyed?
PATIENT: Yes it does. I think "Why doesn't she just say what she thinks?"
CLINICIAN: You are right that I was just uncertain. So it makes you think I don't really say what I think? That I am really certain?

PATIENT: No, not really that. It is more that you don't value what you are say-
             ing, and on the YouTube video you did not value what you had
             done in your research and so on.

CLINICIAN: So what is it about my not valuing my own work enough that has
             been annoying you so much? And what did it do to you last night?

The fourth step is working jointly in an exploratory process to arrive at the fifth
step, which is to establish, agree, and characterize an alternative perspective,
which must be arrived at in the same spirit of collaboration as any other form of
integrative mentalizing. The metaphor we use in training is that the clinician
must imagine sitting side by side with the patient, not opposite them. They sit
side by side, looking at the patient's thoughts and feelings, both adopting an
inquisitive stance. Thus, the patient's annoyance in this session becomes a target
of joint enquiry. The question the clinician is asking now is not about whether the
perception is a distortion or not, but more "So what?" Taking the current clinical
example of the "too modest clinician," what does it matter to the patient that the
clinician is hesitant and does not stand up for herself when challenged?

In this example, the patient informed the clinician that she had cut her arm
superficially shortly after watching the YouTube video. This act indicates that
the video had an important effect on her. So the clinician focused on the feeling
of annoyance that had led to personal dysregulation. The clinician hopes that
the patient will engage in this process, but of course often the patient may just
repeat what she has already asserted. This reaction, however, can in turn become
a subject of enquiry.

PATIENT: Well, don't you think that the work that you have done is worth
             defending and you should stand up for its importance?

CLINICIAN: Yes I do, and I can see that you want me to do that more than I did
             on that occasion. But what was the annoyance that was so strong
             that you ended up cutting yourself?

PATIENT: [Silence for a time.]

Following some probing around this area, the clinician works toward the fifth
step, which is for the clinician and patient to define, characterize, and agree an
alternative perspective. This is not an interpretation of the situation but a more
detailed "look" at what was happening with a different nuance. The key aim is to
mentalize the patient's "transference" experience—all is not as it seems, and the
reactions and counter-reactions have "baggage" attached, giving us a current
sensitivity. In the specific example we are considering, it transpired that the
patient admired her clinician's work and had read about some of it. She believed
that the clinician's work was well beyond anything she had ever accomplished,

and yet she felt that she had some good achievements that she valued. In a distorted affective logic, the patient felt acutely that if the clinician did not value her achievements and they were so much better than the patient's, then it meant that the patient was deluding herself: her own achievements were of no importance. It appears that watching the YouTube video had undermined her sense of self and she had collapsed. It left her feeling that she was a nobody. The "alternative perspective" here is that the problem has not been about the clinician being too modest, but about the vulnerability the patient has to losing a sense of personal pride in her own achievements when she is in a relationship with others. The other person overly influences her autonomy.

After this level of clarification, the clinician cannot sit back and admire his/her cleverness. The sixth step, of monitoring the patient's reaction, is essential. Do they acquiesce easily to the detailed discussion? Do they reject it? Does it lead to further constructive dialogue? The reaction will reveal the validity or otherwise of the mentalizing process that has been going on (see Box 10.5). The gravest danger is that the whole process triggers pretend mode or has even taken place "within" pretend mode. The clinician needs to be alert to this possibility, particularly when a patient seems to agree. Disagreement or the triggering of additional information and emotion suggests that the patient is able to consider what is being said and redirect the conversation to more meaningful elements.

At this sixth stage the clinician is in reality back to the first step of the process of mentalizing the "transference" and has to restart the whole process by validating the patient's reaction. It is the journey rather than the destination that is important: it is engaging the patient in the process of uncovering the way the mind works that is relevant.

Box 10.5 Dangers of mentalizing the relationship

- Avoid interpreting experience as repetition of the past or as a displacement. This simply makes the person with BPD feel that whatever is happening in therapy is unreal
- Patient may be thrown into a pretend mode:
  - Patient elaborates a fantasy of understanding with clinician
  - Little experiential contact with reality
  - No generalization.

Mentalizing the counter-relationship or mentalizing the feelings in the clinician

This topic has been covered to some extent in Chapter 6. Here we are concerned with the technical way in which the clinician marks and uses constructively the feelings he/she has during a session. As we have stated in the discussion on "transference," it is not for the clinician to decide that the feelings that he/she experiences are arising from the patient. Nevertheless, they may be relevant to the interaction with the patient: explicitly mentalizing the experience of the clinician in relation to the patient is an important part of the interpersonal process in MBT. In principle, the MBT clinician carefully monitors his/her feeling of puzzlement and confusion because these contribute to an authentic not-knowing stance (Box 10.6).

But it is more complex emotional responses that need to be harnessed. The patient needs to be able to accurately monitor feeling states in other people and recognize his/her part in creating those states. To encourage this process, the clinician openly communicates what is in his/her mind when it is relevant to the patient–clinician interaction. This is especially the case when something in a session or across sessions interferes with treatment progress. For example, the clinician's mind may be taken up by overprotective wishes for a patient or by fearfulness of or dislike for a patient. Such feelings will occupy his/her mind and prevent a focus on the patient, and may also be of particular relevance to how the patient relates to others. So we recommend quarantining these feelings initially, while they are identified, then talking about them openly but in a way that shows it is the *clinician's* mind that is the subject of scrutiny—that is, to what extent is he/she reacting to the context, content, and process of treatment. Is this

---

Box 10.6 Components of mentalizing the counter-relationship (1)

◆ Monitor states of confusion and puzzlement

◆ Share the experience of not-knowing

◆ Eschew therapeutic omnipotence

◆ Attribute negative feelings to the therapy and current situation rather than to the patient or clinician (initially)

◆ Aim at achieving an understanding of the source of negativity or excessive concern, etc.

just him/her, or is this relevant to the patient's way of functioning? It has not been our experience that patients take this as permission to ask personal questions about the clinician's life; nor is it authorization for the clinician to indulge in self-disclosure in the sense of talking about his/her life and problems; and nor is it approval for the clinician to say what he/she likes about his/her feelings. "Quarantining" feelings means the clinician has to consider the relevance of his/her experience to the patient's problems, the content of the session, and the process of the session. Done skillfully, discussion centered on some of the experience of the clinician is instructive and heightens the patient's sensitivities to interpersonal process.

We recommend a number of steps to mentalizing the feelings in the clinician in relation to the treatment and to the patient (Box 10.7). First, the clinician must identify the feeling itself or, at least, be able to talk about it coherently while working it out. Second, he/she anticipates the reaction of the patient to what he/she is about to express, and openly states this. This is essential if what is going to be said is likely to be difficult for the patient to hear. Third, the clinician marks carefully what he/she is saying, that is, he/she ensures that the patient understands that what the clinician is about to say is non-contingent and is expressing his/her own state of mind and not his/her representation of the patient's state of mind. Finally, he/she keeps in mind the aim of focusing on his/her feelings, which is primarily to identify emotions that may be affecting the treatment relationship and to show that minds influence minds, or, less often, to maintain his/her own mentalizing, for example, if he/she is frightened.

There are a number of common feelings engendered in the clinician, loosely related to the nonmentalizing modes. These are summarized in Box 10.8.

Box 10.7 Components of mentalizing the counter-relationship (2)

- Anticipate response/reaction of patient
- Mark your statement
- *Do not* attribute what you experience to the patient
- Keep in mind your aim:
  - Reinstate your own mentalizing
  - Identify important emotional interaction that affects therapeutic relationship
  - Emphasize that minds influence minds.

Box 10.8 Typical counter-relationship emotions

- ◆ Pretend mode:
  - Boredom, temptation to say something trivial
  - Sounding as if being on autopilot, tempted to go along
  - Lack of appropriate affect modulation (feeling flat, rigid, no contact)
- ◆ Teleological:
  - Anxiety
  - Wish to *do* something (make lists, coping strategies)
- ◆ Psychic equivalence:
  - Puzzlement, confused, unclear, excessive nodding
  - Not sure what to say, just going along
  - Anger with the patient.

Do not be overly persuaded by these suggestions, as nonmentalizing modes are not linked to feeling states so specifically. But the presence of any persistent feeling should alert the clinician to think about nonmentalizing modes and to consider using his/her feeling as a way of addressing the problem.

Part 3

Mentalizing groups

Chapter 11

MBT-Introductory group (MBT-I)

Introduction

This chapter outlines the introductory process to mentalization-based treatment (MBT-I), which has been developed in conjunction with Sigmund Karterud in Oslo. The introductory group is the precursor to the MBT program. It has a number of aims:

1 To inform/educate patients about mentalizing and personality disorder and associated areas of knowledge

2 To prepare patients for long-term treatment

3 To increase motivation

4 To elicit more detail about mentalizing capacities

5 To confirm the initial assessment and diagnosis.

In summary, the primary purpose of the introductory phase is to ensure that patients entering treatment do so with reasonable understanding of the process they are engaging in, that they are aware of the focus of treatment, and that they appreciate the expectations placed on them as well as the expectations they can have about treatment. Patients with borderline personality disorder (BPD) have 10–12 MBT-I sessions to introduce the treatment and to socialize them to the model. People with antisocial personality disorder (ASPD) have 6–8 sessions; recommended adaptations to the core modules to make them more appropriate for working with people with ASPD are discussed in the following sections. The absolute number of sessions is not the essential factor of MBT-I; imparting knowledge, increasing understanding and motivation through empowerment, and developing a therapeutic alliance with clear goals are more important.

At the end of MBT-I, all patients have a meeting with a senior member of the team to review their experience of MBT-I and plan further treatment.

Format of MBT-I

MBT-I is organized as group psychoeducation for a maximum of ten patients in a group. The sessions are organized over 12 weeks and each lasts for 1.5 hours. Some modules contain more content than others and may extend over two sessions if necessary. Importantly, patients must attend a minimum of two-thirds of the sessions to progress to further treatment in MBT. However, if both patient and clinician decide that the intervention is inappropriate for some reason then a review is offered and alternative treatment considered. We do not expect that all patients will fit into the MBT-I treatment model; the treatment model needs to be relevant to the patient's difficulties.

Each group session follows a similar pattern:

◆ Welcome to patients

◆ Summary of previous session's material

◆ Feedback from previous session's homework

◆ Introduction to new topic

◆ Discussion and process work on the topic

◆ Final summary and discussion of homework.

The sessions are built on certain principles:

◆ Exercises are arranged in a sequence, progressing from emotionally "distant" scenarios to some that are more personalized

◆ Discussions are related to participants' personal experience only when the group has developed a cohesive atmosphere and some trust has been established between participants

◆ New exercises and illustrations are encouraged if they increase the psychoeducational understanding of the topic

◆ Homework is voluntary and generally requires the participants to increase their focus on their mind states.

◆ Over the course of the sessions, build up a "directory" of indicators of nonmentalizing—for example, use of words, certainty of opinion

◆ Build up a similar directory of indicators of good mentalizing—see leaflet at http://annafreud.org/training-research/mentalization-based-treatment-training/mbt-i-leaflets/.

Each topic is accompanied by a handout and worksheet. These are available to download from http://annafreud.org/training-research/mentalization-based-treatment-training/mbt-i-leaflets/.

Role of group leader

The group leader, a clinician, remains "in charge" of the group throughout each session and over the 12 sessions, and takes an active role in structuring the group. "In charge" is used here to not suggest that the group leader is autocratic but rather to imply that the group leader manages the group carefully to ensure that each topic is covered adequately and discussed in enough detail to ensure that patients are aware of the relevance of the topic. The group leader often makes use of a whiteboard and/or flip chart to highlight key points or note down contributions from participants in the course of discussions. Crucially, the group leader models a mentalizing stance throughout any discussion, while maintaining an expert stance in terms of knowledge about mentalizing and personality disorder. This balance is important. A mentalizing or "not-knowing" stance can become confused with being without knowledge or understanding. Nothing could be further from the truth, however. The application of our knowledge to inform our own mental states and to stimulate thought in others is the very essence of mentalizing. The group leader models the mentalizing stance by demonstrating that his/her knowledge, while being that of an expert, can be extended, clarified, and enriched by the contributions of group members. Critically, his/her mind can be changed by the minds of others; the participants' understanding of and ideas about the topic in question feed back to the question itself. Hence, there is an emphasis on the group leader stimulating discussion among group members. Maintaining a balance between providing information on the one hand and learning from the perspectives of the group members on the other is a key skill for group leaders. The group leader should be careful not to be too lecturing in his/her style, as this tends to encourage passivity in the group members. He/she needs to generate some group process even though the group is task oriented. The process engendered should be related to the topic of the group so that there can be a seamless return to task.

There is a certain amount of material that must be covered in each session and the group leader needs to follow the manual closely. Experience has shown that it is easy to digress and get lost, which impedes the completion of the program. It is also important that learning takes place through the participants' own activities, although the group leader maintains a psychoeducational perspective. He/she uses examples given by the patients to illustrate points related to the topic under discussion.

Module 1: What is mentalizing and a mentalizing stance?

The group leader welcomes the participants to the session and introduces him/herself.

The group leader describes the purpose of the group sessions, which is that the members will learn about mentalizing, emotions, attachment, interpersonal interaction, and mental health. The aim of this first session is to understand what the treatment program is about and to appreciate what mentalizing is. The group leader expresses his/her hope that, in order to achieve these aims, everyone will participate as actively as possible.

The new members are asked to introduce themselves and to describe briefly why they were referred to the program. If necessary, the group leader helps an individual to express him/herself while being aware of the natural anxiety the person may well have about being in a group for the first time.

The group leader hands out worksheets and encourages the participants to make good use of them.

The group leader briefly describes the structure of the group . . .

- There are a total of 12 group sessions
- The group leader will give a short introduction each time
- Examples based on the participants' own experiences will be discussed
- The group leader states he/she will continuously summarize what can be learned from the examples discussed
- Some texts will be used
- Some role-playing will be undertaken

. . . and emphasizes other aspects:

- The group is psychoeducational
- Each participant will *not* be asked to go into depth about their personal problems
- The group may be used at times to discuss personal issues that are related to the topic, although time for this will be limited.

The group leader then explains that it is important that everyone attends every session. This is important for group cohesion, and it will allow everyone to gradually become more comfortable with each other. Participants are advised that they will also get to know each other better through the exercises and discussions, and the hope is that everyone can participate actively with their own stories.

Topic: What is mentalizing?

> *Group activity*: The group leader writes "What is mentalizing?" on the board and gives his/her own explanation, writing key points down as he/she does so.

The group leader takes what the participants have understood from this and expands his/her explanation of *what mentalizing is* using examples and comments from the group. He/she can now use a flip chart to emphasize key points. He/she can say that there is nothing mysterious about mentalizing; that it is essentially a very simple concept and that it is something that we all do much of the time.

It is important that the group leader covers specific aspects of mentalizing in a way that the participants can understand. First, mentalizing needs to be defined along the lines of being *a mental process by which we attribute intentions to each other*; it is how we understand each other and ourselves as being driven by underlying motives and recognize that these take the form of thoughts, beliefs, wishes, and various emotions, etc. A precondition for good interpersonal relationships is that we understand each other—and ourselves—reasonably accurately.

Mentalizing is normal. When we interact with others in a spontaneous and natural manner, mentalizing takes place *automatically*. We do not even notice that we are mentalizing (i.e., that we are interpreting other people's intentions and feelings). We simply respond to people reciprocally by making reasonable assumptions about their motives. It is only when they depart from an expected "script" or response that we are surprised. At this point, there is an interruption in the spontaneous interaction. We stop and wonder: "What happened now? Did he really understand what I meant? That's not what I meant. Let me try one more time." Or: "Shit, the same thing is happening again, he won't listen. Fine, if he wants to be like that . . . I've had enough of explaining things to him." Then we resort to *controlled* or *explicit* mentalizing.

In the review of automatic versus controlled/explicit mentalizing, it is not uncommon to discover that someone is overly concerned about what others are thinking and feeling. This allows the group leader to outline another dimension of mentalizing, namely the *self/other* dimension.

Gradually, all the dimensions of mentalizing are outlined:

- Automatic/controlled
- Emotions/thoughts
- Self/other
- External/internal.

The group leader offers examples of each of these to illustrate them and asks the participants if they can think about when they feel that other people have relied heavily on any one of these dimensions. Mentalizing is a balance of these aspects of mental function and using any particular one excessively results in poor-quality mentalizing. Relying too heavily on emotional cues may be unreliable; conversely, relying on cognitive understanding (thoughts) without attention to subjective feelings may also cause trouble. For example, a salesperson may be convincing about what they are selling you and yet, if your feeling is one of distrust, it is probably best not to purchase from that individual.

At the end of the discussion, the flip chart should show all four mentalizing dimensions with some examples of the poles of each dimension identified to illustrate them, preferably provided by the participants. These examples can be added to as the discussion develops further in the course of the other group activities. Usually, a small piece of process work can be done using the dimension of external/internal focus. Patients often watch the group leader carefully and notice his/her facial expressions, often giving them meaning; they may also be vigilant about the other participants' behaviors. So the group leader can use obvious examples to illustrate points.

Finally, there may be an opportunity to discuss how we can overinterpret other people's motives and spend considerable time reading things into their actions. This tendency is known as *hypermentalizing*. Most patients will understand that hypermentalizing is counterproductive and consumes large amounts of energy futilely.

> *Group activity*: What would you think if on your way to the clinic you saw a long queue at a bus stop with a man at the head of the queue talking animatedly to someone who you noticed went directly to the front? Other people in the queue look annoyed. Make some notes about what you think is going on for the man at the head of the queue.

This simple exercise is suitable for demonstrating:

1 That people interpret the same event in different ways
2 That some interpretations are more plausible than others
3 That some statements about the scenario are mentalizing (e.g., "I think the man may be irritated/worried/anxious"), while others are not (e.g., "He has been waiting for ages" [description]; "The person at the head of the queue is late for work and the other person is pushing in so he wants to stop him so that he can make him late for work too as they work together and don't like each other. The first one wants the other one to be sacked" [hypermentalizing]).

The important differentiation to make here is to try to identify how some suggestions are about the man's state of mind, and therefore related to mentalizing, while other suggestions are more descriptive and not related to mental states. Many suggestions might be about the whole scene but not related to the question of considering the mind of the person at the head of the queue.

It may help to clarify things if you say something about *situations in which one does not mentalize a lot*, or that do not require much mentalizing skill, in order to emphasize that in this task we are focusing on our own and others' minds. When someone is, for example, performing math tasks or exercising, or resting or eating, they are not necessarily mentalizing; their focus is not on the mind but on the task itself. It is helpful for the group leader to use aspects of the group activity just undertaken to illustrate the difference between mentalizing as a skill of the mind about minds and use of descriptive narrative, for example. The group leader agrees that the person who comes to the head of the queue could be a friend of the other person, or could have been at the head of the queue already and gone to buy something, and that it is important to register these descriptors and think about them. But they do not tell us what is happening *in the mind* of the man who was at the head of the queue.

Benefits of mentalizing

The group leader proceeds by saying that mentalizing is both advantageous and important. It is beneficial to mentalize, for example, when:

+ You are going to console a friend who is sad
+ You want to rectify a misunderstanding with a friend
+ You are going to calm down a child who is angry
+ You feel like getting blind drunk or smashed on drugs
+ You wish to convince your boss to give you a higher salary
+ You are going out with a new partner. . . .

At this point, the participants can add their own examples to the list.

In summary, mentalizing is important for the following reasons:

+ To understand what is taking place between people
+ To understand yourself, who you are, your preferences, your own values, etc.
+ To communicate well with your close friends
+ To regulate your own feelings
+ To regulate other people's feelings
+ To avoid misunderstandings
+ To see the connection between emotions and actions more easily, so that you can escape destructive patterns of thoughts and feelings more easily.

Mentalizing and misunderstandings

The group leader introduces the next topic: that mentalizing has a lot to do with misunderstandings. "Let's discuss why we so often misunderstand others and ourselves. Any suggestions?"

Group activity: Suggestions about why we so often misunderstand each other.

The group leader notes down all the suggestions and comments on them. The point here is to encourage a discussion about the characteristics of the mind, how individuals have different values and different life experiences, and how people use different strategies to hide aspects of themselves.

Suggestions are commonly related to one of the following issues:

The mind's non-transparency. This is a key point: how can we know what is going on in another person's mind?

Our tendency to *attribute thoughts to others* (e.g., to think that others are thinking the same way as we do). This is also known as *psychic equivalence—* although we do not necessarily talk to the patients about this term unless they express particular interest.

Experience that *others understand without you having to say it yourself.* The group leader also mentions here the importance of *not* succumbing to this wish or assumption in individual and group therapy. Clinicians aren't able to read other people's minds, either.

Layers of the mind. This refers to the fact that it is also impossible to fully understand what is going on in our own minds. It is easy to misunderstand oneself; you may have access to *some* thoughts and feelings, but underneath these lie unclear thoughts and emotions that can be difficult to understand.

Differences in interpretations and actions. Individuals vary with respect to how they interpret things, how they arrive at judgments, and their ability to deal with situations; in short, different people have different perspectives on the world. To acknowledge this difference involves acknowledging that wishes and interpretations depend on perspectives, and that, by wishing and believing differently, an individual can behave differently, even in similar situations. An individual's wish regarding, and interpretation of, a situation is influenced not only by the here and now, but also by his/her interpretation of the situation in light of his/her views about the future and understanding of the past. Wishes and interpretations about specific situations also influence memories, preferences, hopes, and other mental experiences. The significant effect that cultural differences can have on our perspectives, wishes, and beliefs also needs to be emphasized, not least because group members may have different ethnic or religious backgrounds.

Defensiveness. When another person adopts a defensive attitude or position and holds back feelings and/or thoughts because he/she is afraid of something (e.g., of being embarrassed or judged) then this will inevitably affect one's ability to understand what is going on in their mind.

Having difficulty finding words to express inner thoughts and feelings. We all have this experience at times, especially when we are anxious.

Deliberate concealment or "playing mind games." If the other person is hiding his/her intentions, playing a game, or being dishonest, it adds to the difficulty of interpreting their mental states. It is the mind's non-transparency that makes it possible for people to hide things in this way.

This discussion is then followed up by a new group activity.

Group activity: The group leader asks for examples involving someone misunderstanding him/herself.

This exercise emphasizes the "self" component of mentalizing and the strong feelings that can result from misunderstanding oneself. Two to three examples should be sufficient here. The group leader helps to clarify possible reasons for the misunderstandings. The group leader may bring up his/her own examples from everyday life and even personal experience, in order to convey that mentalizing problems and misunderstandings are not just something that apply to patients. These could be a misunderstanding in a shop, during a meeting, etc. For example, a person assesses her current state as being angry with her boyfriend, so she shouts at him and he walks out. In fact, her feeling is not so much anger but more related to feeling hurt and misunderstood. These feelings are not best managed by shouting, and if she had understood herself better she might have reacted differently.

Group activity: The group leader asks for examples in which the person has misunderstood others.

This exercise focuses on the opposite mentalizing pole, namely, "other," and how misunderstanding others can cause problems. Again, a few examples will suffice. The group leader assists by relating the points to key words on the flip chart and by discussing possible explanations for the misunderstandings.

Mentalizing stance. With reference to what has been discussed, the group leader suggests discussing some typical examples of poor mentalizing skills. For example: arrogant claims about other people's motives; black-and-white thinking (i.e., without nuances and uncertainty); thinking without taking account of emotions and overlooking the fact that people influence each other.

Group activity: The group leader asks for more examples of poor mentalizing abilities.

After the participants have come up with some more examples, the group leader then defines a *mentalizing stance* as being markedly different from these examples. Instead, it is characterized by curiosity about the other person's experiences, thoughts and feelings; it is a not-knowing, exploratory stance.

Group activity: Two patients are invited to role-play. One will be interviewing the other. The task is for the interviewer to find out how the other person was yesterday afternoon, using a mentalizing stance.

Patients, especially new patients, may sometimes be reluctant to participate in role-play at this stage. If nobody is willing to be the interviewer, the group leader can take this role; often other patients will feel more able to take over once the role-playing has started. The experiences are then discussed. How was it to apply a curious and not-knowing stance about another person's state of mind? How was it to encounter this type of attitude? Does it help to mentalize, that is, to become more aware of one's own state of mind?

The group leader explains that in treatment clinicians will try to take this attitude when considering the problems of the patient.

> *Homework*: Practice using a mentalizing stance. Those who are able to are encouraged to find a friend or someone in their family to interview in the same way as in the role-play, that is, about how the other person was earlier in the day or yesterday. Patients are encouraged to ask questions in a curious, not-knowing, and nonjudgmental way and to try to bring out as many moods, thoughts, and emotions as possible from the person they are talking to. They should note how it makes them feel and also ask the other person how it made them feel.

Adaptation for ASPD: What is mentalizing and problems with mentalizing

It is important that the group leader covers specific aspects of mentalizing in a way that the participants can understand. As a generalization, the MBT-I sessions on mentalizing allow more discussion in MBT-ASPD than in MBT-BPD, with a greater focus on antisocial interaction, aggression, and criminality. Specific detail is given about the dimensions of mentalizing to facilitate structure when considering specific problems brought to the group.

Initially, the group leader begins in the same way by defining mentalizing. Mentalizing is when we attribute intentions to each other, when we understand each other and ourselves as driven by underlying motives, and recognize that these take the form of thoughts, wishes, and various emotions, etc. A precondition for good interpersonal relations is that we understand each other—and ourselves—reasonably accurately. Similarly, we need to have some understanding of institutions and their roles, and try to have some acceptance of their strengths and weaknesses. It is always disappointing when our expectations and hopes are not met by public services, for example, and we need to develop ways of getting the most out of these services constructively. We can do this only if we are aware of their limitations.

> *Group leader*: Outline the dimensions of mentalizing. Give examples to illustrate the poles of each dimension. Draw out the dimensions on a flip chart or whiteboard. If possible, give positive illustrations of the poles and make them relevant to ASPD.

Self: Perhaps consider an example showing that we can all be selfish and consider our own needs above others. When we are like this we do not care what others want or think and we have no time for what is going on for them. We can expect them to do what we want and even insist on it by becoming coercive and intimidating. Sometimes our wishes are frustrated by others and we become preoccupied by our own loss. As an example, when we are prevented from caring for our child, perhaps if the child is in care or our partner will not allow us access to our children, we feel bereft and unable to get pleasure in our role as a parent.

Other: We can focus too much on others at times and we need to consider why we are doing this because if this focus dominates we sacrifice our own needs. On the other hand, it can make us supportive of others and helpful to them by thinking about their requirements. We often do this with our children.

Finally, we can consider other people's needs very carefully and identify them. But, rather than helping them with their problems or simply enjoying the moments with them, we can have other aims—for example, if we have a good understanding of someone we can get them to do things for us; we can even use them for our own purposes without them realizing. In these circumstances there is no real sharing in a relationship; rather, there is exploitation.

Implicit: When we interact with others in a spontaneous and natural manner, mentalizing takes place *automatically*. We do not need to exert ourselves and do not even notice that we are mentalizing (i.e., that we are interpreting other people's intentions and feelings). We simply respond to people reciprocally by making reasonable assumptions about their motives. It is only when they depart from an expected "script" or response that we are surprised due to an interruption in the spontaneous interaction. We can have two reactions to this. First, we can stop and wonder: "What happened then? Did he really understand what I meant? That's not what I meant. Let me try one more time." This is likely to lead to the interaction continuing in a constructive manner.

Second, we can react with emotion, for example, frustration, annoyance, or anger, interpreting the other person as not listening or being stupid, becoming obstructive, and dismissing them. This will end the interactional process. Yet, more often than not this will be based on a misunderstanding that could have been rectified.

> *Group leader*: Emphasize the importance of not making assumptions about other people too quickly.

Explicit: We can think about ourselves or others quite openly. We do this by verbalizing our reflections on what we feel and what we think, taking into account the context. In the group, we ask that all of us are as explicit as possible about our current states. In addition, we ask that all participants consider others' states. It is best to be explicit at points of misunderstanding or uncertainty.

> *Group leader*: Point out here that at times it will be necessary for the group leader to stop the group and to ask everyone to engage in an explicit mentalizing process. This will occur

at times when one or more members of the group become so emotional that they are in danger of "reacting" rather than thinking.

Cognition: Discuss slow and fast ways of appraising events and interactions with people. The slower method is more cognitive, meaning that we think rationally and consider the evidence for something in a relatively dispassionate way. We use this method when we want to solve a problem. So, for example, if we want to work out how to get to an appointment and what time we need to leave home, say, to arrive at the group on time, we consider things such as the transport, time needed to walk, regularity of the buses and trains, waiting time, and so on. We put all the information together and allow some additional time in case of problems, and make a reasonable assessment of the time we will need to leave. We can do the same about other people, to some extent. Some people are good at working out other people and understanding how their minds function, while others are not so good at this.

Affect: Subjectivity, or "gut reaction," is a much faster way to appraise situations. It is not necessarily worse than deductive reasoning (i.e., thinking); the group leader needs to emphasize that both ways of functioning are necessary, and one might be more appropriate than the other depending on the context. For example, if I have a feeling that a situation is dangerous, it is probably best to get out of the situation as soon as possible rather than spend time working out exactly why it is or is not dangerous. On the other hand, if I "lose my head" I may become too emotional to make sensible decisions. We require a balance of cognitive and affective process.

> *Group leader*: Make sure that the group members appreciate that both ways of functioning are helpful and that neither is better than the other. In addition, emphasize that both can be used appropriately or inappropriately.

External: Discuss the focus we all have on external and behavioral information. We tend to notice eye movements, body posture, expression, tone of voice, and facial expression, and make a judgment about someone's state of mind on the basis of this information. When we do this we are often accurate. But we can also misread external cues. People with ASPD are thought to have some general difficulties in reading emotional states, most likely fear and also possibly others. In general terms we improve our understanding of others if we take into account their internal state as well as their external appearance and do not assume that their external presentation necessarily indicates an internal state of mind. To do this we often have to use explicit mentalizing—"You sound like you don't believe me. What is it about what I am saying that you don't believe?" A disjunction between what is being expressed externally and what is going on in the interior of an individual can be made clear by discussing how we can often choose not to let people know how we are feeling and instead "put on a front." We might try to appear confident when we are anxious, we are brave when we feel frightened. So the misreading may arise because the person does not want others to know how he/she feels or because the "receiver" has misread the situation for some reason.

> *Group leader*: Make sure that the group understands this distinction. An individual might come across to someone else in a particular way but this is not necessarily how they feel. For example, someone might come across as angry because they are shouting, but actually they just "want to be heard." Treating the individual as angry might make them feel misunderstood. The way to address this is to suggest that it might help for the person to explain more about the internal state that he/she is experiencing. This is encouraged in the group.

Internal: This refers to our current internal state, how we feel and how we are thinking about something. We can express this to others or cover it up so they cannot know how we are feeling or what we are thinking.

> *Group leader*: Suggest that if we are to feel understood by others and if we are to get help it is important to begin to express how we are inside ourselves. If we cover it up we are more likely to feel misunderstood, to be less involved with others, and to be unable to obtain meaningful support.

At the end of the group, the group leader summarizes the session and makes the following suggestion to the participants:

> *Group leader*: Over the next week, make a note of an interaction between people in which you think mentalizing has been lost and report back about it next week. I will be doing the same and will also report back to you. We can also make a note of when we think we ourselves might have lost mentalizing, and if possible work out how that happened.

Module 2: What does it mean to have problems with mentalizing?

During the first meeting, the group leader will have noted who was active and who was withdrawn. In this group he/she should address sensitively those members who have been quiet so far, with the intention of getting them more involved if possible.

Summary

The group leader starts by briefly summarizing the last meeting. The main points to reiterate are:

- Mentalizing is an ability that everyone has
- Mentalizing makes us meaningful to each other

- We interpret each other automatically and do so more explicitly at times, particularly when we are muddled or uncertain. Even then, we can easily misunderstand others and ourselves because of the mind's complexity and lack of clarity

- We react differently to the same situations, our minds are multilayered, and these layers can be in conflict with each other. We often do not recognize or appreciate that others misunderstand, we can have difficulties expressing our own unclear thoughts and feelings, we may become defensive, and we deliberately hide aspects of ourselves

- Examples of poor mentalizing ability were discussed, such as an arrogant and stubborn attitude and black-and-white thinking, and use of certain words such as "just" "clearly," "always"

- End on what typifies a mentalizing stance, that is, curious exploration and a not-knowing attitude.

> *Group leader*: Ask if the group members were able to do their homework and, if so, how they found it.
> *Group leader*: Ask if anything that has been discussed so far is unclear, and whether there is anything that the group members have thought about since the last time that they wish to discuss in the group.

If patients give examples from their homework, these are discussed briefly and positive aspects of the work are identified. Similarly, if patients are unclear about what has been covered so far, this is pursued briefly. Some questions may be covered later in the program and so are covered only briefly now; rather than discussing them in any detail, the leader confirms that the questions will be answered at a later date.

Topic: Problems with mentalizing

The group leader explains that in today's meeting there will be further discussion about good and poor mentalizing abilities and the consequences of each. First, however, the group is going to undertake some mentalizing exercises. The first task is written on the worksheet for the session (as follows):

> *Group activity*[*]: It is Sarah's birthday. She is planning to celebrate with Mike, her boyfriend, and has invited him home for dinner. She has bought wine to go with the food, and is looking forward to him coming after work. When Mike arrives, he does not have a gift with him, and he says to her "Wow, what a dinner you have made, and on a Tuesday." During dinner, Sarah is quiet and drinks most of the wine herself.
> What happened? Why do you think Sarah behaves the way she does?

---

[*] This exercise was provided by Randi Kristine Abrahamsen, Clinical Psychologist, Bergen Clinics, Norway.

The group leader makes a note of all the suggestions on the board. At the end, he/she summarizes that there are several possible motives that could underlie Sarah's behavior and that these are not mutually exclusive but can complement each other. However, some motives are perhaps more important than others, and there are some interpretations that are less likely than others. Answers like "Sarah usually drinks on Tuesdays" or "Sarah usually doesn't talk when she drinks" are examples of low mentalizing. An interpretation such as "Sarah likes the wine better than Mike" also represents a low level of mentalizing. These are all descriptions and facts rather than statements about her mental state.

An interpretation that Sarah is upset and is trying to manage her feelings represents good mentalizing, not simply because it is likely to be more accurate, but also because it tries to establish Sarah's mental state in relation to her behavior. Some patients may think that Sarah should have said something; if this is the case, the group leader should ask the patients to consider why Sarah did not express what was going on in her mind. The raising of this issue is very positive, not because the patients seem to "know" how someone "should" behave (this would be a nonmentalizing position because it included knowing and absolutes), but because discussion of this issue can stimulate further mentalizing about Sarah's state of mind.

The example serves as a "warm-up" exercise and an introduction to the theme of the consequences of poor mentalizing skills. The group leader summarizes again what was discussed the last time with respect to what typifies poor mentalizing:

◆ Feeling certain about other people's motives

◆ Thinking in black-and-white terms (i.e., without nuances)

◆ Poor acknowledgement of accompanying feelings (little empathy)

◆ Overlooking the fact that people influence each other

◆ Interpretation of others without careful consideration may be irrelevant, be off the point, or even be very concrete (i.e., that first this happened then that happened, etc.)

◆ Little curiosity about mental states

◆ Lots of words are spoken with unelaborated content—that is, no real meaning

◆ Speech is filled with clichés and fancy words that do not seem to have been digested and that tend to alienate the other person

◆ External factors are emphasized at the expense of mental states, for example, that it was raining, or that one had a headache, or the situation is described as being "just how it was," without any more explanation.

Group activity: The group leader asks about possible consequences of poor mentalizing:

1 In relation to others
2 In relation to oneself.

The group leader writes the suggestions made by the group members on the flip chart or whiteboard. Typical answers include:

- It is easy to misunderstand each other and this can have negative consequences (e.g., others feel overlooked, not heard, or wrongly interpreted, and become upset about it, etc.)
- One's actual behavior may differ from the other person's expectations, which can confuse the other person
- One may react in a very emotional way based on misunderstandings, and become afraid, angry, disappointed, etc.
- Poor mentalizing of one's own thoughts and emotions means that one does not always understand one's own reasons for acting the way one does and may cause one to second-guess oneself
- Feeling insecure or needing constant confirmation from others
- Becoming overwhelmed by emotions or acting without reflection (i.e., letting the surroundings or one's own impulses govern one's actions, etc.).

Some patients may give other responses such as "I can always understand other people" or "I find that no one understands me." The group leader has to take such suggestions sensitively and empathize initially with such experiences, but should do this for only a short time and may close the conversation by suggesting that it is something that can be explored further in later treatment. The emphasis should be on using such statements as examples of early warning signs of compromised mentalizing—the use of the words "always" and "no one" are the key. The group leader can suggest that being alert to such words might help to prevent a collapse into nonmentalizing by making the individual "think twice" about what he/she is saying and experiencing. Could there be other possibilities? Is it likely that someone will *always* be right? Are we sure that we understand others *perfectly*?

The group leader summarizes that poor mentalizing leads to:

1 Recurrent problems in relationships with other people
2 Insecurity, an unstable sense of self, poor emotional control, impulsivity, and compromised personal potential.

The group leader says that he/she now is getting a bit ahead of the program since this is a topic for the next session, but that it is important in this context to emphasize that the most important cause of poor mentalizing is strong emotional activation. When emotions are intense, a person's mentalizing ability is undermined, and may even be shut down completely, exemplified by expressions such as "I went into the red zone and that was it," "Everything turned black," "I just froze up," "I couldn't say a thing," "I wasn't able to think." Additional phrases suggested by the group participants can be listed.

Group activity: The participants are asked to think through their own experiences and make some notes about what their own typical reaction patterns are when they become emotional.

The group leader asks if anyone would like to share their own experiences. These are then discussed.

The group leader draws up a curve to illustrate the connection between mentalizing and emotional activation and the transition to the fight/flight response.

The group leader emphasizes four important points:

1 Feelings are activated faster and more strongly in some people than others

2 The most common activating factor is sensitivity in relationships and attachment stress (it can be pointed out that in BPD the sensitive area is mostly that of interpersonal interaction, and this will be discussed more in the sessions on attachment)

3 The fight/flight response can kick in at different times for different people, depending on the individual's personal threshold

4 The time it takes to return to a normal state after intense emotional activation also varies among people.

Group activity: Participants are asked to reflect and make notes on the worksheet about what they think about themselves with respect to emotional activation. What is their sensitive trigger? What is the threshold of their fight/flight response? How long does it take for them to regain their normal state of mind after intense emotional activation?

The group leader asks if anyone wishes to share their reflections. These are discussed.

The group leader emphasizes that these four points are important themes for the treatment: emotional intensity can be controlled, relationships can be influenced positively, the threshold for activation can be raised, and the time it takes before someone gets back to their normal state can be reduced. These issues will be discussed in later sessions.

Homework: Make a note of a situation during the week in which you have noticed that your ability to mentalize was undermined.

Module 3: Why do we have emotions and what are the basic types?

Summary

The group leader summarizes the topic from the last session. The session addressed problems with mentalizing that typically lead to problems in interactions with others. Some key points were:

◆ Indicators of good and poor mentalizing
◆ Difficulties reading one's own and others' minds

- ◆ Problems regulating emotions and impulsivity
- ◆ Interpersonal sensitivity.

The most important reasons for poor mentalizing are:

- ◆ Interpersonal sensitivity in a close relationship
- ◆ Emotional activation, which can make a person unable to function
- ◆ The intensity of emotions, which varies between individuals
- ◆ The threshold for the fight/flight response, which also varies
- ◆ The variable time it takes to regain one's composure after strong emotional activation.

The group leader reminds the group about the homework assignment and asks if anyone was able to make a note of anything that they wish to share.

Topic: Emotions

The group leader introduces the day's topic. He/she invites everyone to brainstorm the topic and writes down the emotions they suggest on the board or flip chart. He/she also asks participants to think about why emotions are important. People with BPD find emotions hard to manage and tend to try to get rid of them, but in doing so they reduce their capacities to mentalize—that is, to understand their own states of mind and those of others.

As the participants name different emotions the group leader writes them down in two columns, but without explaining why. In one column he/she writes the emotions that are later to be defined as *basic emotions* and in the other he/she writes those that are *social emotions*.

> *Group activity*: What types of emotions are there? Why are emotions important? Any suggestions . . . ?

Basic and social emotions

When the activity starts to ebb, the group leader adds some emotions if the lists written down are insufficient. The group leader suggests that *there is a difference between basic emotions and social emotions. This is why he/she has written the emotions down in two columns.*

Basic emotions are emotions that exist in all mammals, while *social emotions* exist in more developed primates and humans. Basic emotions are localized in the same area in the brain, evoke the same physical reactions, and each of them is linked to a set reaction pattern.

The group leader asks the members to suggest other basic emotions that are not already on the list. If no further suggestions are made, he/she then identifies the missing emotions. The group leader explains that there is some disagreement about which emotions are basic, and that we have chosen to present one version (following Panksepp (1998)).

An emphasis is placed on the basic emotion of *curiosity* and playful exploratory behavior. These are key to mentalizing but are almost never suggested by participants as basic emotions—and yet without them life is untenable. We illustrate the importance of these basic emotions, which may have been understandably "lost" during childhood and adolescent development as a result of trauma and neglect, in the following way:

1 Ask the patients who has a cat (in the MBT-I for MBT-ASPD, we instead ask who has a dog). Often a number of patients raise their hand.

2 Ask them what their cat/dog was like when he/she was a kitten/puppy.

At this point the pet owners are likely to describe continuous play and curiosity. This is how young mammals like kittens and puppies (and children!) learn about the world; discovery propels development. Once we lose curiosity, we close our minds down and fail to learn; when we cannot play, we lose creativity. Participants understand this and yet may find it difficult to rekindle such emotions and may even be cynical about their usefulness, which is understandable given their experience. But the group leader persists in emphasizing their importance for everyday life and relationships, and underlines the necessity for the patients to anticipate that clinicians will be curious about their experiences throughout treatment, and that the patients will need to be curious about their own and others' experiences.

The group leader summarizes the seven basic emotions as follows:

1 Interest and curiosity, exploratory behavior

2 Fear

3 Anger

4 Sexual lust

5 Love/caring

6 Separation anxiety/sadness

7 Play/joy.

The group leader asks if anyone has any comments and if anyone is surprised that other emotions are not on the list. The group leader reminds everyone that there is a certain degree of disagreement about this list. And the list is not meant to diminish the importance of emotions like envy, jealousy, greed, gratitude, guilt, shame, pride, etc.

The group leader asks, rhetorically, *why would these basic emotions be important for us?* He/she confirms any suggestions that are related to evolution (e.g., that these feelings have been shown to be important with respect to survival and reproduction) and that they represent an innate preparedness to react to certain triggers. We do not need to learn these emotions or reaction patterns because they are determined by nature (but we can still distance ourselves from them—a topic that will be discussed later). They supply us with automatic responses that have been important for human survival over the course of millions of years.

The group leader then describes the main purpose of the seven fundamental emotions, as follows:

1 *Interest and curiosity/exploratory behavior.* This motivates us to find out useful information about our surroundings (e.g., what resources are available, where food and water can be obtained, whether there is a safe place to hide, whether there are any sexual partners around, etc.).

2 *Fear.* This stimulates us to ask ourselves questions such as: Is what I am facing dangerous? Can it injure me? Could it kill me? Is he/she a rival who is stronger than I am? Is he/she an enemy? When the fear becomes intense enough and the source seems stronger than oneself, it prompts our decision to flee or submit. Fear can also prompt us to freeze/play dead if the threat is overwhelming and we are in mortal danger.

3 *Anger.* If we identify someone or something that is standing in our way, we may show anger and see whether he/she submits. If the person resists, the intensity of anger will increase, which may possibly lead us to attack.

4 *Sexual lust.* This encourages reproduction and the continuation of one's genes.

5 *Love/caring.* This motivates us to care for our children, family, partner, and friends.

6 *Separation anxiety/sadness.* These emotions function as an appeal for others to take care of us. They signal to potential caregivers that one is in danger/in need of protection or that one has become isolated from the group/family, or that one has lost someone close who one depends on.

7 *Play/joy.* This stimulates interaction with others so that one remains a "pack animal" rather than a hermit, increases our skills of interacting with others, introduces the limits to one's own excitement, and enables children's development of strategies for dealing with anger through rough-and-tumble play.

The group leader discusses reactions to this description. As the seven descriptions suggest, basic emotions are essentially different action programs.

Primary and secondary emotions

It can be helpful for patients to consider the basic and social emotions as some-times being *primary* and *secondary* emotional states. The basic emotion comes first in response to something and the secondary emotions tend to come after-wards and block the experience or expression of the first emotion. As we have suggested, the basic emotions are survival and adaptive experiences, which are essential and inform action and reaction. Many patients will try to avoid them but in doing so will diminish their ability to appraise situations and themselves. In other words, emotions are to be relished as part of the information that helps us mentalize; without them our capacities are reduced.

An example is that we might feel angry in a situation and this leads us to feel ashamed. The anger may be an appropriate emotion in the circumstances but becomes overshadowed by our secondary experience of shame, which is a social emotion. Patients often become tortured by the secondary emotional state, which in many circumstances is maladaptive and unhelpful. In addition, clinicians can become distracted by the secondary emotional state and not attend to the primary emotion (anger). In full empathic validation in MBT, it is important to target the primary emotional state if the patient is to feel under-stood and to begin to recognize the complexity of his/her state of mind with feelings being intertwined.

The group leader explains that humans, unlike other animals, have the ability to suppress the feelings of emotional reactions. That is why the relationship between emotions and feelings sometimes seems obscure. The distinction that we mention here should be used only if any participants ask about the difference. Many groups do not have the capacity to discuss feelings and emotions at this level and, if not, it is best to consider feelings and emotions as synonymous.

If appropriate, the group leader emphasizes the difference between:

- *Emotions*, which are the individual's bodily reaction, as action programs, to specific stimuli
- *Feelings*, which are the conscious experience of the body state during emo-tional activation.

The group leader explains that because of their upbringing and socialization, peo-ple can be distanced from their natural, emotional reactions. This means that peo-ple can react emotionally, but that they do not necessarily feel their emotions. Emotions can be suppressed. You can therefore be emotionally activated, but at the same time be unaware of the specific nature of the emotions involved. One can, for example, feel heart palpitations or bodily unease without knowing why. The group leader explains that the reason for this will be addressed and discussed later.

Group activity: The group is encouraged to discuss the emotions listed earlier in relation to themselves and their individual differences. Questions to be considered include whether everyone in the group feels these emotions, and whether each person experiences them with equal frequency and intensity.

The participants discuss their different reactions and experiences. The group leader reminds them about the importance of a mentalizing attitude (i.e., an openness and curiosity in relation to people's differences).

Homework: What emotions have been the most prominent in the past week? Or has the emotional activation been diffuse, that is, more of a physical unease?

Module 4: Mentalizing emotions

Summary

The group leader summarizes the introduction to emotions discussed in the last meeting. He/she highlights that everyone has a wide range of emotions and they can be divided into basic and social emotions and considered as primary and secondary. All mammals experience basic emotions, and they are as follows:

◆ Interest and curiosity

◆ Fear

◆ Anger

◆ Sexual lust

◆ Love/caring

◆ Separation anxiety/sadness

◆ Play/joy.

The emotions are triggered by specific stimuli and consist of physiological reactions. Feelings are the conscious awareness of these bodily reactions. It is possible for people to become emotionally activated without having a conscious awareness of the feelings.

The group leader then asks if anyone has made any notes about emotions and/or feelings they have experienced in the past week that they wish to share with the group. These are discussed.

Topic: Mentalizing emotions

The topic this time is how to deal with emotions and feelings. As we have discussed earlier, this is a very important mental health issue. First of all, the question of how we recognize and name different emotions needs to be addressed.

Group activity: How do we register emotions:
1 In others?
2 In ourselves?

The group leader encourages discussion, with an overall aim of identifying two primary ways in which emotions are registered.

The ensuing discussion commonly gradually identifies the first of these, namely, we register others' emotions by *interpreting* their facial expressions (the "soul's mirror"). This is consistent across all cultures and, to some extent, across animal species. We also interpret others' body language, what they do and what they say. This is *external mentalizing*, which was discussed in Module 1. People vary in their ability to be sensitive to others' emotions, and sometimes people can understand how someone else feels even when the other person is not yet fully aware of it.

The second pathway by which we understand others' emotions is via *identification* with the other person. There are nerve cells called *mirror neurons* in the brain that enable us to experience what someone else is experiencing when we observe them doing something or expressing a feeling. For example, when we see another person feeling sad, we can become sad ourselves. This is part of the basis of *empathy*.

Self and emotions

The discussion can then move on to the ways in which we register bodily reactions (examples of these should be given) and feeling states (which can also be referred to as *affect consciousness*) in ourselves. The group leader can remind members that they touched upon this in the previous session, when they discussed how people differ with respect to their feelings and how they register their emotions—some people do so more easily than others.

Most often, the group participants will be better at giving examples of how feelings are expressed by others than how they feel themselves. The group leader can offer some examples, such as "lump in your throat," "pressure behind the eyes," "weak at the knees," "hairs standing on end," as being indicators of how we feel in ourselves.

The group leader then introduces a group exercise that stimulates thinking about emotional awareness. Some improvement in understanding our emotions can be made simply by being more aware and "being more present in one's own body"—that is, being more vigilant and self-reflective about our internal states.

Group activity: The group leader asks the members to close their eyes and forget the surroundings and focus on themselves. He/she directs their attention inwards, asking such questions as:

- Is there any place in your body that attracts your attention?
- What do you feel?
- Try to feel if there is any trace of emotional activation. Perhaps not, but there often is.
- What types of feelings are you experiencing? (If it's very uncomfortable, leave it alone, but if it's comfortable, try to stay with it.)

This should not last long and the leader should be clear that the most important thing is that each group member is turning his/her attention toward his/her inner experience.

Participants' experiences are then discussed. For some, this exercise may evoke feelings of anxiety, and this should be acknowledged by the group leader. Occasionally, a patient may be unable to do the exercise at all and may even have a paranoid reaction (one patient said that he thought the group leader was trying to control him). Redefine this as fear, which ensures that it is on the list of basic emotions, and emphasize that the person can retain control after all. Some people will report that their physical experiences blocked feelings during the exercise (e.g., that they were too busy breathing to pay attention to what they were feeling), while others may report different emotional states.

Others and emotions

The group leader then turns to the subject of *emotional regulation through others and how others can recognize how we feel*. He/she briefly introduces the topic and says that they are going to do an emotional regulation exercise that everyone is likely to be familiar with: namely, consoling another person.

> *Group activity*: Role-play about emotional regulation through others. The group leader asks one of the participants to act being emotionally upset, perhaps a mixture of disappointment and anger. If none of the participants feel comfortable taking the role, the group leader him/herself can play the role. Another group member is given the following assignment:
>
> 1 To find out what feelings the person has
> 2 To find out why he/she feels this way
> 3 To try to console the person.

The participants' experiences are discussed with a focus on the issue of the patients' willingness or unwillingness to let someone else console them. The group can then discuss, based on other experiences, what behavior/actions by another person they have found most consoling (e.g., empathic understanding, emotional resonance, physical contact, etc.), with an acknowledgement that each person will be different.

> *Group activity*: The group leader asks the participants what it is like when other people tell them how they feel: "Let's discuss what it is like for you when a close person tells you how you feel. Do they often get it right or do they seem to miss how you feel, and if so, are you able to explain your feeling to them?"

The group leader tries to identify that some patients feel profoundly misunderstood a lot of the time and this makes them feel alone, abandoned, hurt, etc. Often, people react to these feelings with anger, which is a secondary emotion in this context but is also a primary emotion as it increases the chance of survival of the self—"I am someone." New ways of reacting are needed to manage this response—these can be discussed.

Emotional regulation

The group leader now brings up the topic of impaired emotional regulation. Impairment of emotional regulation means that one is stuck in a painful, uncomfortable, and often unclear emotional state and may resort to dramatic means (such as getting high or self-harming) to escape from it.

> *Group activity*: The group leader asks the group members to suggest names for such unpleasant emotional states and writes these on a flip chart. The group leader then asks for examples of what the participants have done to get out of such emotional states.

The group leader labels such emotional states *unmentalized feelings* and emphasizes the importance of talking about such experiences in therapy. While in such a state, one can do very self-destructive things. It is important to try to reduce the time spent in such a state, and to practice some of the positive ways people have suggested to manage their emotional states.

Initially, it is useful to suggest that many helpful techniques are simply ways of reducing bodily tension, as the basic emotions are felt with changes in the body—for example, fearfulness and anxiety are signaled by a change in heart rate, sweating, and feeling short of breath, as well as suddenly becoming vigilant and wary mentally. Managing these bodily sensations of over-arousal is a first stage that takes precedence over developing ways to cope with interpersonal sensitivity. The group leader can inform the group that interpersonal sensitivity will be discussed at a later stage, in the module on anxiety.

- Discuss relaxation techniques that they can use:
  - Progressive muscle relaxation
  - Breathing skills
  - Silence and meditation stance
  - Mindfulness.

Some practice of these techniques may take place if the group leader is skilled in the techniques and time allows. Many patients find this useful, and it is necessary for the group leader to return again and again to the practice of relaxation techniques in the groups and to do so at times of tension in the group itself. The group leader needs to be comfortable with running brief relaxation exercises and be able to motivate the patients to practice them at home.

- ◆ Outline other basic strategies used for anxiety:
  - • Distraction by engaging in other activities: Clinicians teach that distraction, by definition, avoids emotion experiencing, and so should be used as little as possible. However, it can be used to prevent a destructive downward spiral
  - • Recognizing that anxiety can arise from automatic thoughts: if an emotion occurs, the patients are asked to consider the associated feeling as a stimulus to thinking about what they are feeling—"What am I thinking right now or what was I thinking just before I had this feeling?"

Homework: Make a note of at least one occasion during the past week when you managed to effectively regulate a problematic emotional state.

Module 5: The significance of attachment relationships

Summary

The group leader summarizes the contents of the last session, including how we register feelings in ourselves and others; interpreting inner emotional signals in ourselves and emotional expressions in others; self-regulation of feelings and how others can help regulate our feelings; unmentalized feelings that are very uncomfortable; and how we can manage such emotional states.

The group leader asks if anyone would like to share an experience of positive emotional regulation from the previous week.

Topic: Attachment

The group leader then introduces the day's main topic: attachment. He/she links this immediately to feelings and emotional regulation, and defines it as follows:

> Attachment is a positive feeling and emotional bond toward another human being.

The first attachment relationships are with your parents/caregivers and other family members. These attachment relationships will later influence your relationships and interaction patterns with others, for good and for bad. Attachment is a phenomenon shown by all mammals. Its purpose is to protect vulnerable offspring against dangers and promote affectionate bonds between relatives. When a young child experiences something uncomfortable (e.g., hunger, thirst, frustration, or fear), he/she instinctively turns toward the attachment person, with an expectation of being comforted by them. The attachment person has an equally instinctive reaction to the child's signals of unease (e.g., whimpering and crying), which show that the caregiver needs to attend to the child in some way. For the child to become emotionally regulated in this way—to be given food or something to drink, to become less fearful, smiled at and comforted, and so on—leads to the establishment of an inner image of the attachment person that is associated with well-being (reward). So eventually just the thought of the attachment person can be enough to calm oneself initially. This is the standard path to emotional self-regulation. But, before one has achieved the ability to self-regulate, being separated from the attachment figure may lead to feelings of unease and fear, which are known as *separation anxiety* and *sadness*.

The group leader summarizes that the attachment process means we learn to understand and regulate our emotions "through" someone else. This process continues throughout life, even though we begin to regulate our emotions ourselves.

Humans can have different *attachment patterns*. In children, this can be tested by observing how a child reacts when he/she is separated from the attachment person, who is most often the child's mother. The test situation begins with the mother and child being together in a room. The mother leaves the room after a while and leaves the child alone; then, an unfamiliar person (an observer) enters the room. The situation of being both abandoned and in a room with a complete stranger triggers separation anxiety and fear in most children. The observer watches how the child deals with this situation and how he/she reacts when the mother enters the room again after some time. Children with so-called *secure attachment* react with unease and protest when the mother is about to leave them, but relax after a while and start to play with some of the toys in the room. When the mother returns, the child goes to the mother and will often cry a bit, but will quickly calm down, possibly by sitting on her lap. After a short time the child will usually resume playing.

Some children, however, have what is called an *insecure attachment pattern*. There are two types of insecure attachment patterns: an *ambivalent/overinvolved* type and a *distancing/avoidant* type.

In the ambivalent/overinvolved pattern, or "clinging attachment," the child is insecure about his/her attachment person—in all likelihood with good reason, because the person has behaved unpredictably toward them (i.e., the attachment person has been erratic in response and presence). In order to attract the attachment person's attention, the child has learned to exaggerate his/her emotional expressions (e.g., they express an excessive amount of unease and crying). When such a child is abandoned in the test situation, he/she cries loudly and clings to the mother when she is about to leave the room. The child then has difficulty quietening down and playing while the mother is away. When the mother returns, the child is ambivalent in relation to her, and cries and protests when she goes to pick the child up, but quietens down gradually. It takes longer for the insecurely attached child to start playing again after this experience. It is as if the child needs to hold on to the mother for fear that she will leave again. In other words, the child takes some time to recover from the emotions triggered by the separation.

The other insecure pattern, distancing/avoidant, is in many ways the opposite of the ambivalent/overinvolved type. While ambivalently attached children have exaggerated emotional reactions, distancing/avoidant children show little response; they are "detached." They do not seem to react at all to being abandoned by their mother in the test situation. It is as if they do not care whether the mother leaves or returns. When these children's physical responses are measured, they have been shown to be stressed in the situation, but they *express this stress to a very little degree*. They have learned to over-regulate their feelings. These children may have experienced their feelings commonly being overlooked, or consistently misunderstood and thought to be something else, or they may have been ridiculed or tormented for what they were feeling, or experienced other negative consequences from expressing their feelings.

Attachment patterns are thus dependent on, and develop from, interactions with one's early attachment persons. Since these interactions have much to do with how the child attracts attention, one can also call them *attachment strategies* on the part of the child. This is not to be confused with the idea of "attention-seeking" behavior. Some patients and their helpers see certain symptoms of BPD as ways of deliberately trying to get attention—for example, taking an overdose. Nothing could be further from the truth, however, and it is important that the group leader emphasizes that the idea of "attention-seeking" behavior is *not* part of the mentalizing framework of understanding.

It is also possible for the insecure attachment strategies, to be mixed. For example, a person might sometimes act ambivalently, and at other times be distanced.

The attachment pattern influences individuals from childhood. However, it is not fixed, and it can change during childhood. It also exerts an influence on one's relationship patterns as an adult: it determines to a large extent how one deals with close relationships, and particularly with situations that cause pain or when there is a danger or fear of being abandoned. Is the other person a source of security and enjoyable experiences, or is the relationship characterized by insecurity and drama, or is it distanced and emotionally "flat"? *The way a person regulates his/her attachment relationships is of major significance for his/her life.*

Group activity: Tom and his girlfriend, Sara, meet again after the university holidays. During the holidays, Tom has not called Sara, and when she called or sent a text message he did not answer. Sara did very little during her holidays, but when Tom asked her about it she answered: "I had a fantastic holiday with plenty to do. I wish the holiday had lasted longer."

Discuss this episode in light of attachment strategies for Tom and Sara.

Finally: Why does Sara answer as she does?

This exercise serves as a kind of run-up to the next exercise, in order to activate the participants in thinking about attachment and so that the group leader can correct any misunderstandings.

Group activity: Think about a relationship with an important person in your life (e.g., girlfriend, boyfriend, family member, or friend) and think about whether the relationship is secure, ambivalent, or distanced.

This activity occupies the main part of the session. Here, the participants are trying to chart their own attachment pattern. They are asked to decide whether their main pattern is secure, ambivalent, or distancing, and to give evidence for why they have alighted on a particular pattern. Many patients give examples that suggest they are both ambivalent/clinging *and* distancing/avoidant. Participants' recognition that they have a mix of attachment strategies is encouraged by the group leader. This recognition means that participants are thinking about themselves in detail and also beginning to recognize that their responses might depend on the different interpersonal contexts of the relationships they are thinking about. The group leader clarifies question about attachment through the examples of the participants.

Homework: Make notes on what is typical for you in your attachment relationships.

Module 6: Attachment and mentalizing

Summary

The group leader summarizes the last session:

Attachment refers to a positive emotional bond with another person. Our typical attachment strategies as an adult are influenced by the attachment pattern that was established in childhood. Typical attachment strategies are *secure* and *insecure* attachment patterns. The insecure attachment patterns can be described as *ambivalent/overinvolved/clinging* and *distanced/detached/avoidant*.

Each of the participants was encouraged to explore a relationship with an important person in light of their different attachment strategies.

The home assignment involved thinking more about what has been typical of one's attachment relationships. The group leader asks if anyone wishes to share the homework. This is discussed.

Topic: Attachment and mentalizing

Growing up in a mentalizing culture promotes secure attachment, which facilitates a person's mentalizing abilities.

A *mentalizing culture* implies a culture with frequent discussions about people and why they behave the way they do, for example, why people do what they do within the family. A mentalizing culture is necessary to help manage any significant events that affect anyone in the family. Discussion about experiences needs to be done with a reasonable degree of open-mindedness, minimal certainty, and without triggering any oppressive family taboos.

The group participants are informed that the treatment program strives toward a mentalizing culture. In the groups and in individual MBT sessions, for example, there is a constant effort to find out about one's own and others' minds and their transactions. This will be re-emphasized in Modules 8 and 9 of MBT-I.

> *Group activity*: What characterizes the family culture of each individual participant with respect to mentalizing?

The group leader leads the discussion on this topic. There are likely to be examples of oppressive silence, anxious family get-togethers (e.g., at birthdays and Christmas), unspoken taboo areas, chaotic family discussions, and so on. The group leader must be prepared for the possibility that the topic in this session may activate painful memories and strong emotions for the participants. Again, the group leader must emphasize that this is a topic that can be explored further later, especially the consequences for each individual.

More specifically, the family environment and attachment experience during childhood has consequences for a person's mentalizing abilities. There may be many reasons for such a situation. The attachment person (parent/caregiver) may not have been available physically or mentally; the person may not have had the ability to listen, understand, or be empathic. There may have been—and indeed may still be—someone else in the way (e.g., a sibling or other parent); the attachment person may not have had good caregiving skills, or there may have been an environment of mental or physical abuse or substance abuse. The end result is often *attachment conflict*.

Attachment conflict means that one inhibits or exaggerates signals about one's emotional state because one fears or is insecure about what will happen if one seeks out or calls for the attachment person. Attachment conflict means that a person's impulse to get closer to an attachment person is inhibited by something else (e.g., fear of punishment, or own wish to punish).

> *Group activity*: Make a note of your own examples of attachment conflicts.

The group leader leads the discussion about attachment conflicts that have been noted and brings the conversation on to the subject of the likely consequences that this may have for a person's mentalizing abilities.

He/she brings up the idea that *attachment relationships are important in order for a child to become aware of their own emotional states, to be able to put words to these states, find out the reasons for them, and use emotions to orient themselves in a mental landscape.*

There will be negative consequences for a person's mentalizing abilities if their relationship to their attachment person(s) is disorganized and insecure in childhood. The child cannot use the attachment person to understand his/her own feelings and relationships, and so is on his/her own in trying to understand these. In addition, it becomes difficult to think around the attachment relationship itself, because the child lacks mental reference "anchors." This can become easier over time as one grows up and gains other references, and can see things from the outside and compare them with other experiences. It is particularly difficult to think about a relationship if it is characterized by violence and (sexual) abuse—how can one begin to understand why a person who should be treating one with care and love is behaving in such a way, with complete disregard for one's well-being?

Attachment conflicts inhibit a child's mentalizing abilities right from the start, and leave behind emotional scars and confusion. They undermine the child's ability to deal with attachment conflicts later in adult life.

> *Group activity*: Make a note of something you find difficult to talk about in a close relationship and what the reason(s) for this may be.

The group leader takes notes and leads the discussion on this topic.

> *Homework*: Make a note of something that has been difficult to talk about in a close relationship in the past week.

Module 7: What is a personality disorder? What is borderline personality disorder? What is antisocial personality disorder?

Summary

The group leader briefly summarizes the topic and discussion from the last session:

- Growing up in a mentalizing culture promotes the ability to mentalize
- Major attachment conflicts in childhood impair this ability
- Impaired mentalizing ability makes it difficult to deal with conflicts in close relationships (e.g., thinking often becomes black and white, emotions will tend to overwhelm the ability to think, etc.).

The group leader asks if anyone wants to share experiences from their homework assignment relating to difficulties speaking about something in close relationships.

Topic: Personality disorders

The group leader then turns attention to the topic of the day, namely, personality disorders.

At this point the group leader takes a didactic approach, outlining the current understanding of personality disorder. Key areas to cover here are:

1 A person can be said to have a personality disorder when his/her personality shows a certain number of maladaptive (unhelpful) personality traits, which are typical ways of thinking, feeling, regulating impulses, and relating to other people. The traits need to have been characteristic of the person since at least late adolescence or early adulthood and have been relatively consistent since that time.

2 Personality traits typically affect self-image and self-esteem, but also influence ways of thinking about others, and will usually cause problems in schooling, work, and/or family life (e.g., being shy, not self-assertive, extremely suspicious, dependent on others, having an uncontrolled temper, always avoiding conflict, etc.).

3 A personality disorder does not affect the entire personality. One can have many good and positive personality traits and many talents in addition to those that are problematic. For example, the famous artists Edvard Munch and Francis Bacon most probably had a personality disorder, to the extent that they had major problems interacting with others. Nevertheless, they were both extremely skillful and innovative painters. (The group leader might also like to consider some prominent politicians too!)

> *Group activity*: Ask each group member to make a note of:
> 1 His/her own problematic personality traits
> 2 His/her good and positive personality traits and any talents.
> Alternatively, ask each member to write down "What makes me 'me'" (i.e., what are his/her individual characteristics).

The group leader asks if anyone wishes to share the notes they have made about themselves, makes a list of key words on the board/flip chart, and leads the discussion.

Following this discussion, the group leader outlines a positive view of personality disorders in terms of their changeability. Personality disorders are *not* necessarily permanent. Many traits can change with age, which usually results in a person becoming more relaxed, less intense, and learning to deal with situations in a better way. Problems can pop up again during times of stress, for example, in connection with work problems or problems in close relationships (e.g., separation and divorce). Personality disorders improve more quickly with treatment—for example, with MBT. Personality disorders may also have a better naturalistic outcome, in terms of improvement, than depression.

Next, the group leader discusses the origins of personality disorders, but does not go into great detail. Personality disorders arise as a result of a combination of genetic influences (on temperament and vulnerabilities) and negative environmental influences during childhood, such as early loss of a parent, neglect, abuse, or trauma. Depending on the balance of these factors, certain characteristics may come to dominate our ways of relating to others and these, in turn, define the different personality disorders.

The group leader now outlines the classification of personality disorders, briefly reviewing key features of the various types:

1 Schizotypal personality disorder: very shy and suspicious, few friends, bizarre views

2 Schizoid personality disorder: flat affect, little need to be together with others, prefers doing most things alone

3 Paranoid personality disorder: suspicious, uncompromising, and temperamental

4 Antisocial personality disorder: repeated criminal acts, ruthless, aggressive, little capacity for caregiving

5 Borderline personality disorder: unstable relationships, unstable emotions, fluctuating self-image

6 Narcissistic personality disorder: grandiose sense of self, arrogant, lacking in empathy

7 Histrionic personality disorder: theatricality, exaggerated expression of emotions, plays on sexuality, constantly draws attention to self

8 Avoidant personality disorder: anxious, inhibited in new interpersonal situations, reluctant to take personal risks, excessively fearful of criticism or ridicule

9 Dependent personality disorder: lack of self-confidence, goes to excessive lengths to obtain nurturance from others, constantly needs advice and reassurance from others

10 Obsessive–compulsive personality disorder: rigid and stubborn, preoccupied with order and schedules, difficulty delegating tasks to others, perfectionist

11 "Personality disorder not otherwise specified": insufficient traits to meet the threshold for any one of the other listed personality disorders, but has several traits characteristic of many personality disorders.

The group leader now leads a discussion about the different personality disorders; it is at the discretion of the leader how many of the categories of personality disorder he/she discusses.

Borderline personality disorder

The group leader goes through the criteria for BPD with reference to mentalizing. He/she explains that these are the traits that are most often found in people in the MBT program, while emphasizing that many participants may have other personality traits that they have problems with as well.

Criteria for BPD:

1 *Intense and unstable relationships, alternating between extremes of idealization and devaluation*: quickly enters into new romantic relationships, idealizes the other person, and allows him/herself to be seduced or infatuated, which reduces his/her social judgment; does the opposite when disappointment arrives, seeing only the negative in the person where before they could see only the positive.

2 *Has difficulties with being alone and strong feelings associated with being abandoned*: therefore, he/she makes desperate efforts to avoid being abandoned, for example, allowing him/herself to be treated poorly, acting submissively, carrying out dramatic acts such as injuring him/herself, or threatening to commit suicide

3 *Identity problems*: fluctuating self-esteem, unstable self-image, constant changes in life goals, difficulties in holding on to one's inner core self

4 *Impulsivity that can be self-destructive* (i.e., impulsive risk-taking): for example, purchasing things one can't afford, driving recklessly and/or above the speed limit, acting on poorly considered decisions, promiscuity, abuse/misuse of alcohol and drugs, etc.

5 *Self-destructive acts*: such as self-mutilation and suicide attempts (to regulate painful emotional states)

6 *Recurrent feelings of inner emptiness and meaninglessness*

7 *Constant mood swings*: for example, fluctuating between intense dysphoria and euphoria in a single day, or between happiness and sadness, bitterness or anger

8 *Intense anger that is difficult to control* (e.g., that may result in throwing things, swearing or physical fighting)

9 *Reacting with suspiciousness or a feeling of being outside of oneself when stressed.*

We have adapted the formal diagnostic criteria into a series of initial screening questions, in everyday language, that can be asked of the participants to help stimulate the discussion:

1 Are you scared of rejection and abandonment, and being left all alone?
2 Are your relationships with your friends and family unstable?
3 Do you see things as either all good or all bad, 100% right or 100% wrong, as black and white, or in absolute terms, for example, "Everybody is . . .," "All men are . . . "?
4 Do you have trouble knowing who you are and what is important to you?
5 Do you impulsively do things that might damage yourself in some way or without planning or caring about the consequence?
6 Do you self-harm (intentional harm to body, including overdoses) or behave in a suicidal manner?
7 Do you have mood swings that can change quickly?
8 Do you feel empty and feel you need others to fill you up and make you whole?
9 Do you get excessively angry in a manner that is to your own detriment?
10 Do you "numb out" (dissociate) or sometimes feel overly suspicious or paranoid when stressed?

The group leader clarifies and discusses the traits as they are presented. It is important that the group leader maintains a mentalizing perspective during the review and discussion.

> *Homework assignment*: Make a note of the personality traits that are problematic for you over the next week.

A leaflet summarizing aspects of BPD is given to the participants.

Adaptation for ASPD

After the discussion about "What is a personality disorder?" and following completion of the exercise of the participants identifying problem areas of their own personality, many of the features of ASPD will have been identified. The group leader uses this information to outline the key features of ASPD. These features may be discussed in a more general way than the current descriptive characteristics in classification systems:

♦ Tendency to be against authority and to engage in persistent unlawful behavior
♦ Sensitivity to others and their motives, often thinking that people do things deliberately to us

- Feelings of being "picked on" by authority (e.g., the police) and of being unfairly treated by systems such as housing, benefits, and employment
- Often finding it necessary to cover things up or not to be fully honest
- Failure to plan and instead finding oneself "doing things"
- Blaming others for events and for our own actions
- Not feeling sorry when we hurt someone, because the other person was to blame or deserved it
- Not caring about safety of oneself or others when involved in problematic interactions
- General aggressive attitude, sometimes leading to fights.

The group leader points out that this sort of pattern describes people's behavior as well as some of their attitudes, and does not help people think about what makes people behave like this or why they may have developed certain attitudes. Neither does it indicate how they might change. These issues are the subject of the next few sessions, and some of the work in the group will be establishing how to change the important problematic areas defined by the participants themselves.

Now, the group leader digresses to cover aspects of ASPD that interfere markedly with treatment. First, people with ASPD have variable motivation for change, and second, they have a strong tendency to externalize.

Group leader: Discuss motivation.

Changing how we react, how we feel, and how we think is difficult for everyone. We can try to see things differently but we tend to default to the way we have managed best in the world. If we try to change how we have managed ourselves in the world, only to fail, our motivation wanes rapidly and we give up. People with ASPD have adapted themselves to their historical and current experience in a way that they feel gives them the best chance of survival mentally and physically. This "best way" of managing is not going to be given up easily.

Group leader: Talk about change and the difficulties encountered. Suggest that the group focuses on each member in turn for five minutes, exploring one aspect of a problematic component of his/her personality.

The group leader then asks open questions about the problems, to try to get the individual to engage in a process of self-evaluation of the problem.

- How serious is the problem to them?
- Is it other people who are more worried about it and, if so, why are they concerned?
- What would be gained by the problem being addressed?
- What might be lost?

The group leader is modeling "change talk," which is both mentalizing and motivational. Often the patient will ask the group leader what he/she should do: "You tell me? You are the expert. That is why I have come." At this point the group leader has a number of options:

1 He/she can pass the question out to the group. This is not a maneuver that is useful in this phase of treatment and it is not a "first-line" intervention in MBT. In MBT-ASPD, it is important for the clinician to come across as authentic. Avoiding questions is likely to provoke patients into becoming more coercive and demanding answers.

2 He/she can start to give suggestions. This is likely to lead to the patient either saying that he/she has tried the suggestion and it did not work, or finding an unassailable reason why it is not a good suggestion, or stating that it is a stupid suggestion that only serves to show that the clinician does not understand the problem.

3 He/she can answer truthfully with some validation of the question: "That is a good question. I don't know what you should do about it at the moment. We need to explore it more before we can think about solutions. At the moment we need to establish that it is something that we need to work on to change."

MBT-ASPD suggests the third option is taken.

Group leader: Outline the idea of externalization—that is, blaming external factors.

The aim here is not to suggest that externalization is in itself a problem and wrong; it is to suggest that we all need to weigh up our own contribution to events, along with the role of the other. If we attribute too much blame to ourselves rather than others we can be overwhelmed with guilt and self-criticism, for example; on the other hand, if we place too much weight on outside causes and blame others constantly for our problems it interferes with a constructive relationship and often leaves us feeling powerless to change anything.

> A patient described how his housing officer had temporarily placed him in a hostel with others, despite knowing that he found close interaction with others provocative and likely to lead to violence. One evening, another resident had looked at him in a way he did not like, so he hit him. He blamed the housing officer for this event. He told the staff at the hostel to sort things out with the housing officer and not him, stating that he had warned people this could happen.

It is common for people with ASPD to place considerable weight on situational circumstances as an explanation for their own behavior. Of course, this has some validity to it. They often state that the group leaders do not understand their social milieu and the context of their life—"Anyone in my position would have behaved like that"; "You have to threaten people, otherwise they will think you are weak"—and conclude that most of their problems are related to external causes, such as money, social norms, or threats from others. The group leader does not challenge this, but balances it by talking about how we tend to do the opposite when considering other people. We do not take context into account. So if someone is aggressive we tend to see this as arising from a personal characteristic—"They are an aggressive person"—and see them as responsible for their actions. We can underestimate the situational contribution to the aggression in the other person. The point to be made is that when considering ourselves we tend to blame the context, but when considering others we have a tendency to attribute their behaviors to personality characteristics.

> The group leader can point out that often we define the characteristics of other people according to their observable behaviors. This is attributing internal causality to what they do. In general, we do not like it when people do this to us. When people see us as an aggressive person because we become angry, we feel misunderstood. We feel that they do not understand our circumstances. This in itself can fuel more anger toward that person, who is experienced as creating the anger in us. It can be mentioned here that excess emphasis on either the self or the other as the cause of behavior is an example of what is called "poor mentalizing." We need to develop a more nuanced way of relating to others and how we see them.
>
> *Homework*: Make a note of the personality traits that are the most problematic for you over the next week.
>
> Monitor how you explain an "event" to yourself—do you see it as your fault or blame other people/authorities involved, or is it more complicated?

A leaflet summarizing aspects of ASPD is given to the participants.

Module 8: Mentalization-based treatment—part 1

Summary

The group leader summarizes the topic and discussion from the previous session:

- Definition of personality disorders
- What are maladaptive and adaptive personality traits?
- How the course of the disorders fluctuates, the fact that most personality disorders improve with age, and that treatment increases the chances of improvement
- Various different types of personality disorder
- Criteria for BPD/ASPD.

The group leader asks if anyone would like to share notes about any problematic personality traits they noted over the past week or if they have further questions about the diagnosis.

Topic: Mentalization-based treatment

The group leader then addresses the theme for the session and starts with a definition of the *aim of mentalization-based treatment* (MBT).

The aim of MBT is to improve a person's mentalizing ability in close relationships. Improved mentalizing ability means that the person experiences having a more stable inner core self, that he/she is less likely to let emotions get the better of him/her and, when this happens, that he/she is able to regain his/her composure more quickly. That is, the person is more robust emotionally, less vulnerable to interpersonal conflicts and better able to deal with conflicts when they do arise, and less impulsive.

How does psychotherapy enable people to achieve improved mentalizing?

MBT is a form of *psychotherapy*. Psychotherapy means that one talks about one's innermost problems with another person and/or several other people. In this way, one becomes more aware about oneself and one's feelings and how one relates to others. To get the most out of MBT it is necessary to suspend distrust as much as possible, to be curious about yourself, and to accept that the clinicians are not there to judge you. Talking about yourself in this context is a benefit in and of itself, because in general when people are left on their own to figure things out they tend to go astray in their thoughts and feelings. All of us can easily trick ourselves in our understanding of ourselves and others.

But psychotherapy involves even more. It also deals with getting closer to other people—letting others into one's life, that is, daring to trust others and make bonds with others, letting others become significant in one's life. As has been discussed earlier in the group, particularly in the sessions dealing with attachment (Modules 5 and 6), this is not an easy process. It requires careful attention to what is happening in one's own mind and in others'. What is happening in other people? Are they ready to accept me and my mind? Do they understand, accept, and support me?

Remind the participants of the session on attachment and mentalizing (Module 6). Psychotherapy will automatically stimulate attachment feelings; the pattern of attachment that each patient identified in Module 5 is likely to become apparent in therapy. The group leader explains that this is a natural development and that it will be important to focus on how the relationship between patient and clinician can interfere with taking an interest in what is going on in one's own mind and the mind of others. The group participants are told that this topic will be discussed in more detail in the next session.

How the treatment is structured

After agreeing a treatment contract for individual and group MBT once per week for 18 months, each person works with a clinician to achieve the following:

1 Mentalization-based problem formulation
2 Crisis plans
3 Agreement on roles and responsibilities
4 Understanding and agreeing immediate and long-term goals
5 Integration between agencies if they are currently involved, for example, work rehabilitation, probation, and social services.

If necessary, an appointment(s) with a psychiatrist is organized for prescriptions of any relevant medication.

The participants are informed that clinicians meet regularly and exchange information about how the therapy is progressing. The clinicians treating a patient are granted permission to discuss the patient's progress among themselves, but the group clinician does not ordinarily mention anything that he/she has learned elsewhere about the patient in the group. It is up to the patient to decide what he/she wants to talk about, and when. There are, however, some circumstances in which the group clinician can address specific issues directly even if the patient does not want to talk about them, for example, when they relate to violence or threats, serious contract breaches, child protection concerns, or suicide attempts.

When it comes to the other group members, the participants are encouraged not to have contact among themselves, either in person, by telephone/text message, or via social media (e.g., Facebook or Twitter), outside of the therapy sessions. If they nevertheless choose to meet outside the group sessions, they are encouraged to talk about these encounters in the therapy sessions. Intimate relationships between patients attending the MBT program are not permitted, and if such a relationship should develop then at least one of the individuals will have to leave and seek therapy elsewhere.

MBT involves practicing mentalizing skills in close relationships

MBT clinicians provide little direct advice, although they will support focused work to find solutions to immediate problems. They try to engage patients in a *mentalizing stance* and, in doing so, help patients to gradually develop their own solutions having reflected on their problems in increasing detail. As mentioned earlier, the mentalizing stance means being curious about other people's minds, about their experiences, thoughts, and feelings—a "not-knowing" attitude in which one attempts to find out by trying many different alternatives. MBT is a collaborative effort in which the clinicians seek to get the patients to come along on the same mentalizing journey. In short, MBT is based on developing and practicing mentalizing skills together with the clinician and other group members. To be good at something, you need to practice it. In this treatment program, the participants have the opportunity to practice mentalizing skills.

The mentalizing group therapy can be described as a *"training arena" for mentalizing*. It requires the following from each individual participant:

1 That they regularly share and talk about events from their own lives, preferably recent events, that have resulted in poor mentalizing (strong or confusing feelings, impulsive actions, poor conflict resolution, etc.), or discuss circumstances when they have been under stress, particularly in relation to others, and experienced high demands on their mentalizing ability.

2 That they try to understand more about these events using a mentalizing stance—exploratory, curious, open to alternative understandings, etc.

3 That other group members participate in this process by exploring their own problems and those of others through a mentalizing stance.

4 That everyone together tries to find out about events in the group in the same way.

5 That they try to bond to the group, its members, and the clinicians.

> *Group activity*: Discuss whether you have problems with:
>   1 Bringing in events from your own life
>   2 Focusing on events in the group
>   3 Assuming a mentalizing stance.

Use the rest of the time in the session for a discussion of these issues.

> *Homework*: Consider how you usually relate to others when you join a group of people you don't know. For example, think back on your feelings about coming to this group for the first time or note your feelings when you meet a friend who has other people with him/her.

Module 9: Mentalization-based treatment—part 2

Summary

The group leader summarizes the topics of the last session:

♦ Aim of MBT—to enhance mentalizing ability in close relationships

♦ The structure of the treatment program

♦ Training in and practicing mentalizing in the group.

The group leader asks for any questions and if anyone has any reflections from the homework of the week. Discuss this with the participants.

Topic: Mentalization-based treatment

The main topic for this session is *the attachment aspect of MBT*.

> *Group activity*: Discuss the difficulties you think you may run up against when you form a therapy relationship with:
> 1 The individual clinician
> 2 The group clinician
> 3 The other group members.

Common objections to forming affiliative relationships include:

♦ Belief that it is both painful and meaningless when you know that you will soon be separated from the other person

♦ They are doomed to failure

♦ People will always betray you/let you down

♦ Attachment involves caring about another person

♦ You cannot trust people.

Some patients will feel that they might care too much about the clinician, but worry excessively that the clinician does not care about them and that the clinician regards the relationship as "just part of the job" for which he/she is being paid. Others may question whether it is possible to bond with all the individuals listed: after all, one needs to like the people one bonds with, and one may not like the clinicians or other group members. Still others may raise the issue that attachment can lead to wanting more, such as a wish to contact the clinician whenever things are difficult. The question of how you can bond with someone who doesn't say anything about his/her own private life may also be raised. Finally, there may be an issue about why participants are strongly encouraged not to have contact with other group members outside of the therapy sessions.

This discussion activates a wide range of themes, and it can easily turn chaotic. The group leader may, after a while, assist by structuring the discussion. One way to do this is to discuss the relationship with the individual clinician, with the group clinician, and with the other group members separately.

For group members who have participated in other therapies, the group leader can take a short time to identify important differences between the previous therapy and MBT.

The group leader then changes the theme to common reasons for not opening up or telling others about what is difficult. These are feelings of being let down, not understood, overlooked, or misunderstood by the clinician or one of the other group members.

> *Group activity*: Discuss what your typical reaction is when you feel let down, misunderstood, overlooked, or something similar by a friend, a clinician, another person, or someone who is close to you.

Group discussion of this topic takes up the remainder of this session. The group leader emphasizes that this is a particularly important topic to address in therapy. Personal reactions to clinicians and other people often have a tendency to "go underground." Clarifying misunderstandings and sensitive interpersonal feelings is a central element of MBT. Feelings and thoughts that are "underground" are often part of an implicit mentalizing process and they have to be made explicit.

> *Homework*: During the week, make a note of how you react when you experience being let down, misunderstood, or ignored, perhaps by someone close to you.

Module 10: Anxiety, attachment, and mentalizing

Summary

The group leader summarizes the last session:

- The significance of forming bonds with others
- Establishing attachment relationships to the clinicians and the other group members
- The importance of attachment to others and how it activates difficult emotions and represents a challenge to mentalizing
- Difficulties faced in treatment
- How one's reactions to feeling upset by others might "go underground" instead of being spoken about.

The previous session's homework about any interpersonal events that led the individual to feel let down or misunderstood is shared. The experience of one's needs and wishes not being met is a very important and rich pedagogic area to expand understanding of therapy, so the group leader may spend some time on this. According to the MBT model, the distress associated with unmet needs arises from non-contingent responsiveness on the part of the other person— perhaps a friend or, in the context of treatment, the clinician, or perhaps the clinic receptionist.

Topic: Anxiety

The group leader introduces the topic of the day by saying that almost everybody who applies for treatment for an unstable sense of self, unstable emotions, and problematic relationships with others will also have disturbing symptoms in a more narrow sense, and that it is often these symptoms that motivate the individual to seek treatment. The most common symptoms are *anxiety* and *depression*. In this and the next session we will deal with anxiety and depression to the extent that they are related to attachment process.

Anxiety is intimately connected to one of the basic emotions that were addressed in Module 3—fear. Fear is indispensable for survival in a dangerous world; it signals danger and activates a person or animal's "alarm button," stimulating preparedness for "fight or flight."

The group leader explains that the threshold at which fear stimulates a fight/flight reaction and the intensity of the response varies between individuals. To a large extent this is a matter of temperament. Some individuals are more intrinsically fearful than others. When this is the case, it can often lead to troublesome consequences because the individual becomes excessively anxious and "takes flight" behaviorally or mentally when there is no need.

Group activity: Make notes on common situations that make you anxious.

The group leader asks each member in the group what they have written down and leads a discussion of the results. Many of the participants may say that they are intrinsically anxious and the source of their fear is unknown. This makes it much more difficult for them to address the problem. The intensity of fear can be so strong that the person's physical and mental processes may not handle it properly. The autonomic nervous system can become overloaded, causing the individual to experience a *panic attack*; this is characterized by increased heart rate, difficulty breathing, dizziness, and fear of fainting, dying, going mad, or simply losing control, etc.

Group activity: Have you had any panic attacks? If so, note how it felt when it happened.

The group leader asks all group members about any experiences of panic attacks.

Thereafter, he/she proceeds with the theme of panic attacks, leading to a focus on how to avoid the sources of possible triggers. For some people these will be situations packed with people, which are associated with worries about being trapped and the escape route—this may be on buses and trains or in shops, restaurants, cinemas, theatres, at concerts, etc. If one avoids such situations and this leads to significant negative consequences, we would describe the individual as suffering from *agoraphobia* (*agora* being the Greek word for marketplace). For some people, the trigger that leads them to become anxious is meeting friends or going out with other people (or even just thinking about these events); this anxiety may lead these patients to avoid these types of situations involving other people. This is a *social phobia*. In general, the anxieties associated with BPD are more complicated than fitting into such well-structured categories of phobia, and this should be made clear to the group.

Group activity: Make notes on any kind of agoraphobia or social phobia you may have experienced.

The group leader asks all the group members about their experiences of *agoraphobia* and *social phobias*. Social phobias are closely connected to excessive *performance anxiety*, which may prompt the individual to avoid social gatherings such as parties, restaurants, group seminars, or situations where the individual feels a burdensome obligation to perform in some way. There is also *generalized anxiety*, in which the individual is tense and worried about problems with daily living; *obsessive–compulsive anxiety* with its obsessions and rituals; and *post-traumatic anxiety*, in which the individual is exposed to painful re-experiences of traumatic memories.

Treatment of anxiety disorders involves *controlled exposure*. Simply exposing the person to the situation that triggers their anxiety is usually not enough in itself. It is necessary for the exposure to be done in a manner that implies an experience of mastery and control, not defeat. At this point the group leader reminds the participants about what they have learned in previous sessions about emotions and attachment. By default, children's natural reaction when experiencing fear is to *turn to their attachment person* or another "secure" person whom they trust. The natural reaction of this person is generally to take care of the child and calm him/her down. Multiple experiences of this kind inform the child that fear is an emotion that can be handled. However, this interaction will not always be ideal, for different reasons (as we discussed in Module 6), and this can leave the child continuing to feel frightened or feeling that it is useless or even worse than useless to approach others, leading to the conclusion that fear has to be handled by oneself alone, or even that one has to hide one's experience of fear. *The fact remains, however, that the best remedy for anxiety is a calming other person.* Everybody who has experienced anxiety must have realized that it helps to be with another trustworthy person in an anxiety-provoking situation.

This principle of another person helping with anxiety is the key to the interpersonal treatment of anxiety. In exposure therapy, for instance, a clinician treating someone with anxiety about traveling on a bus accompanies the patient on his/her initial bus journey; traveling with someone who makes them feel secure helps the individual to manage their anxiety about travel. The presence of the trusted person reduces anxiety and they can help the individual to relax and manage their symptoms. This gives the anxious person an experience of mastery and control when the journey is accomplished. Thereafter, the person may experience the same feeling of accomplishment while traveling alone.

> *Group activity*: Make notes on how other people have had a calming effect on your anxieties.

The group leader asks all group members about this issue and underlines that the *very act of approaching another person when experiencing anxiety is significant because it is the attitude that patients are encouraged to develop toward the clinicians and the group members in the MBT program*. As will be remembered, we have emphasized the importance of trying to bond with the clinicians and the group members. This requires that everyone talks about their everyday fears, including things that happen within the sessions that activate fear. This is easily said, but may be difficult to do. When trying to be open about personal anxieties, one will often experience a kind of resistance within oneself. This may be related to the fact that fear is often connected with shame, or that one gets an uneasy feeling of being childish and helpless, or that one does not trust that the other has the capacity to be helpful or, worse, may misuse the information to ridicule or shame them. Many patients show hypervigilance when interacting with other people.

> *Group activity*: Make notes on themes or experiences that are difficult to talk about.

The group leader discusses these experiences with the whole group.

> *Homework*: Note if you managed to approach another person (family or friends) during last week with something that made you anxious, and whether it did or did not help. What are your thoughts about the reasons why it succeeded or failed?

Module 11: Depression, attachment, and mentalizing

Summary

The group leader briefly summarizes the discussion in the previous session:

- The close association between anxiety and fear
- Fear can be an appropriate response in some situations but, if it becomes excessive, it can lead to panic attacks
- Fear is a maladaptive response if it begins to be triggered by benign or non-threatening stimuli
- Anxiety can easily generalize to other areas—for example, anxiety about being in lifts becomes fear of enclosed spaces.
- Treatments for anxiety disorders typically involve controlled exposure
- Studies have shown that people are able to manage anxiety better when they approach the triggering situation in the company of a trusted person
- It is important not to respond to anxiety by avoiding the source of the anxiety, but approach it bravely by involving others in your exposure to it
- It is important in therapy that one is brave enough to bring up the issues that are really bothersome to oneself.

The group leader goes through the week's homework assignment, discussing the examples brought by group members about approaching others to help with anxiety.

Topic: Depression

Like anxiety, depression is also associated with a basic emotion—*separation anxiety and sadness*. This is also a natural reaction related to a break in what we call the attachment system. All children who have established an attachment relationship will respond with separation anxiety when they are abandoned, and with sadness when the person they miss does not return when expected. We believe that separation anxiety is a natural part of a type of protest phase and that it is connected to crying and screaming, which are used to attract the parent's attention. Sadness belongs to a later phase in which the protest has not had the desired result. When this is because of the death of the caregiver or a close person, that is, a loss, it is referred to as a *grief reaction*. An intense grief reaction is quite similar to depression, although qualitatively different.

Individuals vary with regard to what they react to in terms of sorrow, how strong their grief reaction is, and how long it lasts. In most people, the emotion passes after a time and the individual is able to adapt to his/her new life circumstances relatively quickly. But when the emotion remains intense for a longer time, we refer to it as a depression. Some people may describe it as a *pathological grief reaction*. In depression, the person is sad and low in mood, tired, has low self-esteem, and has ruminative thoughts, feels profoundly negative about life, and often feels guilty. The person has difficulty concentrating, life seems meaningless, and there seems to be little hope for the future. The thought of giving up on life may not be far away.

The relationship between depression and grief reaction is therefore quite a close one. This hypothesis is supported by research on large populations of people. The loss of someone close is the most common trigger for depression. The "loss" does not need to be a death: it could be that someone travels away for a long period of time, that you yourself are sent away from your family, that the attachment person is ill and unavailable, that one's parents divorce, or that one moves away and loses close friends. Or, rather than the loss of a person, it may involve the loss of social standing and social position, for example, by being disgraced in public in some way.

If a person has experienced a serious loss at a young age that led to a poorly processed grief reaction, that person will be more disposed to depression after a loss in adult life. The more depressive episodes one has had, the more likely one is to experience depression again. It is as if one establishes an automatic response pattern to stress and discomfort. The response pattern—a depressive reaction—may also be triggered by things other than loss, but we think that it is in relation to the loss of an attachment person that the reaction pattern is established, as part of evolution. Other things that can trigger depression are general stress and physical illness, as well as factors of which we are still unaware.

> *Group activity*: Make a note of anything that may have triggered a depressive response in you.

This is a sensitive topic. The group leader must spend considerable time reviewing the examples that are given, not because it is important to hear everyone's depressive episodes in detail, but because everyone should have an opportunity to say something on this topic. It is *not* a good idea to ask everyone to think about what may have triggered their own depressions, and then listen empathically to the stories of two or three group members, not leaving adequate time for all participants. The group leader must say openly to the group that it is important that *everyone* is given a chance to talk about their experiences, and the available time should be divided equally. So, if five minutes are set aside for each person and there are eight people in the group, this activity will take 40 minutes.

After this discussion, the group leader then turns to the topic of *the course and treatment of depression*. Most depressive episodes resolve themselves, while some are never completely resolved. The person can continue in a chronic depressive state, which is not as serious in terms of risk as when the depression is at its worst, but is characterized by constant low spirits in which the person has difficulty feeling happy and is unable to take pleasure in activities. This is sometimes referred to as *dysthymia*. The individual has low self-esteem and is pessimistic in all aspects of life, including about the future. Depressive episodes pass more quickly with treatment, and many chronic depressions can be normalized with treatment. Serious depressions should be treated with medication, with so-called *antidepressants*.

Antidepressants can sometimes also be effective for anxiety and panic attacks, and they can also reduce strong mood swings that are due to general emotional instability. Many people with BPD have taken antidepressants in the past, and some members of the group may still be on medication. When someone takes part in a comprehensive treatment program such as MBT, they should take advantage of the situation by considering reducing or ending the antidepressant treatment, if possible. This should be done only after the treatment is well underway, and when the person feels more in control of his/her life. The reason for this is that with psychotherapy such as MBT, some people are able to learn to deal with life's difficulties without medication and gain enough confidence to do without it.

> *Group activity*: Make a note of any experiences you have had with antidepressant medication.

The group leader brings up and discusses the participants' experiences with antidepressants.

The final main topic is *depressive thinking*. The term "depressive thinking" refers to a set of automatic thought patterns that tend to accompany a depressed mood. These can establish themselves as part of an individual's "normal" thinking after repeated depressive phases or when a depressive state lasts for a long period of time. Depressive thinking refers to thoughts that quickly pop up with content such as "Everything is hopeless," "Nothing helps," "It's impossible for me," "I am useless," etc. Depressive thoughts such as these, which are often the result of adverse life experiences, may in themselves sustain a depression or a depressive tendency.

The group leader explains that the mentalizing approach to understanding the difficulties of individuals with depression is to view these thoughts—which often represent cognitive distortions rather than reality—as acquiring overwhelming potency because of mentalizing failure. The low mood acts directly on mentalizing capacities, thereby shutting down the mental processes that are needed to recover from the depression. Being able to question fixed negative thoughts is an important part of mentalizing, and to recover from depression patients need to begin to mentalize.

> *Group activity*: Make a note of your own tendency toward depressive thoughts, which you may have either experienced in the past or be experiencing now. Do you question such thoughts or do you assume they are accurate?

The group leader reviews the participants' notes about depressive thinking and underlines that awareness of the nature of one's own thoughts is an important aspect of mentalizing. In addition, the leader notes when participants' thinking is rigid, fixed, certain, and unquestioned. These qualities suggest that non-mentalizing is playing a part in maintaining the depression.

> *Homework*: Make a note if you had depressive thoughts during the week and how you dealt with them. Were you able to stimulate some doubt in yourself about them?

Module 12: Summary and conclusion

Summary

The group leader briefly summarizes the last session on depression:

◆ Depression is closely connected to the basic emotions of separation anxiety and sadness

◆ This attachment response system has developed through evolution, because it turns out to be beneficial for the relationships between children and their attachment figures

- Loss of attachment figures leads to grief
- Strong grief reactions are similar to a depressive state
- Other events may trigger grief/depressive reactions, such as loss of social position, loss of self-esteem, stress, or physical illnesses
- After a person has had a first depressive episode, they are more likely to have another one. If someone has suffered recurrent depressive episodes, or a milder chronic type (often referred to as dysthymia), depressive thinking may have developed, and that in itself may sustain the depression
- Depressive thought patterns indicate a loss of mentalizing.

The group leader then asks if there is anyone who wishes to share their notes from the homework assignment the previous week, and leads the ensuing discussion. As this is the last session, the group leader makes a decision about how much time he/she can allocate to the homework. This will depend to some extent on the group's activity level. It may also be the case that the group leader has put aside a few topics that he/she has not had time to address in earlier sessions and that could now be reviewed. The group leader must simply improvise a bit more in this last session.

Topic: Summary and recapitulation

At the appropriate time, the group leader says that the group will now spend some time clarifying things that have been discussed during the entire course. He/she asks if there is anything that anyone has on their mind at the moment—something they wish to learn more about, comment on, or discuss further. If nobody brings anything up, the group leader summarizes the subjects that they have been through in the group. He/she starts with the first session, about mentalizing, and brings up the main points, including the group exercises. Through this type of reminder, the group members usually get quite involved, both reflecting on what they have been through and wondering about things they may not have fully understood.

Of course, ending the group can be linked to the loss of attachment processes that have built up over the course of the group. Patients will have feelings about the end of the group.

> *Group activity*: The group leader asks the group to consider their current feelings about the ending of the group. These are discussed.

Approximately 20 minutes before the end, the group leader asks the participants for their feedback:

> *Group activity*: Jot down a few key words about what you think has been particularly educational for you (a topic, a discussion, a homework assignment, an event) in the group. Make a note of any suggestions you may have for improvements to the program.

The group leader brings up particularly educational experiences and makes a note of any suggestions for improvement. At the end, he/she thanks the members for their active participation and wishes everyone the best of luck.

Reference

Panksepp, J. (1998). *Affective neuroscience: The foundations of human and animal emotions.* Oxford, UK: Oxford University Press.

Mentalizing group therapy

Introduction

Group psychotherapy is a powerful context in which to focus on mental states of self and others. It stimulates highly complex emotional and interpersonal interactions, which can be harnessed for patients to explore their subjective understanding of others' motives while reflecting on their own motives. Yet group therapy is one of the more difficult aspects of treatment for BPD patients, who have the task of monitoring and responding to six to nine minds in the group, rather than being able to focus on only two as in individual therapy. Herein lies the danger of group psychotherapy. The level of complexity and the sophistication of mentalizing required for group interaction means that conditions are optimal for emotions to fly out of control as attachment systems become overstimulated and rigid schematic representations of others are rapidly mobilized. Nonmentalizing can become the norm. As such, group psychotherapy may become highly iatrogenic, stimulating mental withdrawal, maintaining collapse in mentalizing, and facilitating action rather than verbalization—the very antithesis of its aim. First and foremost, the clinician has to ensure that such iatrogenic effects are minimized. This is done initially through the careful structure of the MBT group and through the authority of the clinician as "manager" of the group. This is discussed in detail later in this chapter. First we will outline the aims of the MBT group intervention (MBT-G).

Aims of MBT-G

The group is a "training ground" for interpersonal mentalizing, with the primary aim of facilitating mentalizing process between all participants (Box 12.1). Yet mentalizing is *about* something. In MBT for BPD and ASPD it is about the core problems and emotionally salient events of everyday life faced by patients with borderline or antisocial personality disorders. As such, the group process cannot be left to the group. The clinician "manages" the group to ensure focus and to prevent the process collapsing into nonmentalizing modes.

There are a number of ways to manage a group. A common way is to dictate tasks and organize around psychoeducation and skill acquisition, but this will undermine the primary aim of the MBT group—to facilitate learning of the

Box 12.1 Aims of MBT-G

- Primary task of the group is to provide a "training ground" for mentalizing
- Closer to (American) psychodynamic group psychotherapy than group analysis
- Clinician maintains authority and manages the group—does not wait to see how the group "deals with it"
- Some individual-oriented focus
- Clinician actively promotes group interaction
- Attention to implicit–explicit dimension of mentalizing.

process of interpersonal mentalizing. Another way is to allow the group process to dominate on the basis that the group will develop a culture and cohesion over time. The benefits of free association in understanding unconscious process are well known. However, for this to be useful for understanding and addressing problems, patients have to have a good mentalizing capacity. They have to be able to link the emotional significance of their internal processes and associations with external indicators and find meaning of personal significance in this process. This is a tall order for people with BPD, so it becomes important not to leave things to the group. So MBT clinicians must navigate between the Scylla and Charybdis of over-management and under-management, authority and benign neglect, over-control and possible chaos, in the group. A balance is required between structuring the group process with leadership and authority on the one hand, and facilitating development of the milieu or matrix to allow interpersonal mentalizing to flourish. There are a number of consequences for group therapy as a result. We summarize some areas for discussion, which might differentiate MBT-G from other group work focusing on interpersonal process, in Box 12.2.

In clinical practice, this means constant attention on the part of the clinician to the explicit–implicit dimension of mentalizing. Implicit process is made explicit and patients are asked to work on focused process; explicit processing shifts to implicit understanding until further psychological work is needed on the same process but in a new context.

As a reminder, implicit mentalizing is automatic, procedural, natural, and below the level of consciousness. We are not aware that we are doing it and yet, when asked, we know that we are constantly monitoring ourselves and others intuitively, without actively thinking about it. We base our opinions of others on

Box 12.2 Differences between MBT-G and other interpersonal focus groups

- No interpretations are made about unconscious processes
- Group matrix is not a feature of MBT-G
- Clinician refrains from making interpretations "about the group"
- Clinician is an active participant adopting a "not-knowing," non-expert stance
- MBT-G encourages a group culture of relational curiosity rather than suggesting complex relational hypotheses
- Clinician makes his/her own thinking explicit, transparent, and understandable
- Therapy relies on an "active" clinician maintaining the flow and structure of the session rather than adopting a position secondary to group process.

our subjective experience of them as much as on our rational deductions—"He seems very nice but there is something about him I don't trust." There is a balance that we naturally draw as implicit and explicit mentalizing intertwine together—which can be thought of as being more like the "double helix" of DNA than a continuum in its complexity—forming a multifaceted psychological understanding of ourselves, coding our relationships, representing and re-presenting them as we interact.

When we mentalize others we monitor their mental states, taking in their point of view, their emotional states, and a sense of their underlying motives. We intuitively reflect on these and, when things go smoothly, our mind states change in tune with theirs; we take pleasure in the interaction as it progresses and we see that not only have we changed them a little but we, too, have been changed. We respond to the other's presentation of themselves and to their re-presentation of us. If we tried to do all this explicitly, operationally, and methodically, we would stumble and become like an automaton, emotionless and nonhuman. Nobody would like us or feel warm toward us, instead experiencing us as hollow and without depth, and we in turn would be unable to feel close to them. Communication of our inner self would have been interrupted.

But when we mentalize *ourselves* implicitly we are in more treacherous territory, as we are in a position to remain unchallenged and subject to distortions via our defenses, or even dominated by our explicit rationalizations. Yet we are aware that there is something about us that we know *is* us—a sense of being self-rooted in our emotional states. This is the "I" that can represent "me." To reflect on our emotional states we have to remain in them, and to do so we have to maintain an experience of our sense of self, otherwise our emotions will overwhelm us. We need to identify the inner experience, modulate it, and understand its narrative—where has it come from, what is its meaning?—and express it.

Achieving this description of implicit mentalizing of self and other as described here is human perfection, achieved only occasionally by most people for any length of time and rarely in a group of patients with severe personality disorder. Nevertheless, the aim within this dimension of mentalizing is to promote continual movement between explicit and implicit functioning for all patients.

A patient, Rose, was discussing a problem she had with her boyfriend. Another patient, Kate, suggested quickly that she should leave him.

KATE: Dump him. I would not put up with that sort of behavior.

ROSE: I can't do that. I don't want to.

KATE: Well, then it is your problem.

ROSE: I know, but I don't know what to do.

KATE: Well, I said that the best thing to do is for you to dump him.

This style of conversation continued for a few minutes until the clinician intervened.

CLINICIAN: Wait a moment, because I think Rose is still trying to work out a problem. Kate, that was a pretty quick answer. Giving her a final solution might make it more difficult for her to work it out. Let's try not to come to solutions too quickly. Rose, can you work out what makes you not so sure it is a good thing to finish the relationship?

Here the clinician is attempting to keep the focus on Rose's emotional dilemma, to explicitly pick up on the rapidity of Kate's solution, and not to allow the suggested solution to become implicitly accepted as the answer to the problem. Finally, within the interaction there is implicit process between Rose and Kate that needs exploration, for example, a sense that Kate thinks Rose is being weak, perhaps.

There is nothing complex about this intervention, but it prevents the group following an implicit view that the solution has been found and it facilitates greater explicit focus on mental states and interpersonal process. In this example, Rose moved on to discuss the difficulty she had when people gave her quick answers. She tended to think that any suggestion from others was the only answer, but it confused her because she had no idea what she herself thought. Kate's quick response had led to confusion rather than clarity. This was gradually made explicit by the clinician, along with an exploration of the underlying assumptions made by Kate that had led her to conclude that Rose dumping her boyfriend was the only answer.

Clinician stance in group

A focus on the generation of a mentalizing process about and around areas that are affectively salient for people with BPD requires the clinician to follow a number of principles in his/her stance toward the patients and the group (Box 12.3).

First, the clinician, at times, has to take authority in the group (Box 12.4). He/she must be able to do this while remaining part of the group. To this end he/she demonstrates that he/she is a participant in and not an observer of the group. This may appear to be a move away from the not-knowing stance but is in fact in the service of the not-knowing stance, which can be effective only in the context of emotionally balanced interpersonal process.

Second, the clinician maintains focus for the group. The content of the group is not given free rein, and the clinician frequently returns to the topic or interaction under discussion.

Box 12.3 Clinician stance

- Authority without being authoritarian
- Maintain focus and do not allow persistent nonmentalizing dialogue
- Monitor arousal levels and nonmentalizing modes; beware of hypermentalizing
- Work in current mental reality when possible
- Maintain clinician mentalizing and model mentalizing.

Box 12.4 Clinician authority

- Clinician openly and repeatedly explains the primary task of the group
- Maintains structure and states group principles
- Maintains an active and participating stance
- Praises the group by pointing out and acclaiming mentalizing when it happens
- Maintains focus and paces the group.

Third, the clinician actively monitors the anxiety levels of the whole group and of each individual in the group to ensure they are optimal and become neither too high nor too low. Over-arousal results in the group or an individual becoming uncontrolled, while inadequate expression of emotion and over-intellectual discussion—especially hypermentalizing—prevent the development of mentalizing in the context of "hot" attachment interactions. Both situations are to be avoided, and it is to this end that the clinician maintains control of the group.

Fourth, interventions that aim to increase mentalizing within the group in the immediacy of the moment form the key to constructive development of the group. But while we stress that most of the work takes place within current mental reality, this does not mean there should be no consideration of the past and future, both of which may be a part of current reality as a patient explores his/her own meaning and considers him/herself in future situations. Full mentalizing transfers hindsight to foresight, allowing us to predict our future responses and those of others; current sight allows us to understand the past within a new frame, allowing what was implicit to become explicit. So the clinician needs to keep an eye on each patient's history as it is played out in the group and on the trajectory of the group itself as it develops its own history.

Finally, the clinician's own mentalizing is important, as it serves as an exemplar of mentalizing. Identification by the patients with a clinician and with the therapeutic process is an important aspect of all therapy. The clinician overtly engages in mentalizing process, openly asks him/herself questions, actively takes a not-knowing stance, authentically listens and takes an interest, and shows that his/her mind can change. If two clinicians are in the group they talk to each other, in turn elaborating or questioning what the other says, and even challenging each other. This models the mentalizing interactive process and shows that disagreement can be a positive step toward better understanding.

A number of handy hints for clinicians in terms of their focus in group work are summarized in Boxes 12.5, 12.6, and 12.7.

Box 12.5 Handy hints for clinicians (1)

- *Active* stance (very active at times!)
- Able to take control when needed
- "Stop," "Rewind," and "Explore" *early* when there is evidence of non-mentalizing in the group
- In a group with two clinicians, talk to co-clinician and question them
- Participate using concordant affective experience.

Box 12.6 Handy hints for clinicians (2)

- ◆ Give attention to each member of the group (not just the one speaking)
- ◆ Aim to gauge understanding/mentalizing of each member at all times
- ◆ Role is a hybrid of "floor manager" and "dinner party host."

Box 12.7 Handy hints for clinicians (3)

- ◆ While being attentive to the group member who is speaking, keep a scanning eye on the rest of the members
- ◆ Be alert to concurrent activity in the group that may indicate an emotional response to something going on
- ◆ Put the current group discussion "on hold" while the group is invited to attend to the concurrent activity before it gathers momentum and becomes unmanageable. Once the concurrent activity is resolved, return to the "paused" group discussion.

Format of MBT-G

MBT groups are held weekly and each session lasts 75 minutes (Box 12.8). This length of time was chosen after extensive consultation with patients and clinicians; both groups concluded that 90 minutes was too long to concentrate, to work effectively given problems with attentional control in BPD patients (and perhaps in the clinicians too!), and to manage the level of emotional stimulation safely. A time of 75 minutes was agreed as optimal—long enough to allow the generation of mentalizing process around interpersonal problems and to give time to challenge excessive use of avoidant interpersonal strategies, but short enough to prevent overstimulation of emotional states.

MBT-G is organized as a slow open group, partly in the interests of clinical efficiency but also to harness the mentalizing processes that are necessary when a patient leaves and a new patient arrives. The process of engaging a new patient in the group is discussed later in this chapter. The culture of the group is maintained over time by "older" patients passing on the history of the group and inducting new patients into the process.

Box 12.8 Format of MBT-G

- Slow open group
- 1–2 clinicians
- 6–9 patients
- 75 minutes per session
- Agree principles and restrictions:
  - Attendance
  - Attitude
  - Use of drugs and alcohol
  - Focus
  - "Extra-group" contact among group members
  - Reiteration at times of information provided in MBT-I group
  - Principle of "advice-free zone"—explain carefully!

Number of clinicians in the MBT group

MBT-G sessions are run with either one or two clinicians. Naturally, the number of clinicians makes a difference to the process in the group, but there is no evidence to suggest that having either one or two is superior in terms of group process, retention of patients in treatment, or outcomes. Each may have advantages and disadvantages. As a rule of thumb, two clinicians may be necessary if the patient group is severe in terms of comorbidity and the patients engage in frequent self-destructive behaviors. Having two clinicians allows them to model a mentalizing process when they question each other and engage in dialogue; it means that one clinician can manage a patient who is anxious or distressed while the other continues with the focus of the group and tries to generate the interpersonal mentalizing process; and it will reduce the likelihood of cancellations of the group due, for example, to holidays or sickness. On the other hand, the presence of two clinicians can feel overpowering to the group members who already have an individual clinician as well; there is also a risk of alliances developing between one clinician and patient(s) against the other clinician, and so on. Having only one clinician encourages a consistent and focused group culture and, on a practical note, is likely to be more cost-effective for services. In the end, the decision on the number of clinicians allocated to running a group is likely to depend more on practical issues of cost and staff numbers than on well-evidenced clinical processes.

Number of patients in the group

To some extent the number of patients in a group is determined by its purpose. MBT-G is most comfortable for clinicians and patients when there are six to nine patients. This allows complex interpersonal interactions without participants becoming overstimulated. The decision on the number of places in a group may also be dictated by the clinician's experience and training. A lone clinician may find six patients more manageable than a larger group.

Restrictions of the group

Any group needs to agree principles of involvement and engagement. Manifestly all have to agree to attend regularly, to commit to the overall aims, to have a clear mind when attending (and thus not to be under the influence of drugs or alcohol), to focus on the problems of each other, to share, to be considerate of others, and to manage their behavior in the group. More difficult, though, is the question of patients meeting each other outside the group—not just before or after group sessions, but also at other times. Patients naturally realize that they are not alone with their difficulties and may well share problems and want to support each other. They inevitably experience greater companionship and closeness with some members of the group than others. Both can lead to contact in person between patients outside the group—extra-group socializing. In addition, there is the increasing availability of digital contact through social networking sites, text messaging, e-mail, and picture sharing, among others. Often these activities are construed as boundary violations, yet they may also be a way for some patients to sustain their membership of the group. The effects may be positive for some individuals but less so for other group members, who can feel excluded, talked about behind their backs, resentful, and may even demand that the clinician puts a stop to it.

Not surprisingly, managing contact outside the group exercises the minds of all group clinicians, whether they are running psychoeducational, cognitive behavioral, or psychodynamic groups. As a rule, all recommend that patients do not contact each other outside the group unless it is part of a treatment plan, for example, peer support in a community-based therapeutic program. While this recommendation of no or only limited extra-group socializing is common irrespective of the type of group, it is less clear how to respond when patients report meeting up outside the confines of the group. Meeting up beforehand and chatting afterwards is usually tolerated and ignored. It is the between-group contact that is more problematic.

It has already been mentioned that in MBT-G the clinician takes a level of authority in managing the group. This should not be interpreted as becoming authoritarian. Yet, if there is extra-group activity between group members, the clinician may feel that his/her authority is being challenged, the group process is being undermined, and treatment is being compromised. Of course this is, in part, correct. But if the response is authoritarian—for example, stating that this is a boundary violation, that it should stop forthwith, and that if it continues it will possibly lead to discharge from the group—the overall purpose of the group has been undermined as no mentalizing work is being done around the "problem," which, in this case, is patients meeting up outside the group. The moralistic and totalitarian clinician will become seen as a controlling figure who is to be deceived by the patients. So, in MBT-G the "pre-group" and "post-group" group are open for discussion, at least to the extent of considering the form of this extra-group activity and the effect that it has on individuals' feelings and how it influences the relationships in the group itself. Contact *between* groups is taken to be a "problem" that needs additional discussion, which includes the clinician presenting his/her views openly.

Structure of MBT-G

The clinician outlines the structure and purpose of MBT-G at the beginning of treatment. In a new group, this is done by informing the patients that each session will follow a specific pattern over the 75 minutes to ensure that everyone has a chance to talk about themselves in the group, especially if they have a problem that needs to be addressed that week. Over time, the structure becomes part of the culture of the group and new members who join the group can be quickly introduced to the pattern.

Clinician introduction in a new group

> First I want to let you know that we have a pattern to the group each week. We start with a brief summary of the previous group. This allows anyone who was unable to attend the previous session to catch up with the main themes and it acts as a reminder for all of us. One of us [the clinicians] will do the summary, but it is often helpful if any of you have something to add. We can easily miss something very important. After the summary, we go around to ask each of you if you have any problems or concerns that you want help with from the group this week. We don't want any of you to leave the session feeling that you have not had the chance to talk about something that is causing you distress, or perhaps something that has given you pride and pleasure that you want to let us know about. We want you to take your opportunity to talk in the group and we need to know early on rather than at the last minute if there is something that we all need to focus on in the group for you. We will only take 10 minutes for this "go-around" and then we can open the group to discussion.
>
> Now, let's move on to the purpose of the group.

Purpose of group

It is important that both clinicians and group members understand and agree the purpose of the group right from the start. Patients rightly ask questions— "What is the point of this group?" They may do so at any point in the long-term trajectory of the group. If this occurs, the purpose of the group must be restated and reworked, and the immediate trigger for the question explored—what was assumed or was implicit has to be made explicit again because it has been lost. The purpose needs to be as clear as possible throughout the "life" of the group and, at times, it may be necessary to revisit some of the information provided in the MBT-I group (see Chapter 11), which is a useful technique to focus exploration about a complex question.

At the beginning of the group, the clinicians outline the mentalizing process and emphasize the reciprocity of mentalizing, how we learn from each other, and how attachments can allay anxieties and are a context to explore personal concerns safely. The purpose of the group is for studying these processes between people, as well as focusing on problem areas that are very common in BPD and/or ASPD. The clinicians explain that the group members (with the clinicians) need to organize the mentalizing process around their problems and seek to find solutions in terms of managing mental processes, not becoming dysregulated when they become sensitive, or becoming physically aggressive when they feel humiliated. All agree to focus on the detail of the personal interactions in the group and to focus on the core relational processes identified in the individual formulations developed jointly with the clinician in the individual sessions (see Chapter 5). This requires turn-taking, a balance between generosity and self-centeredness, consideration of self and other, and acceptance of alternatives—all of which are essential in constructive social and personal relationships.

It is essential to restate and agree the aims of the group whenever a new patient joins. Working on agreement is in itself likely to facilitate the primary aim of the group to act as a training ground for mentalizing. The new patient has to state what they want from the group, discuss how that is going to take place, ask others what they think, accept that their aims may be different from others', and listen to others' problems when they wish to talk about their own.

Trajectory of each group

Each group session follows the same basic trajectory (see Figure 12.1):

◆ Summary of the previous week and feedback from participants
◆ "Go-around" to establish any key problem areas to be covered in the group

- Synthesis of problems if possible
- Focus on the problem areas in turn
- Close of group.

Trajectory of group session

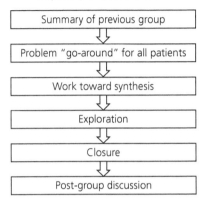

Fig. 12.1 Trajectory of group session.

Summary of previous week

The MBT group clinician engenders a culture of continuity in the group by beginning each group with a summary of the previous session. This is a brief statement about the main themes that were discussed, including the clinician's perspective of the discourse and an outline of any unresolved problems. If there are two clinicians in the group their perspective will have been formulated in the post-group meeting and agreed between them (Box 12.9).

The first part of the summary focuses on content, but the second part sensitively emphasizes any problems within the group, for example, problems

---

Box 12.9 Summary of previous group

- Developed by clinicians in post-group discussion
- Develops culture of patient contribution
- Includes examples of successful mentalizing
- Identifies self–other mentalizing problems
- Maintains overarching themes.

between participants. It is helpful for the clinician to keep in mind three major aspects to include in the summary:

1 Good aspects of mentalizing around particular topics
2 Important components of self and other mentalizing
3 Overarching themes.

The aim of the summary is to enhance the continuity of mentalizing across time, to facilitate cohesion, to initiate patients to the themes in the context of erratic attendance, and to organize the clinician's own mind.

Once the clinician has completed the summary he/she can ask the group members if it is accurate and whether there is anything they would like to add:

> Last week we discussed the difficulties people had in getting others to do what they asked. We had examples from Robert with the housing department, and from Wayne with the benefits office. When people do not respond constructively to our requests we tend to get angry, and in these examples it led to both Robert and Wayne each "cutting off their nose to spite their face." They both walked out having insulted the people concerned. So we had a discussion about managing anger in this situation. We also talked about Pete not turning up enough and what was happening with him—just to say that we rang him last week and he said he would be here this week. Finally, we were talking about the tension between Rachel and Robert, as Rachel feels that Robert talks a lot of bullshit. This was not resolved and I think it would be helpful to return to it today. Roshanne, you were fairly quiet last time and perhaps we should give you more time this week.
>
> Is that a fair summary, and are there other important themes that I have missed?

It may become possible for the group members themselves to provide the summary if the culture of linking themes across groups becomes embedded in the implicit mentalizing process of the group.

"Go-around" of problems

Next, the clinician instigates a "go-around," asking each patient if there is anything they would like help with from the group during the current session.

> Rose, let's start with you. Is there anything that has happened over the past week, or any aspect about yourself, that you would like help with from the group today? As you know, we don't want anyone going away from the group saying that they have not had time to address an urgent problem.

The clinician manages the "go-around" by clarifying the problem(s) the patient brings and then moving on to the next patient. The clinician does not explore the problems of each individual at this point; he/she does so only once all the patients have been asked if they have a concern they want to discuss. Similarly, during the "go-around" the clinician does not allow the other patients to comment on the problems, offer advice or give solutions, or talk about their own experience of the problem. Control of this process and maintaining the task of the group is a further example of the authority of the clinician.

There are a number of reasons to undertake a "go-around" at the beginning of the group. First, as we have just mentioned, it allows the clinician to maintain some authority within the group process; he/she controls the group by allowing the process and content to unfold gradually rather than rapidly and/or explosively. It prevents the group collapsing rapidly into nonmentalizing. Second, it prevents the group becoming unfocused. Focus is further assured if the clinician works toward a synthesis or sharing of some of the problems identified by the patients. Third, it encourages the patients to listen to each other and not to make rapid assumptions about each other. Finally, it encourages mentalizing as a fundamental part of the group culture right from the outset of each group.

The "go-around" can become beset with problems. It can take too long. It is easy for the clinician to lose control of the process and for the task to become diverted so that it is never completed. To avoid this, the clinician can keep to a time limit that has been agreed with the patients but, more importantly, he/she must maintain charge of the process skillfully. There is an ever-present danger that the "go-around" can interfere with the mentalizing process rather than enhance it by concentrating too much on events. This is the reason to ensure that it is given limited time. A common complication is the patient who just says "Yes, I just want to die" or "I don't want any help from anyone here" or "I don't have any problems." In each of these circumstances the clinician takes the response seriously, quickly clarifies what the patient has said, and finds something to validate in their statement.

CLINICIAN: Hannah, have you any problems to bring to the group this week?
PATIENT: I just want to die.
CLINICIAN: Can you tell us a bit more about that problem so we can be clearer about it?
PATIENT: Yes, I want to die.
CLINICIAN: When did the feeling come on so strongly?
PATIENT: I always have it.
CLINICIAN: What is it about it today that makes you want to talk about it?
PATIENT: I don't.
CLINICIAN: It sounds a serious issue though, but is the immediate problem that I keep asking you to say more about it?
PATIENT: Don't want to talk about it.
CLINICIAN: OK. But let's put on the table that you have serious feelings at the moment and are not sure if you can talk about them, and that is the problem for us as a group.

The clinician is attempting not to be distracted by the suicidal statement and, given that the responses are initially oppositional, he tries to identify the immediate problem that he is contributing to. The clinician reduces the interaction as he thinks it might be harmful, and tries to empathize with the patient's struggle to manage a statement to others of "wanting to die" and her difficulty in talking about it. He can return to Hannah later, either at the end of the "go-around" or in the group—"Hannah, can we come back to your sense that you want to die? Is it possible for us to hear a bit more about how it has developed so strongly?"

A patient who says that they do not have a problem is asked a few probing questions to see if they can identify anything, but if this fails the clinician moves on to the next patient, leaving the first patient for a few minutes to think about it. The clinician can then return to the "no problem" patients later. If they still say they have no problems, there are two options. The first is to accept this and move the group on to the core work around the mentalizing process surrounding some of the difficulties brought to the group. The second is to give the patient a problem to consider. This is useful when there are concerns about a patient, for example, related to risk or nonattendance. This can be done compassionately but firmly—"Catherine, could we put your difficulties with getting here as a problem? I think we might see if we can help you get here more regularly if we can." Manifestly, giving the patient a problem has to be done skillfully and in the context of an alliance, and the clinician needs to judge this carefully. Nevertheless, if there are serious problems in the treatment of a patient it is necessary for the clinician to insist that the problems are raised.

Synthesis of problems

Often patients bring similar or overlapping problems, for example, if two of them have harmed themselves, become angry or emotionally dysregulated, or had fights. If participants of the group bring so many problems in the "go-around" that the clinician realizes that it is going to be impossible to focus adequately on all of them, working toward a synthesis is useful. We therefore suggest as a general principle that clinicians work briefly toward a synthesis of the various problems presented in the "go-around." This is a powerful mentalizing process. It increases sharing between participants of personal problems, increases affiliative process, and maintains the authority of the clinician over the group process.

The clinician needs to take charge of this process, orienting him/herself around the shared characteristics of people with BPD—interpersonal problems, difficulties with emotional control, risk-taking behavior, and impulsivity—or ASPD—aggression, irresponsibility, impulsivity, and risky behavior. Most problems can be considered within one of these areas.

Wayne, you want to talk about what happened when you "lost it" with the benefits office. Pete, you have a problem with your girlfriend when she looks at other men and you feel jealous. So it sounds like it might be helpful to consider how we manage strong feelings when we are with other people. Rachel, you had strong feelings last time about Robert, so perhaps we can think about this as well. Shall we see if all these things join up around emotions and how we manage them? Wayne, do you want to start?

In this example, one of the participants is selected to start, organizing his problem around the synthesis of patient problems if there has been some agreement on this.

Focus

Commonly it is obvious who should start; one patient is manifestly distressed, for example. Often the choice is made by the other patients, who recognize that one individual has a pressing matter and quickly point to him/her as the person who should begin; at other times one patient immediately starts without deferring to the others. If no one seems to be coming forward to start, the clinician takes authority to identify who starts by asking one of the patients to begin exploring the problem he/she identified during the "go-around." From this point in the group, the clinician must "pace" the discussion to ensure that all the problems identified in the "go-around" are addressed to some extent. This will be made possible as long as the clinician uses the focus of the synthesis to work on some problems jointly. Of course, some of the responsibility for making sure time is used appropriately remains with the group and the individual patient. If the clinician is aware that a patient is naturally reticent to put him/herself forward and likely to sit back and not demand that his/her problem is discussed, this itself is the problem that needs to be addressed. For example, the patient may have avoidant attachment processes and so have a tendency to retreat even if he/she has defined a problem. Work needs to be done on this through identification of the relational pattern and making the problem explicit when the individual identifies a problem in the "go-around."

CLINICIAN: Alice, that is really helpful. So you have an issue about your sense that you are no good as a person and want to consider what goes on that makes you dislike yourself and feel uncomfortable when people are nice to you. So, like we have found before, we also need to look out for your tendency to defer to others rather than put yourself forward. Can you keep an eye on that and we will too?

Some clinicians suggest that a set time is allocated to each problem; this is known as "turn-taking" and ensures time is shared equally. However, this may create nonmentalizing by embedding teleological processes within the group—"I must have my 10 minutes even if I have nothing to talk about. Otherwise I will feel that no one is interested in me and I am not wanted in the group"—so it needs to be done cautiously. It also distorts the normal social interactive process of moving around and across topics and may prevent the linking of problems by which one person's difficulties may inform another's dilemma. In other words, it may reduce the facilitation of mentalizing process through excessive structure. In addition, it may result in individual therapy within the group. Too many groups default to working with one individual and are oriented around the content of his/her problem. Again, this will reduce the opportunity for interactive mentalizing. So, overall we caution against excessive adherence to this method, because an MBT group is attempting to facilitate an *interactive* mentalizing process.

If a synthesis of some of the problems has been agreed, the clinician uses the synthesis to focus the discussion around the stories the patients have brought. So, returning to the earlier example, both Wayne and Robert can talk about their stories but with reference to the problem of managing emotional states in interpersonal contexts. In other words, the stories themselves become exemplars of the primary problem of managing difficult feelings.

Once some of this work is underway, the clinician can consider guiding the group discussion toward current processes in the group that serve as exemplars of the same problem. In this example, Rachel has strong feelings about Robert, so this can be woven into the discussion. This makes the discussion immediate and aids learning about how emotions can be expressed constructively in a relationship.

Within this work on a problem, the clinician continually works toward mentalizing the relationships in the group through clear identification of the affect focus when necessary. We discuss this later in the sections "Identification of patient relational patterns enacted in the group" and "Mentalizing interpersonal process in the group."

Close of group

The clinician needs to indicate to the group that the allotted time is coming to an end while enough time remains for important topics to be "closed" safely. One way of managing this is for the clinician to outline a summary of the work the group has done so far and focus on some of the residual problems, asking the patients to focus on those areas for the remaining time. This also allows the clinician to emphasize important learning points and point toward areas to be addressed later.

> We only have 15 more minutes, so shall we take stock of what we have talked about? We have discussed this problem of not getting what we want from others and how that also occurs in the group when we feel the group is no good and that we don't get helpful feedback. On the other hand, Kate in particular feels that expressing how she feels in

the group gives her relief as she can "get rid of frustration," and some other people feel this too. I think we need to continue this idea of whether we get something good or something bad most of the time from other people—either now or keep it in our minds for next time. I am aware that we have not spent much time yet on your worry, Roshanne, that you never get what you want from your mother when you visit. This sounds like it links with what we are talking about. Shall we spend a bit of time on it now?

After the group

Following the group, the clinician or clinicians consider their experience of the session and may wish to talk to another clinician if they are facing a serious clinical problem and need advice. This discussion may focus on a number of areas:

- Absence of members—who is to contact them, and how (phone, letter, text message)?
- The overall process of the group—was there interactive mentalizing? Who participated in this?
- Were there any persistent indicators of nonmentalizing and are any patients more identified with nonmentalizing process?
- Risk issues and how to address them
- Feelings in the clinicians directed to the group as a whole and any individuals in the group
- Clinicians' interactive process
- Final agreement about the summary to be fed back next week.

Creating a mentalizing training ground to facilitate epistemic trust

People with BPD are unable to learn from others easily, being naturally uncertain about others' motives in the light of their previous experience. So they are inevitably wary when starting in a group. To address this, the clinician(s) must develop an atmosphere in the group that encourages appropriate *epistemic trust* (i.e., trust in what the clinicians and others are saying and that it is personally relevant to the participants, so they can learn from it) in the participants (see Box 12.10). This is done in part by managing the trajectory of the group and taking authority for controlling the pace of the group, as described earlier. This forms the frame for the mentalizing "training ground." But it is the authenticity of the clinician's curiosity—which generates a mentalizing attitude toward personal problems and establishes a culture of enquiry—that is the key to creating a mentalizing training ground. The role of the clinician is akin to a dinner party

Box 12.10 Facilitating epistemic trust in the group

- ◆ Authentic clinician curiosity
- ◆ Culture of enquiry about mental states
- ◆ Exploration of stories
- ◆ Clarification of problems
- ◆ Mentalizing the detail of the problems
- ◆ Mentalizing interpersonal process in the group
- ◆ Identification of relational patterns
- ◆ Mentalizing relationships within the group.

host, introducing the guests, finding commonality and shared experience between them, stimulating discussion, and reducing unnecessary conflict.

The "culture of enquiry" is not simply an interest in what happened during important events in the patients' lives. It is more about the underlying motivations, that is, what makes someone do something or say something. It is about becoming aware of what feelings and thoughts contribute to decisions and choices; about respecting others' ideas and allowing them to hold a different perspective; about minds changing minds. To reach this laudable aim of creating a culture of enquiry, the clinician must not only promote mentalizing in the group but also tackle nonmentalizing quickly. He/she needs to be alert to the common indicators of nonmentalizing—dismissive statements, use of stereotypes, generalizations, absence of curiosity, over-inclusive talk, excessive detail about events, behavioral change, and so on. Equally, the patients need to be aware of nonmentalizing process in themselves and others. To this end, the clinician repeats, when relevant, information that was discussed in the MBT-I group (see Chapter 11). In other words, he/she uses some elements of psychoeducation in the group to address areas of nonmentalizing.

Exploration of stories about events

We have mentioned that following the "go-around" and development of a synthesis if possible, exploration of difficulties can begin. Commonly, these difficulties are expressed in stories that involve recent interpersonal events, but this is not necessarily the case. It is a generalization to suggest that discussion of recent events is more fruitful in generating affectively mentalized discussion than discussion of historical events. While this is often the case, it is not inevitably true. Patients need to be allowed to choose what they want to talk about with the proviso that, if the clinician is aware of current events that are endangering therapy or life, these events will take priority and be introduced by the clinician.

Differentiating between events told as a narrative on the one hand and exploration of accompanying mental processes on the other is a key element of MBT. Too often, patients describe what happened, complaining about others as they do so, and fail to reflect on the mental world of themselves and the protagonists of the story as the narrative unfolds. In MBT-G it is expected that the clinician will stimulate discussion between group members around the interpersonal events, with a focus on affective reflection. This will include understanding others' motives if the individuals in the group show moderately stable mentalizing. Developing a coherent narrative may be the first step toward mentalizing the stories. The gravest danger for the clinician is to make sense of a narrative that is incoherent. Other patients in the group will naturally complete the blanks in a story, usually by taking the side of the patient, and not concerning themselves with inconsistencies. It is important that the clinician does not do the same but continually tries to generate authentic interest between members of the group in the detail of the stories *and* the underlying mental experiences of all involved (see Boxes 12.11 and 12.12).

In doing so, the clinician moves the discussion between members, ensuring that the group avoids what has become known as the "dead cat process" following a discussion in a group about the death of a cat. In summary, this is a situation in which all the patients describe a similar story, which on the surface looks like an interpersonal dialogue but is in fact each patient remaining in a "silo"

Box 12.11 Culture of enquiry: exploration of stories (1)

- Encourage patients to be aware of what they are thinking and feeling as they tell a story
- Ask other patients to consider the thinking and feeling of themselves and the narrator
- Suggest that patients consider why they/others think/feel as they do in the story:
  - I heard X saying that he is angry, but I think he is hurt about not being taken seriously
  - What am I feeling, what are they feeling, and why?

Box 12.12 Culture of enquiry: exploration of stories (2)

- Encourage patients to articulate explicitly what would otherwise be privately ascertained/assumed about mental states of others
- Support patients to make explicit their working through of their story (detail) so that the rest of the group (clinician and patients) can identify when mentalizing and nonmentalizing has occurred.

and talking only from their perspective, with no interest in the mental states and experience of the others.

Dead cat process

HELEN: I don't know how I am going to manage. My cat died last night. She was my life. I knew that she was ill and I had been looking after her but in the end she just died. It is terrible. If it was not for my other cat I would kill myself.

[Helen continued with further detail about her love for her cat.]

RACHEL: I had a cat that died. I know what you feel. It means that life is not the same. I couldn't cope at all and when it happened I could not move her. I left her in her bed for days. I cried and cried. Cats are what make life worth living for me.

DEBORAH: I don't think I could manage if any of my cats died. I have three at the moment and they are my closest relationship. They care for me and love me in a way that no one else does. They are my reason for living most of the time. Your cats are family.

Each patient continued to reiterate their own experiences of their cats over the years without any of them really focusing on the current emotional turmoil of Helen, who was distressed about the loss of her cat the night before. The topic in the group, namely loss, was consistent. But genuine interest in each other's emotions and authentic sharing was absent. Each patient remains focused on herself, with little turn-taking in the interaction. It is as if they all want to tell their own story about the loss of a cat without concern for the others. It is the task of the MBT clinician to prevent this kind of collapse into self-oriented silos (Box 12.13).

This is done through clarification of the story, exploration of the experience, and active stimulation of interpersonal interactions, with identification of any nonmentalizing responses.

> ## Box 12.13 Culture of enquiry: exploration of stories (3)
>
> ◆ Generate a group culture of enquiry about the motivations of people in the story
> ◆ Insist that patients consider others' perspectives and work to understand someone else's point of view
> ◆ Clinician should directly express his/her own feelings about something that he/she believes is interfering with understanding of the story.

Clarification

Clarification of events

Initially, the clinician attempts to clarify the sequence of events that the patient describes—what led to what, who was involved, how did the interaction unfold? This level of clarification is at the level of "facts" as told by the patient. Some patients give excessive detail, outlining intricate interactions while attributing complex motives to others. If this is the case, the clinician needs to consider whether the patient is hypermentalizing, which is a pernicious nonmentalizing mode that commonly serves to dispel considerable anxiety on the part of the patient. Hypermentalizing needs to be challenged as soon as possible to prevent it becoming embedded in the process; challenge is discussed in Chapter 9. At times the clinician will need to ask the patient to provide an "edited" version of their story if excessive detail is being used—"I don't mean to cut you off, but I think the story is becoming clearer. Could you just give us the main points so that we can start to think about the important areas with you?" While this might sound too challenging to some clinicians, it is necessary to disrupt continuous storytelling if mentalizing is to be stimulated.

Clarification of the problem

The next step is for the patient to clarify the problem (Box 12.14). Stories do not necessarily indicate the problem. At each stage it is useful for the clinician to maintain a not-knowing stance to encourage the patient to identify the exact nature of the problem—"Can you describe what was so difficult about that? What did it feel like at that moment?"

A patient complained that he had phoned the unit to talk to his individual clinician but she had not been available and had not rung him back.

Box 12.14 Clarification of problem

- ◆ Identify the problems within the story
- ◆ Stimulate alternative perspectives from patients
- ◆ Facilitate discussion of managing mental states as the problem
- ◆ Beware of defining the problem based on physical reality and development of teleological solutions.

PATIENT 1: I was told that she would ring me back "before lunchtime." Which lunchtime exactly was that [said sarcastically]? She did not ring me until late afternoon and then I could not answer the phone and anyway it was too late.

PATIENT 2: They are all like that. People don't do what they say they will do. I agree that when they do respond it's always too late. You need them when you ring, not later.

This patient is naturally coming to the support of the first patient and confirming that this experience is something she understands. But it is notable that she has not really clarified with Patient 1 what the problem was. She has merely agreed that when you ask for something you don't get it.

CLINICIAN: I can see that it is a problem if you are told something and then it does not happen, and that when you feel there is some urgency it is even more of a problem. [Beginning empathic validation of the experience.] Can you say what was so difficult about her not ringing you back by lunchtime? [An attempt to define the problem more clearly, rather than leave the patient simply repeating the story.]

PATIENT 1: I needed the help before the afternoon, which is why I had rung in the morning. I didn't want anyone else to speak to me as she at least knows me.

CLINICIAN: Can we focus on what the experience was that meant you needed to talk to her, so that I can understand better what you were struggling with as you became increasingly aware that she was not calling you back by lunchtime?

PATIENT 1: It is the idea that we are promised something and then it does not happen. I cannot bear that.

By this point the problem is becoming a little clearer—the patient is understandably sensitive to being let down by others, particularly those he has trusted to some degree.

The clinician continued to explore this aspect to ensure that the problem was defined. Being let down had led the patient to become angry. This was followed by urges to abandon therapy altogether. So the affect related to a late return of his phone call had undermined the alliance he had with his individual clinician and with the treatment team. This was indeed a problem in treatment and needed to be urgently addressed.

It turned out that the problem had additional complexity. The patient believed that the clinician had deliberately not rung him back because she did not like him. This indicates affectively driven nonmentalizing, which is the target of MBT. The patient needs to learn to maintain mentalizing at these points of sensitivity. Only by trying to define the detail of the problem could the point of nonmentalizing become better defined. In this example, it is becoming multifaceted and ready for exploration. The patient has experienced a need to seek help. Telephoning to speak to his clinician may have increased his personal vulnerability. As his attachment demand is not met, he has to struggle with emotions that destabilize him and he then reorganizes himself in the only way he knows how, which is to angrily withdraw while devaluing the person he wanted to talk to. Even so, though, the original problem that led the patient to phone the unit has not yet been identified and explored. This needs to happen if the full extent of the problem is to be defined accurately.

Mentalizing the problem

Once the sequence of events—the story—is established, the clinician can "rewind" the minds of the group members, asking them to focus on what they have been told. The group members, with direction from the clinician, need to "micro-slice," clarifying the mental experiences of the patient as the events unfolded and bringing their own affective responses and thoughts to the problem. To encourage this, the clinician actively questions the group for their thoughts and experience of what they have been listening to. Some participants will already have responded to the content of the patient's story, and the clinician asks them to elaborate on their points. Often, the members of the group who respond initially are recruited to support the "cause" of the index patient; in this situation it is important for the clinician to clarify whether the alliance is genuine and, if so, to elicit more detail about what is being supported. Alternatively, the clinician identifies difference if it is there, to increase the index patient's reflection on his/her problem. Reflective difference, that is, contrasting perspectives between group members, tends to stimulate mentalizing; in contrast, oppositional difference, arguing about truth and who is right, tends to reduce mentalizing.

Mentalizing the problems brought by the patients is the core of the group work. Once discussion has gently been expedited about the presenting problem, the clinician needs to:

- Listen for indicators of nonmentalizing
- Monitor the arousal levels of individuals in the group
- Facilitate interactive process between all members
- Engage in active participation from a platform of the not-knowing stance
- Deploy interventions from the hierarchy of intervention: empathic validation, clarification and exploration, affect identification, affect focus, and mentalizing the interpersonal relationships between group members and between them and the clinician (see Chapter 7).

Cautions

There are a number of pitfalls for the group clinician when mentalizing the problem (see Box 12.15). The first is gradually becoming trapped in individual therapy in the group. MBT-G cautions against individual therapy within the group. It is all too easy to become sucked into exploring a serious issue with an individual patient to the exclusion of the others. Indeed, when there are two clinicians in the group, both can become wholly focused on one patient, particularly if he/she is at risk. Other patients tend to sit back and leave the work to the clinicians, partly because they feel inadequately prepared to help someone in immediate distress. When this occurs, it is important to "triangulate" (see later).

The second is to work too hard on making sense of interactions. Group process tends to confuse, and the natural response of the clinician is to make sense of the confusion on behalf of the participants. This is antithetical to the core

---

Box 12.15 Clarification of problem: cautions

- Easy to become trapped in individual therapy in the group
- Excessive use of clinician's mentalizing to make sense of the story and to assume understanding of the problem
- Hypermentalizing and rapid interaction about the problem can masquerade as interpersonal process.

focus of MBT, which is to stimulate mentalizing processes in the patients; it is *not* to take over mentalizing on their behalf or to deliver understanding formed through the clinician's superior mentalizing process.

The third trap is to become convinced that interaction is progressing constructively when the group members are interacting freely. Rapid interaction leads to loss of reflection and tends to lead to nonmentalizing or becomes a forum for advice. The clinician needs to maintain control through the constant use of "stop" and "rewind" with clarification. Allowing the group to rush encourages superficiality, embeds implicit assumptions, and obviates reflection.

Identification of patient relational patterns enacted in the group

A key component of the assessment process for a new patient is the identification and discussion between patient and clinician of recurrent patterns of relationships. In essence, these patterns reflect the attachment processes of the patient. If these are to be harnessed in treatment, they have to be readily recognized by both patient and clinician as they become exampled in treatment. The assessor itemizes the patterns in the formulation, which is available for the patient and group clinician. When patients start group treatment the initial discussion between the clinician(s) and the patient necessarily includes statements about these patterns (Box 12.16).

The group clinician needs to be sensitive about this but, when introducing a new patient to the group, the clinician may ask the patient to talk about his/her relationships and support him/her in talking about the relational patterns that he/she has. For example, when a patient comes to his/her first session the clinician may begin by saying: "Would you like to introduce yourself and let people know a little about the problems that have led you to come for help?"

Box 12.16 Identification of relational patterns

- Open sharing by all patients of the relational aspects of their initial formulation
- Focus on attachment processes in the group during individual sessions
- Identification and definition of relational pattern in "stories" given by patients
- Work to delineate benefits and drawbacks of this pattern.

The clinician helps the patient outline some of his/her difficulties and later, perhaps over the next few groups, will ensure that the patient talks about the formulation that has been developed prior to treatment.

We would like to emphasize here the importance that is now attached to explication of the attachment patterns in MBT. This is done collaboratively and explicitly at all times. The patient knows that all clinicians are aware of the patterns and will be looking out for them in treatment; necessarily, the patient needs to have accepted that the formulation about his/her relationships has traction and not simply agreed it.

Nigel was a 26-year-old man who was self-destructive and constantly getting into arguments with others that resulted in violence. He had been arrested on a number of occasions. He recognized that his temper was out of control and stated that he wanted to do something about it. In the assessment, a number of violent episodes were explored with him. One aspect seemed to stand out—most of his arguments began by him stating that he wanted something from someone who then failed to give it to him. This ranged from a request to a friend to borrow some money to demands to stay overnight with people. This was embedded in his formulation as an attachment process in which he seeks proximity to someone for a need he has, only to find that he is rejected, which makes him feel worse. This results in him trying to get what he needs by forcing the person to give it to him. However, currently this pattern involved his constant requests to his former girlfriend and to social services to visit his daughter. All requests were declined, and in response he threatened them on the phone and during meetings. In the group, he voiced his frustration and anger with his girlfriend and the social services.

On one occasion he arrived a few minutes before the end of the group and requested some time to talk about recent events with social services. As the group was nearly at an end, the clinician said that there was very limited time so perhaps Nigel could summarize quickly or even wait until the following week.

NIGEL: Oh, I see. So you think there is no time, do you? Well, I will make sure that there is time. I am not leaving the group until we have discussed it. So you sit down and listen to me.

OTHER GROUP MEMBERS [stating that they could stay for a time]: We have got a bit of time so why don't we go on for a bit?

CLINICIAN: So let's try to use what time we have left.

NIGEL: You are not interested. The only thing you want is to get out of here. You don't care about our problems. Fuck you.

OTHER PATIENT: He is at least staying to listen, so what happened?

NIGEL: Social services won't let me see my daughter. They say I am threatening and won't be good for her. She is my daughter. I should be able to see her. I went yesterday and they threw me out. I am going back to sort them out.

CLINICIAN: Nigel, can I say something here. Is this about your asking them again after you have tried really hard to manage your feelings and then being rejected, with them not understanding your honest wish to see your daughter?

NIGEL [A little calmer from this validating statement]: Yes. I am going to get them and make them listen.

CLINICIAN: Didn't that just happen here? You were going to make us listen by keeping us here.

NIGEL: Well, you are listening now.

CLINICIAN: I hope so. Is that better?

A little later in this discussion, the clinician brought up an element of the problem that had been considered in the group before.

CLINICIAN: Maybe the problem is now that we have been forced to talk with you and so it is not quite the same as if we had given it freely.

NIGEL: I don't care about that.

CLINICIAN: Are you sure? Because we have talked before about your sense that what you want is for people to "really" want to help you and that the only help you get is when you force people to give it.

In this discussion, Nigel became calmer. This allowed the clinician to take up the attachment process that had been enacted. In essence, Nigel had made a request to the clinician, with whom he had a positive alliance, and this had been rebuffed. This triggered his pathological rigid attachment processes as he struggled to maintain emotional stability: he attempts to control the other person through threats in order to manage his experience of rejection and loss of control. The response of the clinician was to retreat to some extent by pointing out that there was not much time left, which increased Nigel's attempts to control him. It was a clinical error. It triggered Nigel's habitual response pattern, illuminating his interactions with others. This had been identified in the assessment and was now being activated in the group process. The clinician correctly tried to reduce his arousal and then start exploring the relational process, developing an alternative perspective about what was happening. In the end the group managed to clarify that Nigel wanted to express his desperation but was unable to set up a facilitating context to do this. The result was that Nigel found himself rebuffed, leading to his natural coercive response. After this pattern was defined again and related to his formulation, it was possible to explore his sense that once he had forced people to do things it was ineffective in meeting his need because it was not given freely. This was worked on later in further groups and his individual sessions.

Mentalizing interpersonal process in the group

Mentalizing models are uniquely valuable in complex interpersonal situations involving, for instance, care and concern, conflict, potential deception, or irrationality. All these situations are very likely to arise during group interaction. But, as we have suggested, nonreflective internal working models come to dominate the behavior of people with BPD in any interpersonal situation that calls forth relationship representations derived from their primary attachment relationships. Group therapy stimulates internal experiences of earlier representations, and relationships are jeopardized because patients divide their mentalizing resources unevenly between their external and internal worlds, becoming hypervigilant toward others but uncomprehending of their own states. All these factors distort the interpersonal interactions in the group.

The juxtaposition of need for support and understanding from others with fear of intimacy and distrust of their motives leaves the person with BPD beleaguered and insecure. Relationships become unstable and rapidly changeable, and a supportive friend can suddenly be experienced as malevolent and dangerous. Therapy must therefore attempt to embody a secure base and aim not to repeat this unstable pattern of interpersonal interaction.

It is important to differentiate the work on interpersonal interactions in the group from interventions using mentalizing the relationship. The two may complement each other and the clinician may be able to move from one to the other, often starting with the manifest interpersonal life of the patient, working on the patient's relationship pattern as exemplified in the group, and deepening the intervention later. In contrast to mentalizing the relationship from a transference perspective (see Chapter 10 for discussion), interpersonal work explores the processes *between* people rather than focusing on the mind itself (Box 12.17).

It is concerned with the individual's family relationships, friendship patterns, work interactions, and community relations, and how they impinge on the patient's life, both constructively and destructively. It is about how the patient

Box 12.17 Mentalizing interpersonal process

- Initiate careful step-by-step explorations of crucial intersubjective trans-actions (implicit to explicit)
- Stop the group process when it is off task or is missing important oppor-tunities for mentalizing interpersonal process in the here and now
- Challenge inappropriate certainty and rigid representation
- Demonstrate and explain the primacy of the here and now
- Link to attachment patterns identified in formulation.

brings these patterns and the underlying attachment patterns into the group itself. So, working on mentalizing interpersonal processes as they are demon-strated in the group takes the manifest aspects of the patient's relationships and looks at how they help or hinder the patient or are harnessed to give support in times of crisis. Only once the interpersonal patterns have been clarified is it pos-sible to work in greater depth by mentalizing the relationship, taking into account developmental components.

In order to achieve a mentalizing exploration of the interpersonal interaction between patients, the clinician needs to:

- Keep in mind the interpersonal network of each patient
- Identify patterns in external relationships that are repeated within the group; this should have been considered in the original formulation
- Balance exploration of relationships between the members of the group with consideration of their relationships outside treatment
- Explore the satisfying and dissatisfying aspects of relationships, both within the group and outside
- Link the patients' experience in the group to their relationships outside it.

It was apparent from the initial assessment and formulation of a patient, Jean-nie, that her tendency was to try to please others. If she felt someone did not like her or was critical of her, she tried to adopt their view and to behave in a way she believed they wanted her to. As a result, she was vulnerable to exploitation. During the group she rarely talked about her own problems and focused on helping others. Whenever they talked about a problem, she would ask them questions and be supportive. Once an alliance was established between her and the clinician, he decided to try to work on this aspect of her manifest behavior in the group. He did so by bringing it up as something for her to consider when she said that she had no problems to discuss during the "go-around." Initially, he was positive about her helpful attitude to others' problems and asked her if this was a role she found herself taking in her everyday life.

CLINICIAN: Jeannie, you are always helpful to others in the group and you have just been really helpful to Peter. Do you find yourself helping people in everyday life?

Jeannie agreed with this, and it was established that she had many examples of being helpful to others. In many aspects this confirmed the validity of the initial formulation.

CLINICIAN: It occurs to me that you don't talk about yourself so much and you often say that you don't have any problems for the group when we go around at the beginning. It makes me think that you might be deferring to others. Is there any mileage in exploring that?
JEANNIE: Yes, it would be a good idea.
CLINICIAN: Are you deferring to me now? [A small challenge; this surprised Jeannie.]

Jeannie hesitated and said that maybe she was and that she did not think it was a problem for her. So the clinician allowed the group to continue, concerned that she had agreed too easily (suggesting that she was in pretend mode). The initial exploration of the interpersonal process and other preparatory work had not been done to indicate a move toward mentalizing the relationship with him and others in the group.

A bit later in the group, Jeannie said something in response to another patient, Leslie.

LESLIE: No, Jeannie, that's definitely not right. What made you say that?
JEANNIE: Oh, I can see that it is not right. Sorry about that. You are right. I got that wrong.

Jeannie continued being self-deprecating, and so the clinician said that this was an example of what he had been trying to identify earlier in the group. Was she really changing her mind, or simply agreeing with Leslie "for a quiet life," worrying about upsetting him? Had she really agreed with the clinician about deferring to others?

JEANNIE: Oh, I don't know. I don't really want to talk about it. I don't want to be forced. I am sorry that I got it wrong Leslie.

In this illustration the clinician is gradually trying to build up a picture of Jeannie's pattern with other patients. Once this is established and recognized by Jeannie and others in the group, she has a chance of working on it in the group in more detail, and the clinician can move from mentalizing the interpersonal process to mentalizing the relationship. Of course, the danger in this sort of interpersonal interaction is that the clinician is confirming his/her own views of the pattern and beginning to force them on to the patient. This breaks the safety principle in MBT of the clinician ensuring he/she does not take over the mentalizing of the patient and force his/her understanding on the patient. But it also implies that mentalizing the relationship may be considered at this point once the clinician has recognized that he/she may be forcing the issue and the collaboration has been lost. Is there a contribution from both the clinician and the patient in the interaction which could be explored to deepen the understanding of the interpersonal process? In mentalizing the relationship, the contribution from the clinician is actively explored. So, in this example the clinician would first have to validate the patient's experience of being forced to talk about something. Following this, the clinician's contribution can be clarified and the patient's tendency to capitulate explored. In fact, in this situation in the group it is possible that Jeannie's refusal may be her first step toward asserting her own wishes. This process between patient and clinician could be focused on and then triangulated.

Triangulation

There is nothing new about the concept of triangulation, nor do we claim any originality in the technical intervention of triangulation. In effect, triangulation is creating a space, an alternative dimension and perspective, in the dialogue between two people by inserting a third person. It is the oedipal triangle revisited; it is a triadic interaction in place of a dyadic communication. Clinicians actively triangulate in MBT-G (Box 12.18).

Box 12.18 Triangulation

- Clinician identifies important interaction between participants
- Notes the observer(s)
- Separates the protagonists
- Actively explores the observer(s)' own experience of the interaction (talk about self) or about his/her/their thoughts about the observed interaction (talk about others).

It is left to the clinician's sensitivity to decide when to do so if two patients are engaged in a dialogue. Involving others in an intimate conversation between two group members too early can be disruptive; too late and the potential for increasingly detailed perspectives and understanding is lost because the minds of the other patients are no longer attending to the issue under scrutiny.

Triangulation is an intervention addressing the collapse or imminent collapse of self–other interaction into self–self interaction. When interaction between two patients, or between a clinician and patient, becomes inaccessible to the rest of the group, the isolation of the interaction from the rest of the group suggests that mentalizing has begun to shift from self–other to self–self, to the extent that the two protagonists are creating a shared representation which excludes alternative scrutiny. Often this is a collusion of sameness and agreement—"I am just the same. I know exactly how you feel. You are right and no one should think differently." Bion (1961) described this process between patients as a component of *pairing*, one of his "basic assumptions," in which two patients take on the work of the group through their continued interaction. In addition, Bion anticipated that pairing allowed other members of the group to listen eagerly and attentively with a sense of relief and hopeful anticipation. However, in patients with severe personality disorder the converse is more common; they tend to sit and watch and slowly drift away. In addition, it is not our contention that the collapse into dyadic interaction necessarily creates something for the whole group, such as the formation of an organizing idea that can be identified or interpreted in a helpful way. People with severe personality disorder are unable to meaningfully recognize such a high level of group and social representation. As a result of this more limited understanding of the process, MBT-G refrains from interpretation of the group process itself but, instead, triangulates by actively inserting "other" mentalizing into the dialogue to prevent collapse into nonmentalizing process.

Of particular significance is ensuring that triangulation takes place when two clinicians become involved with one patient. In this context, the clinicians are viewed as one person; that is, the interaction is psychologically dyadic even though there are three people involved. Involvement of both clinicians tends to occur when one patient is identified as being at serious risk or has been involved in an important personal event. It interferes with the overall mentalizing in the group just as much as two patients joining together to the exclusion of others. The problem is exacerbated because both clinicians may be unaware of the rest of the group for a considerable time. To reduce the risk of this happening, in MBT-G the clinicians have an explicit agreement when working together that if one of them focuses on a patient, the other clinician thinks about triangulation and intervenes either by talking to his/her colleague, directly bringing in an alternative perspective, or by actively bringing in other members of the group. When clinicians talk to each other it draws the mind of the patient away from a focus on "self" to possible interest in "other." Once this is achieved, the clinicians can facilitate group interaction around the focus of the problem.

Who to triangulate to?

In MBT-G, the clinician triangulates to a specific person. Rarely does he/she triangulate to the group as a whole by saying, for example, "What do others think?" "Has anyone else any thoughts about this?" Specifying an individual forces the interactive process and does not allow the group to easily sink into ineffectual silence. In contrast, asking the whole group to comment would enable group members to avoid the question and to remain detached from the problems being discussed. To prevent this, the clinician moves the dialogue to a member whom he/she knows may have some interest in the problem or may recognize the difficulties the other person is presenting. At this point the clinician has two choices. He/she can ask the chosen person to comment on the dialogue between the two other patients—"What is your view about their discussion?"; "Can you help them with this problem?" Alternatively, he/she can ask the person to talk about his/her experience of the dialogue—"What is your feeling in listening to this?"; "What does it make you think about in yourself?"; "Does it trigger any ideas about your own life?"

The slight difference in emphasis between these two aspects of triangulation is whether the intervention focuses the patient who is brought in through triangulation on the mind states of the other protagonists or on his/her own state of mind and reactions formed by observing and listening to the dyadic dialogue— "about them" or "about me in response to them." Often the move to stimulate another patient to consider the effect on him/herself as observer of the dialogue stimulates more interactive mentalizing, but this is not necessarily the case, and the clinician can move the dialogue back and forth between the two using both foci, carefully monitoring the outcome on interactional mentalizing. This highlights both the focus of the dialogue between patients in the group and the experiences of the others that can be projected on to the interaction.

Parking

Problems with attentional control are frequent in patients with BPD and other personality disorders. Patients often find it hard to suppress a dominant desire in order to attend to a subdominant process. This means they may not be able to easily focus on a topic of relevance and importance to another person if they, themselves, have a strong desire to talk about something affecting them. They will try to do so but sooner or later their dominant wish to talk about a topic relevant to them will burst out, usually following signs of increasing tension or even desperation. Yet constructive interaction with others requires good attentional control. All of us have to suppress a pressing wish to talk about something if there is a need to discuss something else or if we are to focus on another person. If people with BPD are to improve their personal relationships, it is important that they increase their capacity for attentional control because this is the "bread and butter" of the to-and-fro of conversations. They need to learn to inhibit their impulse to demand attention or, alternatively, gradually but sensitively divert attention to themselves in a socially constructive way. The aim of the clinician "parking" a patient is to help them generate this capacity, facilitated by the use of a positive therapeutic alliance (Box 12.19).

MBT clinicians constantly monitor the arousal levels of all patients, following the MBT principle that arousal has to be maintained within a moderate range, neither too high nor too low, if mentalizing is to be facilitated rather than impeded. The clinician is constantly alert to indicators of arousal, whether behavioral or psychological. As soon as the clinician recognizes that a patient is becoming agitated, parking him/her may become necessary if the group process is not to be suddenly disrupted by that one patient's excessive anxiety. The patient may show his/her agitation by shaking a foot, moving around excessively or trying to interrupt; alternatively, he/she may be withdrawn, looking down, furtively glancing or appear preoccupied. The clinician quietly notes this and asks the patient if he/she can wait for a short time so that the group can conclude the current focus before attending to him/her. Often, this is best done slightly conspiratorially as this will make the patient feel special and attended to by the clinician. But, equally, it can be stated openly—"Rachel, can you hang on a short time so that we can finish off this with Peter. We will be back to you in a minute." The point here is that the patient must feel they are seen as a person

---

Box 12.19 Parking

- Clinician notes that a patient is unable to maintain attentional control
- Identifies the experience of the patient rather than the content of the problem
- Actively helps the patient focus on a subdominant theme
- Keeps a lid on the dominant desire by momentarily letting off steam
- Clinician must not forget he/she has "parked" a patient—may have to pause the group if the patient becomes excessively anxious.

with a need and that their urgent demand has been recognized. This allows them to temporarily inhibit the urge to talk about their own problem and possibly attend briefly to the problem being discussed.

> A patient, Emma, was clearly agitated as soon as she arrived at the group. During the "go-around" she said that she had to talk about her boyfriend, who she thought was seeing another woman. She had challenged him about this but he had denied it and said that she was being "borderline paranoid." This had enraged her. At the end of the "go-around" she was asked if she wanted to go first but she suggested the group started with another patient, who had taken an overdose. The discussion started focusing on the suicide risk of this patient, but it was obvious to the clinician that Emma was becoming increasingly unable to focus on the difficulties of the patient who had overdosed. Her foot was gyrating back and forth and she was impatient. Quietly, he turned to her, for he was sitting next to her, and said "It is really hard listening to other stuff when you want to talk about your own problems. If you can, can you hang on and I will make sure that we get round to you soon." Emma calmed. As the group continued, her tension returned, so each time this became apparent the clinician turned to her and quietly said that it would not be long. This, again, reduced her tension.

The skill of the clinician is to know how long a patient can be "parked" or placed in the queue. If it becomes necessary to allow a patient to take over the focus of the group, to "un-park" him/her, the clinician needs to state this explicitly and to "park" the active patient and his/her current topic for a time—"Mark, can you hang on to that for the moment so that we can come back to it. I think Emma needs to come in now and talk about her problems as she can't concentrate on your issues at the moment. We will definitely come back to yours though."

It will be apparent that parking is a further way in which the clinician takes some authority in the group. He/she ensures that arousal levels and patient imperatives are recognized and managed. In addition, the "parked" patient feels that they are recognized as an individual and that their needs are recognized. Parking serves as an *ostensive cue* making the patient feel recognized as an "agent," a person who has needs. This ostensive cue signals to the patient that the clinician has a communicative intention addressed to his/her needs but asks that he/she waits for a short time while other concerns are dealt with. This encourages the patient to manage his/her internal pressure to dominate the discourse and to make demands on others.

Of course, it is necessary for the clinician to remember who has been parked and to return to their concerns sensitively when possible!

Siding

Sometimes the clinician may have to actively take the side of a patient during an interaction in the group. This is known as "siding." This is more than simply being supportive to a patient, and requires the clinician to act as the mind

---

Box 12.20 Siding

- Clinician notes that a patient is vulnerable to other patients' actions/comments/focus
- Clinician actively takes the side of the vulnerable patient
- Other clinician (if present) takes the position of antagonist
- Clinician supports the vulnerable patient until mentalizing is rekindled in the group
- Clinician switches sides if necessary when the vulnerable patient is more stable.

---

of a vulnerable patient throughout an interaction in the group. The key indicator for the clinician to start taking sides is if one patient is becoming increasingly vulnerable in the context of a discourse either between him/her and another patient or between the patient and the rest of the group. A patient may inadvertently be cruel to another, make a dismissive remark when a patient is struggling to talk about a problem, or actively attack someone in the group verbally. The clinician rapidly assesses the state of mind of the most vulnerable patient and takes some authority by siding with him/her. He does this by saying something in response on behalf of the patient—"That was a bit harsh, Karen. Can you try to express what you mean a bit differently?" The clinician continues to act on behalf of the vulnerable patient for as long as necessary while ensuring that the other patient does not become vulnerable or feel under attack him/herself. The aim is to maintain reasonable levels of attachment arousal and to reduce the immediate stress of the situation (Box 12.20).

A patient, Andrea, reported that she didn't know what to do about her boyfriend. She wanted to be with him but he was avoiding her and it made her feel unwanted and unattractive. As she talked about this she became increasingly upset. The group members tried to reassure her that it would be OK and gave her all sorts of suggestions about how to deal with the problem. Each time she responded by saying their comments were unhelpful. Suddenly another patient, Catherine, said, "Oh stop moaning for goodness sake. Leave him then so that we can talk about something else. You are being pathetic." Andrea began sobbing.

CLINICIAN: Hang on. What are you saying here? Andrea is struggling with how to manage her boyfriend and talking about how she feels hopeless, and you say this is pathetic. That sounds awfully judgmental to me. Andrea, I don't think this is pathetic. The problem we have is how to help you to feel a bit stronger about it, and that is our problem. Now, Catherine, can you say what it is that is going on for you about this rather than commenting on Andrea?

At this point the clinician has taken the side of Andrea and pushed the focus back to Catherine. This will reduce Andrea's stress. Now the clinician has to monitor the effect on Catherine as she, too, may become vulnerable. Indeed, in this group she did so and reacted by challenging the clinician.

CATHERINE: You always support her. You like her better. We spend so much time on Andrea in every group that there is nothing for the rest of us and it has no effect. She always says that things we say are useless.

CLINICIAN: You may be right about some of that, but I think it is important that we don't dismiss Andrea and her struggle to work out what to do. So I thought it might help if you could talk about what effect it is having on you.

The clinician is keeping the focus on Catherine at this point but trying to ensure that he supports her to some extent. The conversation continued, and as the tension reduced the clinician passed the focus back to Andrea, no longer taking sides.

CLINICIAN: Andrea, while I can see that what Catherine said was hurtful, what do you make of this sense that every time the group try to help that it seems to go nowhere? Is that your experience?

The group then began to focus on the problem of trying to help someone but that person not finding the support helpful. The problem was that Andrea's negativity gradually produced frustration in other members and left them feeling hopeless, a response that was normalized by the group leader. Nevertheless, the group members were tasked by the clinician to make sure that if they were becoming frustrated when talking to Andrea they should say so. Andrea was asked to monitor her negativity and to identify anything that she found helpful, so that she could let the group know.

To conclude with this example, having structured the MBT group, the group process harnesses the initial formulation agreed with each patient to inform mentalizing of the relationships that each one has in the group. Andrea had identified early in treatment that people avoided her and it made her feel that she needed them even more. This led her to contact them more, but doing this seemed to put them off her more. She was lonely, even with her boyfriend. In the group, Andrea is talking about her experience of being unloved by her boyfriend. This leads her to demand support from the group but, as their suggestions are rejected, the people in the group also start to "unwant" and avoid her. After the clinician reduces the arousal levels through siding with Andrea, the interactional process becomes the platform from which the clinician mentalizes the interpersonal relationships she has with her boyfriend and the other patients in the group. This meets the primary aim of the group, namely, to increase the experience of maintaining mentalizing within the emotional interaction of important attachment relationships.

Reference

Bion, W. R. (1961). *Experiences in groups*. London. UK: Tavistock.

Chapter 13

Antisocial personality disorder: mentalizing, MBT-G, and common clinical problems

Introduction

The principles underpinning mentalizing groups for people with antisocial personality disorder (ASPD) are similar to those for borderline personality disorder (BPD), so this chapter should be read in conjunction with Chapter 12. However, the focus of the group work in MBT for ASPD is modified to make it more appropriate for these individuals. These modifications are discussed in this chapter.

Randomized controlled trials of MBT have included people with ASPD. In a trial comparing MBT with structured clinical management for people with BPD (Bateman & Fonagy, 2009), a subanalysis of the data showed that, although the effectiveness of MBT for BPD was attenuated in participants who also had comorbid ASPD, the adverse effect of the comorbidity was less with MBT than with structured clinical management. This led us to consider whether MBT could be modified to improve outcomes for people with ASPD. There are limited data to answer this question. MBT was designed for BPD but it may have broader scope. Mentalizing is a key component of self-identity and a central aspect of interpersonal relationships and social function. Thus, improvements in mentalizing may impact on a range of disordered mental processes, whatever the source of pathology. If personality disorder is conceptualized as a serious impairment in interpersonal relationships, intimacy, identity, and self-direction (Skodol et al., 2011), enhancing mentalizing might ameliorate personality disorder as a whole, regardless of subtype. Yet, adaptation of the basic MBT model is likely to be necessary—not only because the mentalizing problems of people with ASPD differ from those found in individuals with BPD, but also for a number of descriptive reasons (see Box 13.1).

First, people with ASPD are more likely to demonstrate over-control of their emotional states within well-structured, schematic attachment relationships, rather than the under-control in chaotic attachment relationships that are more commonly found in people with BPD. Their dyscontrol may be limited to

Box 13.1 Mentalizing and ASPD: summary

- Individuals with ASPD are unable to develop any real understanding of their own inner world (self)
- Experts at cognitively reading the inner states of others; misuse this capacity to coerce or manipulate others, with no "we" mode of empathic understanding
- Lack ability to read certain emotions (possibly a wide range) accurately—a component of externally based mentalizing
- Cannot generate how they would feel in the other's situation
- Fail to recognize fearful emotions from facial expressions. This suggests a dysfunction in neural structures, such as the amygdala, that subserve fearful expression processing
- There is a robust link between antisocial behavior and specific deficits in recognizing fearful expressions. This impairment does not appear to be attributable solely to task difficulty.

volatile anger. Second, people with ASPD tend to seek relationships that are organized hierarchically, with each person knowing their place; in contrast, people with BPD aim for, but tend to struggle to reach, consensus and shared respect. Third, it is specifically threats to the hierarchical order of relationships that lead to arousal within the attachment system in people with ASPD; this triggers an inhibition of mentalizing, which in turn leads to fears of inability to control internal states. It has been suggested that the internal state most feared by people with ASPD is threat to self-esteem (Gilligan, 2000). People with ASPD inflate their self-esteem by demanding respect from others, controlling the people around them, and creating an atmosphere of fear. This maintains their pride, prestige, and status. Loss of status is devastating as it potentially reveals shameful internal states that threaten to overwhelm the individual, so any threat of loss of status becomes firmly rooted as a dangerous reality that has to be dealt with by physical force. Momentary inability to mentalize—to see behind a perceived threat to what is in the mind of the person apparently threatening them—means that they have no way of keeping out an encroaching rapidly lowering self-esteem and loss of position. Emotional capacities such as guilt, love toward others, and fear for the self may protect them from engaging in violent behavior, but the loss of mentalizing and the attenuated ability of people with ASPD to experience such feelings prevent these inhibitory mechanisms being mobilized. Fourth, if the reduction in ability to recognize others' emotions is more pervasive than being restricted to fear and sadness, then a focus in treatment on recognizing *all* emotions in others is essential. Finally, fear for the self is often absent in these individuals and their violent impulses are uninfluenced by the emotional expressions of others, which frequently go unrecognized. Indeed, the consequences and dangers of aggression become secondary to the need to reduce internal collapse of a sense of self. All this has to be taken into account in formulating the aims and focus of group treatment for people with ASPD.

Group work is crucial for people with ASPD if nonmentalizing and disorganized group behavior in their lives is to be addressed. In such groups, teleological systems tend to dominate (see Box 13.2). Many people with ASPD live within a subculture of barely restrained violence and implicit threats; in this regard they are more likely to be influenced by their peer group than by clinicians whom they see as unlikely to understand the sociocultural context in which they live. More importantly, group work stimulates a hierarchical process within a peer group, which can be harnessed in vivo by the clinicians to explore participants' sensitivity to hierarchy and authority and the ensuing mentalizing distortions (see Box 13.3).

Box 13.2 Nonmentalizing and disorganized groups: teleological systems

- Expectations concerning the agency of the other are present, but these are formulated uniquely in terms restricted to the physical world: only what is material can be meaningful
- Attitudes to ideas and feelings:
  - Focus on understanding actions in terms of their physical, as opposed to mental, outcomes
  - Only a modification in the realm of the physical is regarded as a true indicator of the intentions of the other
  - Only action that has a physical impact is felt as potentially capable of altering mental states in both self and other:
- Physical acts of harm: aggression is seen as legitimate
- Demand for physical acts of demonstration of intent by others: for example, payment, acts of subservience, retributive justice.

Box 13.3 Creating a mentalizing group

- Activate attachment by creating an attitude of compassion and wish to understand
- Enhance the curiosity that members of the group have about each other's thoughts and feelings
- Be careful to identify when mentalizing has turned into pseudomentalizing (pretending to know)
- Focus on misunderstandings (mentalizing is the "understanding of misunderstanding")
- Encourage and develop a culture of curiosity coupled with respectful not-knowing.

Aims of treatment

MBT-ASPD aims to:

1 Stimulate robust mentalizing in all dimensions in the context of hierarchical interpersonal interactions and intimate relationships (see Box 13.4)
2 Reduce aggression as the primary pathway of expression of problematic internal states.

Box 13.4 Aims of MBT-ASPD group

- Increase understanding of self (internal) states
- Develop an awareness of self–other interactional states
- Consider others' subjective experience
- Build up a capacity for considering what someone else feels
- Identify hierarchical and inflexible aspects of relationships.
  In order to:
- Reduce aggression as the primary pathway of expression of problematic internal states.

Problems undermining treatment

Individuals with ASPD notoriously undermine attempts to treat them. This may manifest in a number of ways:

1 Their motivation varies considerably

2 Requesting treatment often appears to have secondary motives

3 Initially they deny problems and blame others

4 Practical problems, for example, crime and dealing with the courts, prison sentences and recall to prison (e.g., for those who reoffend while on parole), and housing.

The clinician needs to make an agreed hierarchy of problems likely to interfere with treatment. Initially, lack of motivation to attend regularly may be the primary problem, as this will interfere considerably with the continuity of sessions. But participants' motivation will not be increased by appeals to a socially collaborative group process, for example, by appealing to their social/group responsibilities not to undermine the process and continuity of the group through nonattendance. Such attempts to induce guilt will not serve to increase motivation. The attenuated capacity for such feelings in people with ASPD means that they cannot be harnessed as powerful organizing factors. It is better to establish with participants a mutual acceptance that you will do what you can to work on their problems from a practical and a psychological point of view and that this can be achieved only through regular attendance.

Focus of MBT-ASPD

In the light of the theoretical and clinical understanding of the roots of violence in people with ASPD outlined in Chapter 2, MBT-ASPD focuses on:

1 Understanding emotional cues—external mentalizing and its link to self and other internal states. Participants are asked to identify how they decide how someone else feels.

2 Recognition of emotions in others—other/affective mentalizing. For example, accepting descriptions of feelings, asking about feelings in others.

3 Identification of affect states in the self—self/affective mentalizing. The clinician focuses on the description and labeling of affects, and the recognition of bodily indicators of feeling states.

4 Exploration of sensitivity to hierarchy and authority—self/cognitive mentalizing. Work in the group identifies competition, attempts to control others, and dismissive statements toward others.

Box 13.5 Key mentalizing components in MBT-ASPD

- Understanding emotional cues—external mentalizing and its link to internal states
- Recognition of emotions in others—other/affective mentalizing
- Exploration of sensitivity to hierarchy and authority—self/cognitive mentalizing
- Generation of an interpersonal process to understand subtleties of others' experience in relation to ones' own—self/other mentalizing
- Explication of threats to loss of mentalizing that lead to teleological understanding of motivation—self/other mentalizing and self/affective mentalizing.

---

5 Generation of an interpersonal process to understand others' experience in relation to one's own—self/other mentalizing.

6 Explication of threats to loss of mentalizing that lead to teleological understanding of motivation—self/other mentalizing and self/affective mentalizing. The clinician methodically links emotions with interpersonal interactions and participants' requirement to take action to control perceived external threats.

See Box 13.5.

Format of treatment

1 MBT-ASPD combines weekly MBT group therapy with monthly individual sessions.

2 Treatment for each individual lasts 1 year.

3 In pilot studies of MBT-ASPD, two clinicians ran the group. Having two clinicians rather than one may be more important when working with individuals with ASPD than with BPD—both to manage risk and to model the ability to work with another person constructively while being respectful of differences.

4 The trajectory of each group session is structured in the same way as for people with BPD:

- Summary of the previous week and feedback from participants
- "Go-around" to establish any key areas to be covered in the group

- Synthesis of problems if possible
- Focus on each problem area in turn
- Closure
- Post-group discussion.

See also Box 13.6. Features of the group are outlined in Box 13.7.

Many MBT-ASPD groups begin with dialogue seemingly in pseudo-philosophical-political mode about how awful the system is, how no one can be trusted, how the police are corrupt, and so on. In essence, this is pretend mode. Contrary to the usual exhortation about pretend mode (challenge it and do not allow it to become embedded), it is important to allow the participants to do this at the beginning of a group to give them a sense of unity. However, the aim is to bring the conversation back to a focus on problem areas and/or on the here and now of how they are feeling as soon as possible.

5. The individual sessions are provided by the group clinicians and are *not* delivered by a separate clinician. The rationale for this is:

Box 13.6 Treatment format

- Treatment for 1 year
- Group therapy once per week for 75 minutes, with initial introductory groups focusing on emotion recognition and understanding of ASPD
- Individual therapy with group clinician once per month
- Integrated psychiatric care
- Crisis planning
- Code of conduct.

Box 13.7 Group features

- Slow open group
- Avoid:
  - Time-out contracts
  - Discharge due to failure to meet attendance contract
  - Exhortation based on the effect on others of an individual's absence
  - Challenging a hierarchical relationship early in therapy.

- ◆ The individual sessions are provided primarily to support the person with ASPD in the group.
- ◆ The peer-group interaction may be more significant as a process for change than individual therapy with a clinician.
- ◆ Having the same clinician minimizes the opportunity for deception about what happens in the group, which may distort discussion about the group work in the individual session.
- ◆ It allows a focus on different perceptions of events and experiences in the group by contrasting the experiences of the clinician in the group with those of the participant.
- ◆ Participants may use the individual sessions to discuss issues that they are reluctant or ashamed to talk about in the group, such as difficulties in their personal relationships, depressed or suicidal feelings, etc. Exploring their sensitivities individually may facilitate the participant to talk about them in the group in future sessions.
- ◆ When new participants join an established group, the individual sessions may also be used to go over the psychoeducational topics covered in MBT-I.

6 Participants are asked to complete brief outcome measures on a regular basis. The core outcome measure is the Modified Overt Aggression Scale (MOAS) (Yudofsky, Silver, Jackson, Endicott, & Williams, 1986). This can be done at the end of each group.

Organization of sessions

Each group session lasts for 75 minutes. The first six to eight groups are organized as an introduction and an engagement phase; this is a modified version of the MBT-I for BPD (see Chapter 11, where the modifications specific to ASPD are described).

It is common for the introductory sessions to be diverted from task by participants with ASPD. They attend for their own reasons and these frequently dominate their requests in the early sessions. Participants often present at a time when they have social, legal, or personal problems, for which they may well request written statements about their psychiatric problems, support with access to benefits, help to see their children and/or partner, and so on. This creates severe problems for the clinicians, who wish to help but can easily begin to feel manipulated and diverted from task.

Suggestion: Tell the participants that you are unable to provide any letters of support with regard to social, legal, and interpersonal problems until the six to eight MBT-I sessions are complete. The rationale for this is that it is not possible to know what can be said in such letters until this assessment and engagement period is complete.

Some group principles

Code of conduct

Developing a code of conduct is a central feature in groups for ASPD (see Box 13.8). Appropriate rules and boundaries need to be agreed for members to function together effectively. It is important that the clinicians do not impose their own code of conduct on the group, but first establish a discussion around the participants' moral values and sense of responsibility and fairness. Commonly, people with ASPD have distinct rules that are rigidly applied. Find out what these are, as they often include many of the common principles sustaining group behavior.

Nonjudgmental attitude

Although the overt reason for each participant's referral has been for acts of violence, the clinician must appear neither to condemn nor condone his/her offenses, but instead maintain a benign attitude of attempting to understand the participant's internal state of mind and mental precursors of violence. Although the antisocial person will defy the laws of society with no apparent compunction, breaking their own internal code of conduct, for example, harming a woman, may induce feelings of shame and wrong-doing in the individual. The clinician takes care not to trigger this feeling of shame.

Clinician requirements

The group clinicians must set certain group principles or rules in order for the group to feel safe (see Box 13.9), but must also permit the expression of

---

Box 13.8 Developing a code of conduct in the group

- Developing a shared code of conduct is a key task but will be problematic for participants with ASPD
- Highlight and explore participants' own code of conduct by discussing their interactions with others and what leads to violence
- Adopt a benign attitude of curiosity and understanding
- Neither condemn nor condone behaviors.

Box 13.9 Group principles

- Regular attendance
- Commitment to thinking about others as well as themselves
- Openness within the group
- Confidentiality outside the group
- Discuss contact between participants outside the group
- Prohibition of threats and violence
- Avoiding inappropriate and offensive comments
- "Advice-free zone."

anti-authoritarian attitudes without these becoming destructive to the group. People with ASPD will predictably react against whatever rules they feel are being imposed upon them. If the clinicians are identified by the participant as agents of social control, arbitrarily imposing "socially acceptable" rules and regulations, the participant will inevitably oppose this and therapeutic work will become impossible.

Clinician principles operating in the group are discussed with the participant early in treatment. This discussion includes agreement about attendance, openness within the group, prohibition of threats and violence, refraining from contact with other participants outside of the group, and commitment to thinking about others as well as themselves. At the beginning of the group the clinicians should also outline the importance of avoiding inappropriate comments that are likely to cause offense. In MBT-I, it is pointed out that racial and sexual stereotypes are manifestly nonmentalized phenomena.

It is important that the clinicians explain the reasons underpinning these principles (see Box 13.10). As we have mentioned, people with ASPD are little influenced by concern for others or for overall group requirements, so explaining your principles by suggesting that, for example, when they do not attend this affects everyone, will be ineffective. Applying pressure through inducing guilt and/or encouraging selflessness are contraindicated. The participants' experience in life has been of coercive methods and sometimes punishment, all of which have had little effect on their behavior; do not recreate this in the group. The reason for encouraging attendance is so that the individuals can address their problems consistently; erratic attendance means that gains will be lost rather than consolidated. Learning from others is also increased with reliable interaction.

Box 13.10 Communication of group principles

- Discuss principles operating in the group with participants early in treatment
- Explain reasons underlying group principles
- Do not appeal to social generosity/selflessness of individuals or the effects of their actions on others
- Do not inject pressure through attempting to induce shame or guilt
- Emphasize necessity of regular attendance for individuals to address their problems consistently and learn from others.

Confidentiality and disclosure

All services have clear policies and procedures in relation to confidentiality, and all clinicians have a duty to protect personal confidentiality and the public where necessary. It is therefore necessary to clarify the limits of confidentiality and disclosure to participants at the outset (see Box 13.11).

In principle, the treatment team respects the privacy of individual sessions, and does not discuss in the groups information that has been volunteered in the individual sessions. However, every aspect of treatment, including the individual sessions, is discussed within the clinical team. The participants are informed

Box 13.11 Confidentiality

- Clarify the limits of confidentiality and disclosure to agencies at the outset
- Frame as "discretion"
- "Team confidentiality"—all information is shared within the clinical team
- Participants are encouraged to talk about violent/aggressive incidents in the group, to mentalize and identify points of mentalizing change
- However, they may be reluctant to talk about current offenses for fear of disclosure
- They may talk about previous offenses if they do not reveal too much detail to warrant disclosure.

about this "team confidentiality" and its aim of maximizing safety and the effectiveness of treatment. Contact with professionals outside the team, for example, probation officers, social workers, and housing officers, is agreed with each participant. All members of the group are required to keep shared information on personal issues within the treatment setting.

Participants should be told at the start of treatment that staff have a duty to report any serious incidents that are described with sufficient detail for the victim and/or offense to be identified. Disclosure will also be considered if there is a current significant risk to self or others, or to children. As far as possible, disclosure will not be undertaken without full discussion and consultation with all those involved in the individual's management, as well as informing the individual participant concerned.

A straightforward guide, to be discussed with the group, is that if they say "who," "where," or "when" about a crime it may lead to a requirement for the clinician to break confidentiality.

Risk

Participants are encouraged to talk about aggressive and violent incidents in group therapy, many of which are related to the antisocial subculture in which they live, so that they can learn to mentalize these experiences by identifying the feelings and thoughts that are associated with the violent behavior. However, in order to do this, an atmosphere of trust must be fostered and maintained by the MBT clinicians. Participants may be reluctant to talk about current violent incidents for fear of being recalled to prison or convicted. One way of managing this is to encourage them to talk about undisclosed past violence for which they have not been convicted, provided that they do not reveal identifying details of offenses (dates, full names, locations, etc.) so that this information does not need to be passed on to the authorities (see Box 13.12). The clinician thus needs to differentiate an acute risk from the chronic baseline risk. The former may need action on the part of the clinician, while the latter requires careful management with agreed safety monitoring.

> A participant reported that he had slashed someone with a knife since the last group. He talked about the circumstances and insisted that his action was appropriate in the context he was in. Other participants agreed. The participant had allowed his flat to be used for the financial negotiations of local drug dealers. He had asked them to finish their transactions and to leave because he had decided to go out. They refused, so he informed them that he would ask them one more time and if they had not gone in 10 minutes they would be responsible for the consequences. The leader of the drug dealers had not left within the given time and so the participant had picked up a carving knife, threatened him, and slashed his face and back as he ran out of the flat. There was discussion about the participant's action and the clinicians tried to focus on the events

---

Box 13.12 Risk and disclosure

- Clinician needs to differentiate an acute risk from participant's chronic baseline risk

- Disclosure beyond clinical team considered if there is a current serious risk of harm to others, or past identifiable offenses/victims

- Need to consider the acute risk of harm to another, *but* with the risk of the participant disengaging from treatment if clinician discloses, versus the participant staying in treatment *and* long-term risk reducing if disclosure is not made

- Do not disclose without full discussion with all involved, including the participant if possible.

---

leading up to the violence and the experience he had had about being disobeyed. The whole group insisted that the actions of the participant were reasonable in the context he had found himself in. It was not possible to get the participant to consider the effect that defiance from a (younger) person had had on him.

The clinicians were able to identify the provocation that the participant had experienced, but remained concerned about his action even though it occurred within the antisocial male subculture in which he was immersed. The clinicians agreed that they would see him after the group to discuss it further with him. On this occasion it was not necessary for there to be any breach in confidentiality as the victim was unknown, the aim had been to warn him about further transgression, and he was reported to be only superficially hurt.

Contact with other group participants

While most participants readily accept the rule that there should be no violence in the group or clinic, they find it more difficult to accept the recommendation that group members should not meet up in the community between sessions. Refraining from social contact with each other may be particularly difficult for participants who are socially isolated and feel that they have connected to others in the group. We may give them a variety of explanations as to why this is discouraged, such as the formation of subgroups of participants from which others might feel excluded, the dilution of therapeutic efficacy within the group, and the risk that participants may disagree and have a confrontation externally, which might lead to them not wishing to return to group therapy. But participants often do not accept these intellectual rationalizations until they have experienced the effects themselves. In practice, clinicians should adopt a flexible stance, for example, allowing participants to have a cigarette and brief chat together after the group session finishes, but discouraging more extensive contact with each other outside the group (see Box 13.13).

In the group it appeared that Stan, a man in his fifties, was becoming increasingly admiring of another younger participant, Tom, who was in his twenties and seemingly better able than Stan to cope with stressful situations. In his history, Stan had a pattern of becoming friendly with younger men, lending them money and asking for emotional support in return. But the relationships tended to end in violent confrontations when the younger man failed to show sufficient gratitude and offer adequate support.

In one group session, Stan inadvertently let slip that he had spoken to Tom during the week. The clinician asked whether they had met up outside of the group. Stan became irritated and said that he couldn't cope with his family's refusal to see him during the past week, and had phoned Tom for support, as he knew Tom was stronger than him and could give him advice as to what to do. The clinician wondered why he hadn't contacted the clinic to speak to one of the clinicians. Another group member said at this point that talking to a clinician wasn't the same: "Only we understand each other, you don't come from the same background, you couldn't understand." The clinician agreed that they may have different backgrounds and therefore different experiences. He said it sounded like Stan had not been able to wait until the group session. Stan calmed down in the group and accepted that he would talk about it in his individual session. He admitted that he'd been disappointed with Tom's response when he rang him, saying that Tom appeared uninterested in his distress. Meanwhile, Tom admitted in his monthly individual session with his clinician that he felt overwhelmed by Stan's demands, and hoped he would never end up as depressed and lonely as him. Both clinicians suggested to Tom and Stan that it might be better for them not to contact each other between sessions.

A few weeks later, Stan and Tom arrived looking complicit and laughing. Stan said to the clinicians that they'd just had lunch together. Stan's clinician looked rather shocked, which Stan commented on, saying that he was "just joking"; he said that both he and

---

Box 13.13 Extra-group activity

- Adopt flexible stance—"firm but fair"
- Promote attitude of curiosity, exploration, and understanding
- Explain reasons behind principles
- Accept minor joint activity, for example, cigarette with each other for 15 minutes after group session
- May explore disruptive activity in individual sessions to enhance reinforcement of group principles.

Tom knew that they weren't meant to meet outside of the group, which was perhaps right, but they had both by chance come early, and had, with two of the other group members, felt the need to "catch up" just now because the sessions weren't long enough for everyone to talk about what they'd been up to.

Nevertheless, the clinicians rightly mentioned the attachment patterns that Stan had identified in his assessment sessions and suggested that it might be helpful to consider his relationship with Tom in that context.

Power differentials

People with ASPD are sensitive to hierarchy and power differentials (see Box 13.14). In MBT, it is recommended that these dynamics are openly discussed with participants. This issue is introduced in MBT-I. In the module on personality disorder in MBT-I (Module 7; see Chapter 11), the outline description of ASPD includes the characteristic tendency to challenge perceived and actual authority. It is openly acknowledged that the participants may see the clinicians as being in authority. While this is true in some respects, for example, in that the clinicians organize the group, the relationship between participants and clinicians needs to be characterized as collaborative and a joint endeavor.

In the MBT group, clinicians need to keep in mind the likelihood that many interactions may contain an implicit rivalry in which they themselves may become involved. The most useful intervention in MBT in these circumstances is to make the struggle for hierarchical structure part of an affect focus (see Chapter 9) to see if "naming" the dynamic interaction can reduce its power to distort the therapeutic work. It is important to avoid power struggles, which in the end can lead to ultimatums from the clinicians.

A critical role for the clinicians is to explicate aspects of the participant's "alien self"—that is, all the aspects of the person associated with weakness

---

Box 13.14 Hierarchy and power

- People with ASPD experience relationships in terms of power and control
- Clinicians should avoid assuming a position of power in relation to participant(s) too early in treatment
- Apologize for perceived errors and accept criticism
- Clinicians' role is to carry participant's "alien self"—this can be explored *only* once the participant feels safe and contained.

and vulnerability that he abhors, disavows, and projects on to others. The clinicians accept being perceived as weak or ineffectual for a long time, and indeed they are "weak" in many ways, but not necessarily those that are noted by the participant. Participants feel safe and contained if the clinicians do not challenge these dynamics, and may even be able to talk about them, albeit readily identifying threats to their self-esteem, being "disrespected" by others, and the resulting unbearable feeling of shame as common triggers for their violence. We caution against the use of transference interpretation when these dynamics are fixed, as such interventions can too easily stimulate feelings of humiliation if the clinicians are perceived as elevating themselves to a position of importance in relation to the participants. Instead, clinicians should readily apologize for perceived errors and accept criticism to counteract the participants' expectations that the clinicians hold all the power.

Differences in the ways in which participants with ASPD relate to male and female clinicians may reveal gender prejudices that inform the power differential in their relationships and the construction of their codes of honor, such as prohibitions against violence toward women. Participants may appear to experience female clinicians as more vulnerable and less authoritative than their male counterparts. At the same time, they may be less comfortable having individual sessions with a female than with a male clinician. The reasons for this will need to be explored when possible.

Ultimatums

It is easy to become embroiled in arguments with participants about their attendance, attitude, behavior, and use of offensive statements about others, for example, comments about race and gender. Ultimatums should rarely be issued (see Box 13.15). If they are, it is better that they are "life" ultimatums rather than "therapy" ultimatums. The participant is warned, for example, that his attitude is unlikely to bring him more satisfying relationships, that his threats to the housing office are unlikely to increase his chance of getting accommodation, that nonattendance of the group means it is less likely that he will learn to manage his emotions better. Issuing ultimatums about discharge from therapy is generally unhelpful and rarely increases motivation or stimulates change. Nevertheless, it may be necessary at some point to talk to a participant about a potential breakdown of treatment and to identify possible ways of addressing the problem. This is done collaboratively by first agreeing with the participant what the problem is. This is no small task, as many participants will deny that there is a problem.

Box 13.15 Issuing ultimatums

- Ultimatums should rarely be issued
- Avoid becoming embroiled in arguments with participants about their attendance, attitude, behavior, and use of offensive statements about others, for example, comments about race and gender
- If they seem unavoidable, they should be "life" ultimatums rather than "therapy" ultimatums
- Issuing ultimatums about discharge from therapy rarely increases participants' motivation or stimulates change
- If a potential breakdown of treatment seems imminent, try to identify possible ways of addressing the problem collaboratively by first agreeing with the participant what the problem is.

A participant talked constantly in the group. He interrupted others. He swore at the clinicians who tried to interject. He walked out, saying he had other business to attend to. The clinician told the group that he would try to talk to the participant about it on his own. The participant was offered an individual session, but when challenged about his behavior and attitude he said that he could not see a problem at all. He said that other participants didn't mind him talking and that this was a problem manufactured by the clinicians. Eventually, the clinician managed to agree with the participant that they would talk about it in the group more, and this was done the following week.

Whenever possible, argument needs to be avoided, although even a calm but firm statement asking a participant to consider a problem can cause a reaction.

Collaborative relationship

All therapies try to develop a collaborative relationship between clinician and patient. This is an essential component for effective treatment of people with ASPD—but it is also a complex task (see Box 13.16). Engaging in exploration of motives for treatment, taking interest in the person's experience, agreeing joint goals, and discussing the diagnosis will all increase the collaboration in the relationship. Initially, however, the individual's motives for coming to treatment may be unclear; sometimes they may be related to depression, traumatic stress, and anxiety, at other times seemingly related to benefits, requests for reports for unfitness for employment or a court summons, and at others related to more personal developmental wishes, such as becoming a better father to a young child.

Box 13.16 Engaging the participants

- Engaging and maintaining individuals with ASPD in treatment is a key challenge
- People with ASPD do not like to think of themselves as "patients"—this label is associated with shame, stigma, and vulnerability
- May need extended period of engagement or motivational work before engaging in formal treatment program
- Address anxieties about diagnosis, group therapy, and confidentiality.

The clinician can sometimes feel manipulated and tricked and so resist the form of relationship he/she feels forced to engage in. This dynamic process can become entrenched, making the joint project of therapy impossible. To make matters more uncertain, the clinician can think that he/she is developing a collaborative relationship and even that he/she has an attachment-based relationship with a participant, only to find that the experience is not reciprocal and, in reality, the participant is still trying to work out what they can get from the clinician and the system. It may not be possible to recognize this and it becomes apparent only when the participant fails to attend appointments and is not contactable.

> A clinician had been working with a participant on his aggressive outbursts, and the participant reported these to have diminished. In addition, he reported that his relationship with his girlfriend had improved. It was only when the girlfriend phoned the department to say that she had taken out a court injunction against the participant that the clinician realized that the positive attitude the participant appeared to have to treatment and to the clinician was part of an attempt to get a positive recommendation about progress in treatment for his probation officer.
>
> The participant continued to attend, so the clinician made explicit the negative effect that pretending to improve had on their working relationship while simultaneously trying to validate his wish to improve. A life ultimatum was also stated—that pretending to people that he was something he was not was likely to lead to misunderstandings, trouble, and damaged relationships.

"Advice-free zone"

At the onset of the group it is worth attempting a discussion about advice. Participants tend to give each other advice, and the participants often welcome it. They may also demand advice from the clinicians. The clinicians can open the discussion by highlighting the difference between the practicality of advice and the understanding of problems in terms of mental processes and personality function. Although there may be times when immediate advice, for example, advice to the participant to visit his general medical practitioner or to attend his probation appointment, is both useful and necessary, the aim of the group is to work on how emotional problems and interactional patterns create interpersonal and social dysfunction. It is *not* to offer practical advice. The aim is to work toward the group being an "advice-free zone."

To some extent this discussion can be done in the MBT-I sessions, but it is necessary to make "giving advice" an explicit topic in the MBT group itself. It is agreed and/or eventually stated by the clinicians that the group is an "advice-free zone" and that it should be respected as such.

Engagement and nonattendance

Engaging and maintaining people with ASPD in treatment is a key challenge, as the majority of individuals with ASPD do not accept that they have mental health difficulties and will not willingly present for help (see Box 13.16). Clinicians treating people with ASPD in the community should anticipate numerous challenges, including lateness or missing planned appointments and therapy sessions, frequent crises, boundary violations, and drug and alcohol abuse. Many individuals with ASPD may need an extended period of engagement or motivational work before engaging in the formal treatment program, and they may be particularly anxious about going into group therapy. Building a therapeutic rapport and collaborative relationship with each participant is essential. Caring, fairness and trust, and an authoritative—but not authoritarian—style should characterize the treatment relationship.

Attendance can be encouraged by:

1 Phoning the participants each week 24 hours prior to the group. This can be done by an administrator or secretary rather than one of the clinicians. This should be discussed with the participants when they start in the group. Most appreciate the reminder, but on occasions a participant may find such calls intrusive and not want the reminder. It is important to get a mobile phone number that the participant will answer: many participants have more than one mobile phone, using one number for friends and another number for organizations or for other purposes.

2 Contacting participants when they miss sessions. The clinician should pro-actively follow them up, such as calling to remind them of appointments or to enquire sensitively why they missed a session, as well as positively reinforcing their engagement in therapeutic tasks.

Breaks in therapy

Breaks in treatment are particularly difficult times for people with ASPD and may be associated with an increased risk of "acting out." Although breaks in the group therapy sessions may be minimized due to the clinicians covering for each other when one is away on leave, inevitably there will be times when the group cannot meet, for example, over Christmas. The potential impact of the clinicians' absence on individuals with ASPD may be underestimated due to the erratic attendance of the participants themselves and their denial of attachment needs. It is important not to collude with the participants' conscious rejection of their need for treatment, and be alert to them becoming more disturbed during breaks in treatment, which they may find difficult to acknowledge. Any awareness of dependence on the clinicians or group may be associated with feelings of vulnerability and humiliation. Similarly, difficult feelings regarding the ending of therapy should be anticipated and discussed if possible, to avert premature dropout.

Common clinical situations in group treatment for people with ASPD

Recruitment to cause

People with ASPD will frequently recruit each other to their "cause." A "cause" is often structured around an experience of being treated unfairly by an organization (see Box 13.17). For example, they:

1 Have a complaint about someone or an organization and wish to "triumph" over that person or organization; they recruit members of the group and the clinicians to agree with them

2 "Explain" their behavior by blaming someone else.

Box 13.17 Recruitment to cause

Participants ally with each other against a "system" or organization, for example, housing, police, and hospitals:

+ Empathize and find point of validation
+ Allow sharing initially
+ Nudge discussion to emotions triggered, for example, unfairness
+ Question participants' teleological understanding of the situation.

In talking about the problem they gradually enlist other members of the group to their cause and, in doing so, the group members organize around the problem, eventually challenging the clinicians either to get something done about the problem or to recognize that no other response to the problem was possible once all the circumstances were taken into account.

Example 1

In a group session, a participant discussed how the housing department had not answered his question about his application for a flat. He had asked whether a medical officer had assessed his application. He was told that a senior housing manager had seen the application and that it was not being sent to the medical officer because it was deemed unnecessary. At this point he told them that they were not doing their job properly and threatened that he would come to the department to sort it and "them" out. Another participant said that the housing department never did its job properly and the people there were only interested in themselves. Gradually, this developed into a discussion between all the members of the group about how people in the housing department were incompetent and useless. Many examples were given. Finally, the group turned to the clinicians and said that they needed to write to the housing department to get something done about it all.

Example 2

A participant reported that he had stabbed someone, not fatally, but had done it to "wound and warn." He had met with some other members of his peer group in a pub. Other people were making a lot of noise and being "discourteous" to others in the pub. He asked them to keep quiet and use less offensive language. They ignored him, so he asked them again a few minutes later. When they did not desist from using bad language he pulled out a knife from his pocket, threatened the person he thought was the ringleader, and eventually stabbed him in the arm. Others restrained him and the landlord asked the noisy group to leave the pub.

The group clinicians thought that this incident needed careful exploration, but in trying to do so the other participants gradually came to the conclusion that the stabbing had been an appropriate reaction to the circumstances. They pointed out that the participant had given warnings—"That is fair. You give a warning and if they don't take any notice they have it coming to them"; "See, he gave two warnings. That is more than necessary. Only one is necessary." They pointed out that you cannot allow people to ignore you—"They start getting the wrong idea about you and think you are soft." They pointed out that "people like that only understand that sort of lesson." Eventually, they began to try to persuade the clinicians that this reaction was the only sensible way to manage the situation and that the clinicians would understand this if they were living in the same circumstances.

What can the clinician do?

1 Empathize with a number of the points that the participants make. No one likes to be taken advantage of; if you ask someone politely to do something it

is problematic if they challenge that request; no one likes their authority to be questioned.

2 Place the action in an emotional context—what was the emotion that was being triggered? The point here is to try to move the focus on behavioral actions and outcomes in the physical world toward a mental understanding of what happens. For example, the discussion about the stabbing needs to be more about the challenge to authority and the potential humiliation than about the stabbing being an appropriate action in the context.

3 Question their understanding of motives and their assertion that the eventual action was the only response. People with ASPD often become teleological about motives. In these two examples, the group members agreed that the only reason the housing manager did not pass the application to the medical officer was because she wanted to prevent the participant being rehoused, and that the stabbing was the correct and reasonable response because it worked—the other people were removed from the pub.

4 If the response to the previous points has some effect, the mentalizing task is:

   a. To move on to identifying/labeling the affects in the self

   b. Recognizing the sensitivity to that affect

   c. Considering whether the interaction involved a threat to a "position" in a hierarchy.

Defiance

People with ASPD rebel against anyone they see as being in authority, and they tend to see clinicians as being in authority. Their interpersonal relationships are based on control, competition, and domination. If the clinician appears forceful, he/she is likely to undermine motivation by activating a contrary attitude. At the beginning of the group the clinicians may ask the group members to agree aims, for example, to reduce acts of aggression. However, the participants may not have this aim. The more the clinicians try to enforce this aim and insist on it as an area for change, the more defiant the participants are likely to become. The discussion of an aim becomes an interpersonal battle rather than a consideration of a focus for treatment. The participants may argue, for instance, that it is the world that needs to change rather than them. They use cognitively driven arguments to hide their fears about change. For them, change threatens relegation in the interpersonal league table, submission, and experiences of shame. A clinician who insists that the primary aim is to reduce aggression will lose the argument (see Box 13.18).

Box 13.18 Defiance

People with ASPD tend to have a contrary attitude—in life and in group:

- ◆ Argue with participant—*contraindicated*. What do you do if you find yourself opposing the participant?
- ◆ Presentation of clinician's perspective—needs to be skillful and infused with not-knowing attitude
- ◆ Validate but with a nuanced twist (subtle challenge)
- ◆ Use an affect focus on the interaction.

What can the clinician do?

1. Argue with the participant:

PARTICIPANT: I cannot work.

CLINICIAN: What is the difficulty with working?

PARTICIPANT: I cannot work. I feel too depressed. I cannot get up in the morning. If they make me go to work I will fail.

CLINICIAN: Are you able to say what it is that makes it difficult for you to get up in the morning?

PARTICIPANT: I have never been a morning person.

CLINICIAN: What time do you go to bed?

PARTICIPANT: When I am tired.

CLINICIAN: What time is that?

This conversation could go on and on. It is apparent that the clinician wants to focus on the participant returning to work, but the participant is set on his belief that he cannot work. Once the question of getting up early has been exhausted, continuing the conversation in this way is likely to trigger the participant to give additional reasons for not being able to work. No clinician wants to argue with a participant, and yet it is sometimes impossible not to become engaged in a quarrel. As soon as the clinician realizes he/she has become involved in a disagreement, he/she needs to back out. Apologize— "Sorry, I realize that I have not fully understood the exact problem." A diversion can then take place on to an allied subject. In this example, the clinician could say: "Being forced to do something you cannot do is oppressive. Are there other areas in which these things are occurring for you?"

If disagreement occurs around the initial aims of the group, the clinician takes an inquisitive stance, being as open-minded as possible, and asks the group to start redefining aims together.

2 Present his/her own view for the participant to consider. If done skillfully this can be effective. "I apologize, it seems that I am arguing here. I thought that working might be a way of improving your sense of personal achievement and make you feel better about yourself."

However, if this is done less skillfully it can lead to argument or the participant gaining a sense that the clinician does not understand.

3 Validate the participant's perspective but with a nuanced twist. In MBT terms, this is a subtle challenge, but not to the extent of being oppositional. The aim is to give a slightly different vantage point to the same situation, looking at it from a perspective the participant has not considered— "Working is a pain most of the time. I agree. But it is often how we use our talents and feel good about ourselves and gain confidence. Do you feel good about yourself generally at the moment?" Or, if there is discussion over the aims of the group, "We thought that reducing the number of acts of aggression was important, as it is those things that seem to get you into trouble with the law. Are there different aims that you think we should discuss?"

4 Use an affect focus about the interaction you have engaged in—"We seem to be getting into something here where the more I want to think about work and what might be the impediments to it, the more you oppose it. Do you have a sense of that? It might be better for us to consider if this sort of interaction is something that repeats itself."

Escalating threats

Participants may threaten each other within the group or even outside the group (perhaps on social media sites such as Facebook or Twitter). Of course, this is unacceptable. Verbal threats and physical violence are proscribed for all participants in the agreement made at the beginning of the group. Nevertheless, aggression between group members, or between them and the clinicians, may occur. More commonly it is between the participants themselves, often related to misinterpretation of what someone says or how one participant has looked at another in a manner suggesting disrespect. Threats made by one participant to another may also stimulate anxiety and fear in the clinician and undermine his/her own mentalizing. In this situation the key task is for the clinician to retain his/her mentalizing at all costs.

Participant-to-participant threats

As soon as the clinicians sense rising tension between participants it is important to intervene (see Box 13.19). De-escalating impending aggression early is the key task. Initially, the aggression is usually verbal but, as the participants often point out themselves, the time gap between verbal and physical aggression is very small for them:

> I asked the barman for a drink very politely. He ignored me and carried on standing there and did not even look at me. I asked him again very politely. When he ignored me again I picked up the glasses on the bar and threw them at the mirror behind him. You cannot be treated like that.

This level of impulsivity may occur within the group. It is necessary for the clinician to monitor for any indicators of impending aggression.

What can the clinician do?

1 Use any de-escalating technique you think might be useful! Keeping calm verbally and physically, and maintaining a relatively impassive or neutral facial expression with natural eye contact is essential. Do not "stare" at the participant, lean forward, or clench your fists. Maintain physical distance if the participant is not seated, and do not touch him.

> A member of staff came out of a room to ask two participants who were talking loudly in the corridor to keep quiet. In doing so, he unthinkingly touched one of them on the shoulder. The participant stopped and turned on the member of staff, "What did you touch me for? Don't you dare touch me. Who the fuck do you think you are?"

Keep talking quietly and suggest that the group returns ("rewinds") to an earlier subject when mentalizing was present. If necessary, engage in a "broken record" repetition of what you would like to do.

Box 13.19 Escalating threats: participant to participant

Participant verbally and/or physically threatens another participant:

- ◆ Use de-escalating techniques
- ◆ Take authority but do not become authoritarian
- ◆ Maintain a cognitive position in contrast to the affective position
- ◆ Take a participant out of the group for a short time to discuss the problem
- ◆ Co-clinician discusses the problem with the other participant in the group.

2 The MBT clinician has to hold a balance between taking authority to manage the group and a role in stimulating interactive mentalizing process. Escalating threats suggest that mentalizing of self and other has collapsed. This is a point at which the clinician takes authority (as distinct from becoming authoritarian, which would only serve to escalate threat).

PARTICIPANT 1: Come over here and say that.

PARTICIPANT 2: You don't want me to come over there to say it. You are a piss artist.

CLINICIAN: Thank you. We are not here to call each other names. Eddie, thanks for the apology, and Mark, thanks for accepting the apology. Let's now go back to where we were when we were talking about how we work out if someone is trustworthy.

PARTICIPANT 2: I haven't given an apology.

CLINICIAN: No, I gave it for you, and thanks for that. Going back as I said . . .

Here the clinician is trying to manage the situation by reducing the aggression quickly. Keeping some control of the interaction is necessary. It may be possible to revisit the problem between the two participants later. However, this may take time. People with ASPD tend to bear grudges and are unlikely to forgive in a meaningful way. Occasionally, the clinician will be told that they have sorted it out between themselves. This is an indicator to ask how this "sorting out" was done and if they could talk about it as an illustration of how to work out conflict without aggression.

3 If one participant leaves the group in the context of an altercation with another group member, one of the clinicians (if two are running the group) may go out to talk to the participant while the remaining clinician works to calm down the situation in the group. It is not necessarily optimal to persuade the absent participant to return to the group. It may be better that he goes home, to return next week. But if the participant outside calms, the clinician can go back into the group to find out if it is safe for him to return. He can then report back to the participant and negotiate a quick safety agreement between the participants.

CLINICIAN 1: OK. I will go back in to see if things are safe for everyone and check out if Joe is calmer too.

CLINICIAN 1 [on coming back in to the group]: I have been talking to Craig and he is OK now. If things are calmer here, shall I ask him to come back in and then we can go back to think about what has been happening? But I need to know it is safe and that we are not going to start an argument again.

CLINICIAN 2: Joe, do you think you can now manage not to get into an argument with Craig and we can think more about what was going on?

The two clinicians then make a decision. The principle to follow is for each clinician to support a different protagonist in the interaction, and it is for the clinicians to take the authority to decide on reconvening the group. This is known as "siding" (see Chapter 12).

4 It may become necessary to ask both participants to leave a group. In this case, *do not* ask them to leave at the same time. Say that it seems that it would be better if they both left. One clinician takes out one of the participants and has a brief conversation with him to try to maintain an alliance and to de-escalate the situation. The remaining clinician in the group does the same with the other person and then asks him to leave after a suitable interval.

Participant-to-clinician threat

To some extent, threats to the safety of the clinicians are a more significant risk to the continuation of the group. Clinicians will not be able to maintain their own mentalizing in the context of persistent threats toward them or (as may occur) their families. Maintaining mentalizing in the clinician is a top priority for the MBT group. So, the principle in this context is for the clinician to reinstate his/her own mentalizing or to maintain it in the context of personal threat.

What can the clinician do?

First, the clinician needs to ensure his/her own personal safety. If this is unclear then he/she should stop the group and seek support from other staff. Assuming that his/her personal safety is not under threat, the clinician has a number of options (see Box 13.20).

Box 13.20 Escalating threats: participant to clinician

Participant threatens clinician:

- ◆ Use de-escalation techniques and keep primary focus on safety
- ◆ Apologize for creating the difficulty—measured "submission"
- ◆ Affect focus on the hierarchical relationship (if present) or interactional process when the participant calms
- ◆ Address in individual review.

1 De-escalate the situation as described in the section on participant-to-participant threats.

2 Apologize for his/her difficulty in thinking when under threat. The clinician should find a way to say this without becoming overtly submissive: "It is really difficult for me to think about how to help when I feel under threat"; "It will make it hard for me to continue to try to help if I cannot feel safe in developing our work together about your problems."

3 If the threat is not severe but related more to a hierarchical relationship between participant and clinician, this needs to be identified as an affect focus interfering with treatment: "I think perhaps we are getting into a bit of competition between us. Is there something going on for you that does not want to back down about this? From my side I have a sense that I want to prove that I am right. I appreciate that this is not a good way to work out how to manage the problem we were talking about."

4 The circumstances contributing to the threat need to be reviewed in an individual session, in which areas of sensitivity leading to possible violence are explored and potential interference with continuing treatment is clarified.

Idealization of themselves as a "group"

Participants with ASPD rapidly identify with each other early in treatment, seeing their own personal qualities and problems as being shared by others in the group (Box 13.21). This may be the first time many of them have sat down to talk with others who share similar problems, and it is reassuring to them to be able to identify with other individuals. Rapidly, perhaps too rapidly, they begin

Box 13.21 Participants' idealization of themselves as a "special" group of people

Participants integrate and form a cohesive group through paranoid organization:

♦ Allow this early in treatment

♦ Validate the sharing of similar problems

♦ Unity allows exploration of difference

♦ Change the focus from general advice to more personally specific advice—"What is it about Peter that makes you think that your advice will be equally useful for him?"

to think that they understand each other well. When the clinicians start to question a participant, other participants may answer for him and suggest that the clinicians do not understand the person in the way that they understand each other. The clinicians are excluded from the participants' idealization of themselves as a group. Ignoring the clinicians, the participants may even arrange to organize something outside the group, which they frame as mutual support. If the clinicians try to challenge this, they are seen as interfering and failing to understand how the participants can give each other support—"No one else helps us, so we have to help each other." This is a time when giving practical advice to each other becomes the norm.

What can the clinician do?

1 Initially, it may be best to accept the cohesion and unity that idealization of themselves as a group brings.

2 Validate the participants' experience of having similar problems and the sense of belonging that this experience brings.

3 Move from validation to suggest that this unity allows exploration of difference.

4 Work on the general advice that they often give to each other in this context—"I have had that problem. You should do XXXX"—to make it more personal. Here, the clinician should attempt to extract a mentalizing process from the advice: "What is it about Tony that makes you think that your solution might fit him?" Explore aspects of the solution that helped the individual and what it is about his suggestion that makes him think it is useful for the other person. Ask the other person to consider it in detail.

Expression of emotions in the self

We have already suggested that people with ASPD have problems with expressing affective components of their own internal states, particularly within interpersonal contexts. Identifying their feelings—especially those associated with vulnerability, such as shame and humiliation—and expressing them within the current interpersonal context is not something that participants will do naturally in the group. Focusing on others' feelings or problems, rather than expressing one's own personal feelings, is more comfortable for people with ASPD.

There is one exception to this, though—participants will express forcibly how tense they are or how "near the edge" and explosive they feel. They will also express "anger" and issue threats. This is less often related to the current interpersonal context in the group than it is an expression of their baseline state or a feeling about organizations/systems such as the police, housing department, or benefits office.

The aim in the group is to encourage participants to identify their *current feeling in the group* rather than to express their bitterness about external organizations, and to increase their recognition of the way context influences their current feeling. So, for example, an experience that the clinicians are listening and taking their problems seriously can be calming, while a sense of being ignored can be arousing.

Participants may also have a limited recognition of the complexity of feelings, with basic emotions being colored by social emotions. Aggression may be used as part of a survival strategy to cover humiliation or a fear of submission. This is covered in the MBT-I sessions (see Chapter 11) and it may be necessary to remind participants about this.

Finally, an expression of emotion by one participant allows the clinician to focus on whether the others in the group recognize the feelings expressed by the participant. This moves the group to work on emotion recognition in others (see Box 13.22).

> A participant presented as angry when he was talking about people rejecting him. The clinicians asked him to put aside his anger and see if he had any other feeling in him. In his angry statements he had said something about his mother refusing to allow him to stay at home when he was 17 and making him live with his grandmother. Within his anger he managed to identify how hurt he was that a "mother who gives birth to you can reject you so completely." He had no idea how to manage that feeling.
>
> The clinicians empathized with his experience, which had also left him feeling distrustful of others.

What can the clinician do?

1 Ensure that the participants are reminded of the information about emotions given in the MBT-I sessions.

Box 13.22 Emotional expression: self

Participants find naming and expressing the complexity of their current and past feelings uncomfortable or impossible:

- Question the participants' tendency to collapse all feelings into "anger"
- Reiterate information from MBT-I about emotions
- Work on identifying affects
- Increase the link between affect and context
- Link this work with stimulating emotion recognition from self to other.

2 Attempt to identify the complexity of any feeling, as illustrated in the previous example.

3 Specifically work on identifying affects in the group—"How do you feel now?" If the participant is unable to label the affect, ask him to describe his state as best as he can. Does he feel it in his body?

4 Explore possible reasons for the feeling if it is identified—"What makes you feel like that?" Is it related to the interpersonal or relational context?

5 Link a focus on personal internal affect to whether others in the group recognized the emotions. Did they see the individual as only angry, or were they aware of his feelings of hurt and rejection?

Emotion recognition in others

The inner emotional state of a participant may or may not be recognized by other members of the group prior to any obvious expression of the emotion(s). People with ASPD are sensitive to the states of others but they do not empathize with the effect the feeling state has on the other person. At times they may misuse their understanding of someone's underlying state.

> A group participant described how difficult it was for him to identify how he felt. The clinician realized that if he kept asking the participant to say how he felt it made him feel exposed and embarrassed in front of the other members of the group. So the clinician moved the topic of the group. Quickly, one of the other participants said, "Don't move on so fast. I think Alan needs to say how he feels. How do you feel? Come, on tell us." It became apparent that this participant was being cruel to the embarrassed participant and enjoying a sense of dominance and control over him.

In this situation, the clinician tries to rebalance the mentalizing process, "siding" with the vulnerable participant and asking the participant who is tormenting the other person to start describing his own inner state (see Box 13.23).

Box 13.23 Emotional expression: others

Participants may recognize emotions accurately in others but fail to identify with and be compassionate to them—they recognize the *affect* but do not empathize with its *effect*. They can misuse their understanding.

- Ask Paul if he can describe how Peter feels
- How was that inference made?
- Work on moving from this external focus to an internal focus of mentalizing.

What can the clinician do?

1 Work with the other participants to see if they identified how another participant was or is feeling. If not, why not? Is it because the feeling is not being expressed, or is it because they were not alert to the person's feeling? For example, they may not notice that one of the group members is distressed while the clinicians *are* aware of this due to the participant's demeanor and facial expression.

2 Explore the external mentalizing focus and how it adds information to understanding how someone else feels but at the same time can create confusion unless we are careful. The apparent anger from a person's facial expression may not relate directly to his internal state.

3 Work with a specific example in the group about how a participant feels and whether that was apparent to the rest of the group (see Box 13.24).

Moving external mentalizing focus to internal focus—other

Relying on external cues, such as facial expression, eye movements, and body posture to indicate the motives of others is a normal process and underpins many daily interactions moderately well. People with ASPD are sensitive to external cues, particularly related to the way someone looks at them—"the look" is a universal trigger for them and yet it is rarely specified; it is something that people with ASPD recognize when it occurs but cannot describe. It is not simply a "funny look." It is a look that threatens social position and implies a challenge to an imagined hierarchy. This sensitivity to external cues does not translate into interest in the affective internal states of the other or into curiosity about underlying motives. People with ASPD assume that motives are malign unless proven otherwise, and react accordingly to counter the perceived threat.

Box 13.24 Emotional expression: self–other

Participants with ASPD cannot easily engage in a self–other affective mentalizing process. They tend to default to practicality and advice.

- When Peter is talking about a problem, ask Paul to describe how he thinks Peter is feeling:
  - How was that inference made?
  - Check it out—"Is that how you feel, Peter?"
  - If not, "Please describe how you feel"
  - Then pass it back to Paul to reconsider.

Box 13.25 External to internal mentalizing

Participants make assumptions from external mentalizing focus:

- Identify and jointly work on the specific aspects of external mentalizing—facial expression (describe), tone of voice (describe), and body posture (define)

- Practice moving from external to internal focus—use a group exercise if necessary

- Identify disparities between external information and internal states.

The clinician needs first to help the participants take an interest in other people's internal states having identified an external cue, and second, to help them empathize with the other's state rather than misuse their understanding (see Box 13.25).

What can the clinician do?

1 In group work, ask the participants to practice questioning someone in the group about their internal states—for example, "Tell me what makes you shout like that?" Insist that the participants listen to the answers.

2 Take an interaction in the group and focus on elements of the interpersonal understanding within the interaction.

> A participant was saying how angry he was about the child protection social worker who was involved with his family, raising his voice as he told the story of her alleged incompetence. When he paused in his diatribe, the clinician asked him to stop so that the group could explore their understanding of his current feelings and the basis for their understanding. The participants said that he was obviously angry, as he had raised his voice. The clinician said that he could see that but thought the participant also felt aggrieved that he was being misunderstood, and also powerless, giving as evidence the fact that he kept on asking the clinicians to get something sorted out. The clinician then asked the participant to appraise the accuracy of these understandings of his feelings.

3 Generate a process that appraises feeling states and underlying motives as being more complex than the linear form so often insisted on by people with ASPD.

Paranoid reactions

Paranoid reactions may occur in the group (see Box 13.26). These are discussed, in part, in the section on escalating threats, which are themselves often

---

Box 13.26 Paranoid reactions to clinician

Participants may suddenly react without warning to something in the group:

- Quickly identify what the trigger is
- Overtly consider if their understanding has any merit in terms of clinician contribution
- Validate how they could have understood a comment in the way they have
- Explain your own motive while not denying their understanding
- Open the discussion in the group if other members had a similar understanding
- Accept that you will be more thoughtful about how you say something.

---

triggered by misunderstandings, sensitivity, frank paranoid interpretations of something that is said, or through inappropriate reliance on an external mentalizing focus and associated assumptions about others' motives. Occasionally, a participant may react explosively to something that either the clinician or someone else says; in this situation the interventions recommended for deescalating threatening behavior are recommended. However, the reaction may be primarily mental rather than physical, with the participant responding verbally, albeit expressing considerable anxiety, rather than behaviorally.

In a discussion about feelings, the clinician suggested that it might be useful for the group to consider how they begin to recognize they are becoming angry. One participant reacted by saying, "You are trying to control us. You are trying to take us over. I am not doing this. You only want to find out what we have done."

CLINICIAN: I am not sure what you mean. Can you tell me what I was saying or doing that make you think that?

PARTICIPANT: You just ask us to tell us what happens in our minds so that you can control what we think.

CLINICIAN: Please can you describe how I do that? I don't want to do that, so I need to be sure that I don't keep making you react so strongly to what I am trying to do.

PARTICIPANT: Why would you want to know what makes me angry? It is only so that you can do something before I do.

This discussion continued with the clinician trying to expand the conversation and then asking the group for their ideas about the difficulty of trying to explore mental and physical process that alerts us early to becoming angry and potentially stimulating a feeling of being controlled.

What can the clinician do?

1 For a participant-to-clinician reaction, try to understand the participant's perspective. Suggest that his experience of what you have said or done makes his reaction understandable but that there is a misunderstanding of your motive and that you would like to try to understand what it was that made the participant see it the way he does.

2 Explore a participant-to-participant motive/reaction. Outline your own understanding of what a participant meant if another participant is reacting sensitively.

3 Try to find something that you can validate within the reaction.

4 Open the discussion to the group, asking them if they had a similar understanding of the other participant's/clinician's motive. Beware of humiliating the participant who had the paranoid reaction while doing this.

Understanding antisocial behavior from the perspective of problems with mentalizing gives a theoretical platform on which clinical interventions can be built. MBT-ASPD is an attempt to integrate interventions into a coherent clinical treatment targeting mentalizing vulnerabilities. Organizing treatment and providing effective intervention for people with ASPD is difficult but rewarding. There is little doubt that for many of these individuals, being taken seriously and being offered treatment is a new experience. There is evidence that their mental health needs are neglected by services (Crawford, Sahib, Bratton, Tyrer, & Davidson, 2009) and that they may even refuse help when it is offered because they have been rejected from services so many times in the past, leaving their needs unaddressed. Whether MBT-ASPD is effective in addressing their problems remains to be seen and, to this end, randomized controlled trials are underway.

References

Bateman, A., & Fonagy, P. (2009). Randomized controlled trial of outpatient mentalization-based treatment versus structured clinical management for borderline personality disorder. *American Journal of Psychiatry*, **166**, 1355–1364.

Crawford, M., Sahib, H., Bratton, P., Tyrer, P., & Davidson, K. (2009). Service provision for men with antisocial personality disorder who make contact with mental health services. *Personality and Mental Health*, **3**, 165–171.

Gilligan, J. (2000). *Violence: Reflections on our deadliest epidemic.* London, UK: Jessica Kingsley.

Skodol, A. E., Clark, L. A., Bender, D. S., Krueger, R. F., Morey, L. C., Verheul, R., . . . Oldham, J. M. (2011). Proposed changes in personality and personality disorder assessment and diagnosis for DSM-5 Part I: Description and rationale. *Personality Disorders: Theory, Research, and Treatment,* 2, 4–22.

Yudofsky, S. C., Silver, J. M., Jackson, W., Endicott, J., & Williams, D. (1986). The Overt Aggression Scale for the objective rating of verbal and physical aggression. *American Journal of Psychiatry,* 143, 35–39.

Part 4

Mentalizing systems

Mentalizing and families: the Families and Carers Training and Support program (FACTS)

Introduction

Families are in the unique position of being able to support mental health treatment of a family member, but they can do so only if they are aware of what to do and how to manage situations that commonly arise. Borderline personality disorder (BPD) is a particularly challenging condition for families to manage, as the difficulties often present as a problem in the relationships between family members, who often inappropriately blame themselves for the difficulties, and may even be stigmatized by others who erroneously see them as the cause of the disorder. As a result, families of patients with BPD struggle to cope with their own feelings, leaving them traumatized, disempowered, and unsure how best to help their relative or loved one. Yet, support and advice for family members is rarely available and, even when it is, it is often misleading and sometimes offensive, confusing, and unhelpful.

The importance of the family system in maintaining or moderating serious behavioral problems associated with mental health problems has become increasingly evident from research findings. Psychoeducation delivered by mental health professionals for families of patients with the most severe and enduring mental disorders (schizophrenia and bipolar affective disorder) is routinely provided and is grounded in a robust evidence base (Leff, Kuipers, Berkowitz, Eberlein-Vries, & Sturgeon, 1982; Leff & Vaughn, 1985). Intervention reduces the negative effects of family interactions and, by doing so, reduces patient hospitalizations. No such evidence exists for people with BPD, although expert consensus suggests that family involvement may be similarly helpful (Gunderson & Hoffman, 2005). The limited data available suggest that the continued involvement of family members with patients with BPD improves outcomes (Hoffman, Fruzzetti, & Buteau, 2007). Expressed emotion signifies positive family involvement and a wish to help; it does not hinder improvement. Yet, family members of patients with BPD often report feeling too traumatized and disempowered to be of help to their ill relatives (Porr, 2010) and so may withdraw. Families thus need to know how to help their relative with BPD—but this information is not systematically available.

In recognition of the lack of involvement of families in the treatment and support of people with BPD, the National Institute for Health and Care Excellence (NICE) guideline on the treatment and management of BPD (2009) makes a number of statements. These are summarized in Box 14.1.

The section of NICE guidance concludes with the statement that there is an "absence of research into whether family interventions alter the social outcome and welfare of a person with borderline personality disorder." (p. 96).

In recognition of this gap in the care of people with BPD, FACTS—a *families and carers training and support* program based on an understanding of mentalizing and emotions—has been developed. This operationalized program for families contains information about BPD and includes information and training in basic skills on how to manage some of the common problems that people with BPD present to their families. The primary aim of the intervention is to improve the well-being of the family member (or significant other) and to reduce family crises. Importantly, the program is designed to be delivered *by families to families* with some support from mental health professionals if necessary (see Box 14.2). This increases the likelihood of sustainability of family support in clinical services and the voluntary sector. The program is not intended to be delivered by mental health professionals alone; their role is to teach families the information and to train them in the delivery of the program, and to offer support when necessary.

Box 14.1 Families and borderline personality disorder: NICE guidance (2009)

- "When a person is diagnosed with borderline personality disorder, the effect of the diagnosis on carers is often overlooked." (p. 93)
- "Families/carers of people with borderline personality may have needs that are at least equivalent to families/carers of people with other severe and enduring mental health problems." (p. 94)
- "[E]merging evidence suggests that structured family programmes may be helpful . . . " (p. 95)
- "[S]tructured psychoeducation programmes that also facilitate social support networks may be helpful for families." (p. 96)
- "Inform families or carers about local support groups for families or carers, if these exist." (p. 99)

Box 14.2 FACTS: summary

- ◆ Content developed by families
- ◆ Course of five modules:
  - Introduction to Borderline Personality Disorder
  - Mentalizing
  - Mindfulness and Emotion Management
  - Validation Skills
  - Problem-Solving
- ◆ Delivered by families to families
- ◆ Task-oriented group rather than a support group.

The course for families was developed jointly with families and professionals, building on our current understanding of BPD. It was predicated on the idea that families who have a better understanding of BPD will be able to learn safe and helpful responses to common interpersonal and emotional problems associated with the disorder. The course is organized as five modules to be delivered over five evenings. The modules increase participants' understanding of BPD and introduce them to some basic skills in mentalizing and other skills that can be used to manage interpersonal and emotional crises between the family member and the person with BPD.

In the development phase, 18 families were recruited to participate in the five-module psychoeducation and skills development program. Two family members received a brief training to deliver a pilot program. The course was found to be acceptable and useful, and the trainers adhered to the manualized package. The development phase is now complete.

At the time of writing, a randomized controlled trial has been completed but the data have not been unlocked and analyzed. However, the initial pilot project with families suggested that it was well received, increased empowerment, and reduced family crises.

Each module is equivalent to one session of 90 minutes and is fully manualized, with handouts and suggested videos. The initial session includes an additional 30 minutes to enable family members to get to know each other and share some of their difficulties informally. However, as the course is not a support group, it is important to maintain the structure carefully and to deliver all the information and skills suggested in the manual.

The presenter's notes, slides, and handouts and worksheets for family members are available on the Anna Freud Centre website at http://annafreud.org/training-research/mentalization-based-treatment-training/facts/.

Other websites that people have found useful include:

+ http://www.borderlinepersonalitydisorder.com
+ http://www.bpdfamily.com
+ http://www.rethink.org

Family members who deliver the modules are instructed not to worry about covering all the content of a module in a single session. Modules 2 and 3 are long and may run into each other over more than two sessions. This is acceptable as long as all areas are covered by the end of the course. In addition, the order of the modules may be adjusted to the needs of the presenters and participants. Some family presenters have delivered Module 3 before Module 2, on the basis that managing one's own emotions through mindfulness is necessary before good mentalizing can take place. However, mentalizing also manages emotions, as well as placing the focus on both the family member and the person with BPD. So the overall logic to the order of modules is outlined to the families: first, an understanding of BPD is necessary, with an emphasis on the interpersonal and emotional symptoms (Introduction to BPD module); then, the family member has to mentalize him/herself and the person with BPD (Mentalizing module) and be able to manage his/her own emotions if he/she is to help the loved one with BPD (Mindfulness and Emotion Management module) and be able to empathically validate him/her effectively (Validation Skills module); finally, an ability to do some general problem-solving helps to manage difficulties over time (Problem-Solving module).

Preparation

Presenters leading a session naturally take time to prepare notes and ensure that they fully understand the material. The manual contains all the information required to run the sessions. Presenters often do further research on topics, using websites and books. It is important that presenters not only have a good understanding of the material, but also that they can demonstrate to the families that they are able to use many of the skills and techniques themselves. Presenters even use many of the skills to ensure that the course runs smoothly. For example, when families share their personal experiences, presenters use their own validation skills to help participants feel that their experiences are meaningful, important, and understandable in the circumstances. Presenters also use their mentalizing skills during the sessions by actively exploring the group members' experiences, remaining patient and accepting their views, and de-escalating discussions that become heated or emotional. If a presenter is finding a session particularly challenging, he/she might use mindfulness techniques to stay calm and logical, which in turn will help him/her to process and manage the problem at hand. By actively using these skills during a session, presenters not only demonstrate to the families that it is possible to apply the techniques in all situations—they also produce a comfortable and positive environment for the group.

Presenters also make several practical preparations before each session. A projector or screen is needed to show slides and a flip chart or whiteboard is useful to make notes on. It is recommended that the presenters sit at the front next to the screen while family members sit in a semi-circle around the screen. This has been found to be an effective format as the families feel that they are part of a group and that they can all contribute to the session, but the focus is still on the presenter and the slides, therefore maintaining emphasis on this being a learning course rather than a support group. Participants are also given handouts and copies of the slides, and are asked to complete exercises during each session. It is recommended that the participants are given a pack containing the printouts for the whole course at the first session so that if they miss a session they can catch up on the module from home. In addition, participants may like to read ahead, so that when they arrive for a session they are fully prepared.

The recommended length for each session is 90 minutes, except for the first session, which is 2 hours long. The extra half an hour is used to introduce the families to each other and establish a cohesive and comfortable group environment. Presenters make it clear to the families at the outset that, in order to create an open environment where they can share their stories and difficulties, families need to agree among themselves not to disclose each other's personal details with anyone outside the group. Presenters also reassure families that during the course they can discuss as much or as little of their personal background as they are comfortable with. If someone asks another family member a personal question, they are never obliged to answer it. Presenters remind the families that this is a training course and not a support group. Nevertheless, they will have the opportunity to share personal experiences, although this will not be the primary focus of the sessions. Finally, the families are informed that the presenters are not available to provide advice in between sessions.

After the family members have agreed to the principles at the beginning of the first module, the presenters give the families a brief opportunity to introduce themselves and explain why they are attending the course. For many families this is the first time they are among a group of people who are having similar experiences to them, and so the temptation to discuss their experiences extensively can be strong. It is not necessarily a bad thing for presenters to have a good understanding of the family members' backgrounds, but there will not be enough time to cover the content of the first session comfortably if the introductions are too long. Family members can also find it disturbing to describe their background and the problems they face in detail, so presenters encourage the families to keep their introductions short. They do this by doing their own introductions first as exemplars, keeping them brief and not overly detailed. The rest of the group will hopefully follow suit.

Structure of sessions

Each session follows a particular format. At the opening of each session (except for the first session, which opens with the personal introductions), family members briefly say how the past week has been and outline any important events that have taken place with their relative with BPD. Presenters do not allow the family members to linger on this for long, as otherwise there will be inadequate time to cover the content of the session. Presenters then summarize what was covered in the previous session. To gauge whether anything needs to be clarified or revisited, presenters can ask the family members themselves to summarize the previous session and perhaps give examples of times in the week when they have used the techniques they learned in the session. Presenters then summarize what they will cover in the current session, and why the content is relevant to family members of people with BPD (see Box 14.3).

After opening the session, presenters start to deliver the content of the module in detail. Although this is a training course, presenters avoid a "lecturing"

Box 14.3 Structure of sessions

- Introductions (first session)/feedback on past week (other sessions)
- Summary of previous week and report on practice of techniques learned
- Questions about previous week's topic
- Outline of current topic
- Delivery of the relevant material and practice
- Summary, close, and suggested home practice.

style and remain engaged with the group at all times. Contributions and questions from family members are encouraged throughout the session, although presenters maintain control of the group and do not allow too many tangential subjects or excessive focus on one point. Managing a group is not necessarily a skill that presenters naturally have. The brief training for presenters suggests that they take a firm but flexible approach, balancing the primary aim of the session—that is, ensuring that all the relevant material is covered—with elaboration of the content using some examples given by the participants. Occasionally, presenters revisit the content of earlier sessions to show how previously learned skills can be used in the current session.

A 5-minute "comfort" break occurs in most sessions to allow the families to rest and relax. Occasionally, the group will not feel the need for a break, but most of the modules have a lot of content to cover and family members find it too intense if there is not a short break. However, presenters are firm about keeping this break short, as otherwise they will not have time finish the module.

At the close of each meeting, the presenters summarize the content of the session and give the families the opportunity to ask any questions and clarify any points that they did not understand. Presenters also briefly summarize what the next session will cover, and encourage the families to complete any homework. If there is time to spare at the end of a session and presenters feel that the families did not have much opportunity to discuss the relevance of the content to their own lives, they lead a more general discussion on the families' personal experiences and how they can apply the techniques learned in the session at home. However, it is important that presenters end the session on time in respect for the participants' busy lives. Presenters remain mindful of the families' complicated home lives and respect participants' occasional need to leave early or miss sessions without prior notice.

At the end of the course, the presenters take time to summarize the tools learned over the five modules, and give the families time to discuss things they have found especially useful, clarify anything they are uncertain about, and ask any questions. Families are also encouraged to exchange contact details, so they can continue to help and advise each other and keep the course fresh in each other's minds.

Activities

Each session is punctuated with various activities to keep the families engaged and to help illustrate how the course content can be applied in daily interactions (see Box 14.4).

Box 14.4 FACTS methods

- Psychoeducation
- Exploration
- Role plays
- Exercises and worksheets
- Videos
- Identification of skills when they are used in sessions.

Role plays

Role plays are used throughout the course. For a role play, families break up into smaller groups, and provide their own example of a situation or conversation with the person with BPD in their family that they would like to re-enact in order to practice handling situations in different ways. Although this is a useful way for families to apply techniques to situations that they are familiar with, it can prove time-consuming and difficult for families to generate their own role plays; they may also be tempted to start discussing their personal experiences rather than engaging fully in the role play. If presenters think there is a risk of this happening, they give families an example scenario to use instead. Furthermore, rather than breaking the group up into smaller groups, presenters may ask two family members to do a role play for the rest of the group. Presenters listen carefully to each role play, prompt the family members to use different techniques and approaches, and give them the opportunity to try role plays again if they are unsuccessful the first time. If a role play is done in front of the whole group, everyone watches and listens, gives feedback on how they think the role play went, and suggests ways in which they might have handled the situation.

Exercises and worksheets

Activity worksheets for each session are provided to help families understand the material and apply the course content to their own lives. The worksheets are straightforward and easy to complete, but if the families need clarification, the manual contains instructions for each activity and explains their purpose. Presenters can use these activities within the sessions or suggest them as homework. If presenters set an activity as homework, they make time at the beginning of the following session to briefly discuss what families learned from the activity when they did it at home.

Videos

Three of the sessions also have optional videos to facilitate focused discussion and to keep family members engaged. These are most effective if the presenters introduce the video, explain what it is being used to illustrate, and give families the opportunity to ask any questions after the video has been shown. Details of suggested video clips are provided in the presenters' notes for FACTS.

General discussion

The final, and perhaps most useful, activity is allowing the families time to discuss how the content applies to their own experiences with their loved one with BPD. Presenters need to judge when to allow the families to share recent events and when to facilitate discussion between all participants about the event. At all times the discussion needs to focus on how the participants could use the skills being learned in the course to manage the "event" better. If the presenters think the group would benefit from breaking up into smaller groups for discussion, they can do so, although, as with the role plays, presenters need to sensitively prevent families becoming so absorbed by their personal experiences that they fail to discuss the relevant skills and techniques. If families do break up into smaller groups, the presenters ensure that families remain focused by asking a representative from each group to report back on what they have discussed.

As mentioned earlier in this chapter, FACTS is not just a support group but a training group. As part of this, presenters ensure that personal examples are not tangential and that they usefully illustrate the practical applications of the content. Presenters also need to be sensitive to the fact that members of the group will be struggling with a wide range of different problems, and consequently their experiences will not necessarily overlap. For example, some families might have regular arguments with their family member with BPD that turn aggressive or violent, while for other families, the member with BPD is so withdrawn that he/she rarely interacts with them, let alone argues. It is important that presenters reassure families that while they do not have time to directly demonstrate how a point or technique is relevant to every single experience, the skills demonstrated and practiced during this course have been chosen because they can be used in a wide variety of situations. Families need to take time between sessions to consider how the course content might apply to their own lives, and how they can start using some of the techniques to target the problems that their significant other with BPD is having.

The following sections provide a brief summary of each module, outlining their aims, example role plays and discussions, and any particular problems or challenges that might arise.

Module 1: Introduction to Borderline Personality Disorder

The aim of Module 1 is to give the families an introduction to the FACTS program and to outline the history of BPD, how it is diagnosed, and its potential causes and possible treatments (see Box 14.5). Some of the families will already be familiar with the material covered in this module as they will have looked at books or websites on BPD, or sought information from a mental health professional. However, others may not have done much research into the condition, so it is important to cover these topics to ensure that all of the families have some basic knowledge about BPD.

There are several activities during this session to help deliver the content. Through discussion, families identify key problems they are having with their family member with BPD, and decide how they fit with the main problem areas associated with BPD. This is a useful introduction to the diagnostic criteria of BPD, which can be further illustrated using a video clip and a worksheet.

The session then turns to the possible causes of BPD, and families complete another worksheet to speculate about what might have contributed to their family member's BPD. While a large portion of this session is used to discuss the possible causes of BPD, it is a sensitive topic for many families, who often experience intense guilt that their loved one has not developed into adulthood in the way they had expected.

> One family member wondered whether the relationship she had had with her daughter when she was a baby was not suited to her daughter's emotional needs, and whether this had caused her BPD. The presenter quickly pointed out that speculating about this could never reach a conclusion and was likely to lead to self-blame rather than offering solutions to her daughter's current problems.

Box 14.5 Module 1: Introduction to Borderline Personality Disorder

- Outline and personal introductions
- What is BPD? Description of characteristics
- Identification of characteristics of significant other leading to diagnosis of BPD
- Causes of BPD—neurobiology, development, environment
- Treatments—highlighting improvements over time and with treatment.

If a family member is concerned about having been partly responsible for their significant other's BPD, it is important that the presenters use their validation skills, reassure families that they did the best that they could, and encourage the families to put their feelings of guilt aside so that they can focus on learning skills that will help their significant other.

Presenters need to be particularly cautious when addressing the relationship that exists between childhood abuse and BPD, as this topic is very sensitive for many of the families. Several family members may have even been accused of abuse or neglect at some point by their significant other. It is important to emphasize to families that their significant other having BPD does not mean that abuse necessarily took place, and that when family members are engaged with their relative's mental health, they are very unlikely to be the perpetrators of any abuse.

Presenters need to be similarly careful when discussing different treatments that are available for people with BPD. A problem might arise if some people have had access to specialist treatments while others have not. To address this, presenters can emphasize that nonspecialist treatments are being shown to be as effective as the specialist treatments as long as they are delivered carefully and in an organized way. Families often exchange advice about treatment, and recommend self-help books and websites that they have found helpful.

Before ending the first session, presenters encourage families to consider their personal goals and what they would like to get out of the course. This gives the families focus for future sessions, and highlights to the presenters the areas of particular importance.

Module 2: Mentalizing

The aim of Module 2 is to describe and explain mentalizing and demonstrate to families how it can help in their interactions with their family member with BPD (see Box 14.6). By the end of the session, families will understand how to recognize when they or their significant other is not mentalizing, how to maintain a mentalizing attitude, and will have had the opportunity to practice mentalizing techniques through role plays and activities.

There are several activities during this session to demonstrate the importance of mentalizing. Presenters show a video clip from "Everybody Loves Raymond," in which two people experience the same scenario in different ways, or show a video of an optical illusion of a rotating ballerina, which some people perceive as turning clockwise while others perceive it as turning anticlockwise. But perhaps the most effective way for families to see how the same scenario can be perceived in different ways is to ask a member of the group to describe an event

---

Box 14.6 Module 2: Mentalizing

- What is mentalizing? Definition and discussion with video
- Identification of nonmentalizing
- What interferes with mentalizing in ourselves and significant others with BPD?
- Maintaining mentalizing and practicing it at home.

---

that has happened with their significant other, and ask the other family members to brainstorm different ways that the people involved might have experienced that situation.

> One family member described how his daughter's driving often made him feel nervous and uncomfortable, and how when receiving a lift from her recently, he was so distracted by his nerves that he did not engage in any conversation with her. His daughter, annoyed by his silence, became incredibly angry with him, resulting in a row.
>
> The family members then speculated on how the situation might have looked from the daughter's perspective. Perhaps she knew from previous exchanges that he did not like her driving, and so was already feeling defensive when she picked him up. Perhaps she interpreted his silence as him being ungrateful for the lift. Some family members even suggested that his behavior was irrelevant, and that his daughter was in a bad mood from a different event earlier in the day.

This activity is useful to show families that there are numerous ways to interpret any situation they encounter with their significant other, and emphasizes the importance of mentalizing in such circumstances and not making assumptions about others' motives.

Later in the session, a role play is used to demonstrate to family members the importance of pressing an imaginary "pause button" during difficult exchanges. As explained earlier, families can generate their own examples of situations where an imaginary pause button might have been helpful, but giving the families a pre-prepared example to use is just as effective.

In one role play, two family members took on the roles of a daughter with BPD and her mother. The daughter was accusing her mother of loving her brother more than her.

DAUGHTER: Mum, why don't you love me as much as my brother?

MOTHER: I love you both the same. What makes you think that I love you less?

DAUGHTER: You do more nice things for him, you cook him dinner, you hug him lots . . .

MOTHER: I'm sorry to hear you think that. Is there something I can do that might make you feel differently?

The exchange continued, but eventually became too heated, and the mother and daughter reached an impasse. The presenter reminded the mother that if she was struggling to resolve the situation, she could use the "pause button."

MOTHER: I'm sorry, but I'm struggling to know what to make of this. Please can I go and think about it for a while?

DAUGHTER: OK. Talk later.

Another role play can be used to help families identify signs of nonmentalizing, although this exercise can be slightly more difficult as families need to be able to act out nonverbal cues, such as facial expressions and body language. If families are not comfortable with this, presenters use the homework sheet "Reading the Mind in the Eyes" to demonstrate the importance of reading and interpreting nonverbal cues.

When describing common nonmentalizing traps, presenters often refer to their personal experiences with these difficulties, and to explain how they have overcome them. In a brief discussion, families might also be able to think of times that they have fallen into nonmentalizing traps, and decide ways that they could overcome them in the future.

> One family member described how she had struggled with her need to win arguments with her son, but had managed to overcome this by accepting that winning individual battles against him would not help either of them win the war against his emotional struggles. Indeed, winning trivial arguments, such as getting her son to tidy his room, might cause him to become so irritated with her that he would not talk to her for several days. This could turn out to be so detrimental that him having a messy bedroom was preferable.

It is important to let families know that their ability to mentalize improves with practice and that they will not always mentalize successfully, particularly if they do not manage their emotions. Presenters briefly offer families some advice on what to do when mentalizing has failed and a conflict has arisen between them and their significant other. Some of the techniques are covered in later modules. It is more important that families leave this session with a good understanding of what mentalizing is, and with tools and techniques they can use to mentalize in situations that arise with their significant other. There are some worksheets that families can use at home to ensure they have understood the content of the module.

Module 3: Mindfulness and Emotion Management

The focus of this module is to teach families how to process and manage their emotions appropriately (see Box 14.7). By using the mindfulness and emotion management skills taught in this module, families can experience their emotions without allowing emotions to take over difficult situations or interactions that arise with their family member with BPD. One problem that presenters need to be aware of is that some families will be in the habit of interpreting "emotion management" as meaning "emotion *suppression*."

> One family member's daughter with BPD had become angry with a crisis house team because they had made an administrative error which delayed her admission. Although the error had made the father angry as well, he had suppressed the emotion and not expressed his frustration in front of his daughter in case it caused the situation to escalate. After discussing this event with the group, he concluded that suppressing his anger may have caused more harm than good, as it led his daughter to assume that he was unaffected by the problem.

Presenters explain that emotions serve important functions and should not be feared. They are sources of information about a situation or interaction, and mindfulness is a way of managing and attending to emotions. Many of the families will already have some knowledge of mindfulness techniques, which may have been taught to their significant other to help them monitor and understand the emotional difficulties that are often associated with BPD. Some family members may even have received mindfulness training before, as, for example, workplaces are increasingly training their employees in emotion management and mindfulness techniques.

Families are asked to share their experiences of mindfulness and the ways they have found it helpful. Initially some families find it difficult or uncomfortable to practice mindfulness; occasionally their reservations are because

---

Box 14.7 Module 3: Mindfulness and Emotion Management

- What are emotions?
- Emotion management for families
- Emotional control is necessary for good mentalizing
- Positive use of troubling emotions
- Mindfulness—video and practice
- Opposite action to manage troubling emotions.

mindfulness originated from Buddhist practice. It is important to emphasize that while this is the case, the mindfulness exercises that the families will be using are not related to religion, but rather are tools that can help them process and respond to emotional experiences.

Families practice generating mindfulness using circumstances that they themselves have experienced. In a discussion or role play, families have the opportunity to examine and label their emotions in a specific situation.

> One family member described how her daughter regularly tells her when she has cut herself. The emotions she experiences when receiving this information include resentment and frustration, but in order to participate in the situation effectively she acknowledges her emotions while trying to maintain an outward appearance of calmness, asking her daughter questions about what she can do to help.

In later discussion, families return to these experiences and consider how they might have used some other well-known techniques to moderate extreme and disturbing emotions. One such technique is *opposite action*. In the just-mentioned example, the family member forces herself to behave toward her daughter calmly and kindly despite feeling frustrated and angry toward her.

> One family member recognized that she naturally used opposite action when she encountered "road rage" while driving; she always smiled at the person who was frustrated and waved a thank you. This made her feel less anxious.

Presenters emphasize to families that while opposite action is not always appropriate, especially in emergency situations that require immediate action, it is useful for keeping some situations calm.

After learning about the uses of mindfulness, families are given the opportunity to practice it. Presenters either guide this exercise themselves, or use a video or soundtrack that talks the families through a mindfulness exercise. Families are encouraged to practice mindfulness in a range of scenarios during the coming week: the more they practice it, the more they will be able to apply it during difficult interactions with their significant other.

Module 4: Validation Skills

The aim of this module is to teach families the purpose of validation, when to validate, and how to validate skillfully and effectively (see Box 14.8). Some of the families will already be using validation, so the presenters need to ensure that they are using it correctly and in appropriate contexts.

The families themselves need validation from the presenters throughout the program, and only if they feel validated and empathized with themselves (including in relation to their worries that they may have caused their loved one

---

Box 14.8 Module 4: Validation Skills

- ◆ Understanding empathy and validation
- ◆ Recognizing the importance of using validation in everyday interactions
- ◆ Validation of families in the session
- ◆ Practice validation in role plays
- ◆ Discussion of examples when validation may have reduced conflict and increased constructive interaction.

---

to develop BPD) will they be able to learn to validate others. Validation helps them to move away from self-blame and allows them to work on solutions. Suggesting that family members validate their loved one with BPD before they themselves have felt validated can be experienced as invalidating and unempathic. In other words, it could well make them feel guilty, uneasy, and uncomfortable with themselves and with the rest of the group. Hopefully, the families will have been validated at the beginning of the family meetings (see description of Module 1).

It is important that the presenters are clear to the families about how to validate properly; this requires an expression of empathy without accepting or affirming damaging or inappropriate behaviors. Some families express concern that by validating their significant other's experiences, it might encourage them to continue to engage in self-destructive behaviors. However, an attempt to validate should specifically address a significant other's emotional experience rather than their behavior. For example, saying "I understand that you feel anxious" might be an effective way of conveying empathy and validating someone's experience, and is not the same as saying "I think it's acceptable to drink excessively because you are anxious." Families need to learn to validate their loved ones without encouraging behaviors that are detrimental to their own and others' well-being. It is also important that the group members be realistic about what is achievable with validation. It can effectively defuse some situations, but it might take a lot of repeated validation to achieve this. Equally, validation might not improve extreme situations at all, although if this is the case the families can be encouraged that at the very least, they are unlikely to make the situation worse through validation.

Family members are given the opportunity to practice their validation skills through role plays and activities. Given an example scenario, families discuss in small groups how they might use validation to avoid an argument and keep the situation calm. They can discuss interactions they have had with their significant other that have escalated, and speculate on how a more validating stance might have helped. A role play can also be used to give families the opportunity to practice generating validating statements in the heat of the moment. Presenters listen carefully to the family members' attempts to validate, say whether they were successful or not, and offer constructive feedback.

During one role play, a presenter took on the role of someone's daughter, who did not want to meet her friends because she thought she looked ugly in her dress. A family member took on the role of the mother.

DAUGHTER: I'm really nervous about this social event, I don't want to go.
MOTHER: Why are you nervous?
DAUGHTER: This dress is terrible. I look really ugly.
MOTHER: But you look beautiful!
DAUGHTER: No. Forget it. You don't understand. I'm not going.

Upon discussing the use of validation in this role play, the families decided that the reason the attempt to validate ("You look beautiful!") was unsuccessful was because it focused on the daughter's actual appearance rather than validating her emotional experience of her appearance and her anxiety about going to the party. A better approach might have been to validate her nervousness ("Yes, social events you have to dress up for make me feel nervous sometimes. We all want to look our best, and never being sure is so difficult"), or even to validate her experience of feeling ugly ("It's normal to get anxious about your appearance before a big event. Is there something you can wear that might make you feel more at ease?"). If a role play is unsuccessful the first time, family members have the opportunity to try again using the feedback from the presenters or group members. Presenters reassure family members that although validation will not be easy to start with, they can continue to practice it with their families at home for homework; there is a worksheet to help them with this.

Module 5: Problem-Solving

The aim of the final module is to teach families how to solve problems that arise with their loved one with BPD using a calm and logical attitude, and a basic four-step framework that can be applied to any problem (see Box 14.9). By the end of this module, families are able to recognize when they are or are not in the right state of mind to address problems, understand the difference between praise, criticism, and feedback, and know how to use a four-step framework to solve problems that arise with their significant other.

Box 14.9 Module 5: Problem-Solving

- ◆ Outline of problem-solving and the four basic steps:
  - Defining the problem
  - Generating potential solutions
  - Selecting and planning the solution
  - Implementing and monitoring the solution
- ◆ Differentiation between praise, criticism, and feedback
- ◆ Practice with examples, using skills from previous modules
- ◆ Final summary and recap.

Families are given a worksheet that encourages them to consider the differences between praise, criticism, and feedback, and how they each give rise to different emotions and responses. Working on these differences and putting them into practice is a highly mentalizing process, and making the distinction in daily life necessitates an ability to mentalize both oneself and the other person. Listening for whether the other person hears you as praising or criticizing them when you are primarily giving nonjudgmental feedback, for example, allows you to modify your responses accordingly. This is mentalizing the other person. If your aim is to give feedback but their response suggests they hear it as criticism, then your next response to them has to take that into account so that a reflective process is set up between you. The distinction between feedback and criticism or praise is sometimes subtle and difficult to detect. Families are helped to distinguish between them, and learn how to alter phrases to make them sound more like feedback than criticism. They also learn that to some extent the differences between feedback and praise or criticism are dependent on the other person. Some family members feel that even if they do attempt to provide feedback to their significant other, it will be misinterpreted as criticism. Some even feel that praise can easily be misinterpreted as criticism. One family member cited an exchange between him and his daughter: "You look lovely today!" "Are you saying I don't look lovely on other days?" Even so, it is important that family members understand that even though praise or feedback can still lead to an argument, they are much less likely to cause problems than criticism, and so are preferable.

> One family member came home from work to find that the washing up had not been done. Although she found this frustrating, she managed not to criticize her son for

being messy, and instead said, "It would be helpful for me if you did the dishes before I got home." Her son apologized and agreed, and the family member understood that the outcome would certainly not have been as positive had she criticized him instead.

When teaching the families how to solve problems using a four-step framework, presenters refer to skills learned previously in the course and show how they might be useful in the problem-solving process. For example, families can use their mindfulness skills to identify when their emotions are too strong to problem-solve, and use management skills such as opposite action to calm situations to a point where they can problem-solve effectively. Furthermore, the first step of problem-solving (defining the problem) might benefit from mentalizing with the significant other to find the underlying cause of an issue. Families practice getting to the core of a problem, and can use a worksheet to aid this, or the group might like to refer back to examples from previous sessions to speculate about problems that might have been underlying a particular situation.

> Referring back to a role play in Module 4 where a daughter was nervous about going to a social event because she felt ugly in her dress, family members suggested that the real cause of her upset was not her appearance at all. Perhaps instead she was anxious that there was going to be a particular person at the event or that she would struggle to socialize.

Only after getting to the real root of a problem can families start devising strategies to resolve it. Families practice resolving problems at home using a worksheet.

References

Gunderson, J. G., & Hoffman, P. D. (Eds.). (2005). *Understanding and treating borderline personality disorder. A guide for professionals and families*. Arlington, VA: American Psychiatric Publishing.

Hoffman, P. D., Fruzzetti, A. E., & Buteau, E. (2007). Understanding and engaging families: An education, skills and support program for relatives impacted by borderline personality disorder. *Journal of Mental Health*, **16**, 69–82.

Leff, J., Kuipers, L., Berkowitz, R., Eberlein-Vries, R., & Sturgeon, D. (1982). A controlled trial of social intervention in the families of schizophrenic patients. *British Journal of Psychiatry*, **141**, 121–134.

Leff, J. P., & Vaughn, C. (1985). *Expressed emotion in families: Its significance for mental illness*. New York, NY: Guilford Press.

National Institute for Health and Clinical Excellence. (2009). *Borderline personality disorder: Treatment and management. Clinical guideline* **78**. London, UK: National Institute for Health and Clinical Excellence. http://www.nice.org.uk/guidance/cg78/evidence/cg78-borderline-personality-disorder-bpd-full-guideline3

Porr, V. (2010). *Overcoming borderline personality disorder: A family guide for healing and change*. Oxford, UK: Oxford University Press.

Chapter 15

Mentalizing the system

Introduction

A recurrent theme of this book has been the interactive nature of mentalizing. Even in relation to oneself, mentalizing is a highly social occupation: it involves interpreting the mind in relation to the world around it. In Chapter 1, we suggested that personality disorders may be usefully conceptualized as an adaptation to what has been learned from the social environment—in particular about the need for epistemic hypervigilance. In this chapter, we discuss some systemic approaches to mentalizing that indicate how intervening with the social environment of the individual can be relevant in clinical contexts. We will begin by considering the importance of the system around the clinician in the mentalizing approach. In the second section of the chapter, we will discuss an intervention to reduce bullying and violence in schools as an example of a systemic approach to creating a more mentalizing environment.

The system around the clinician

The emphasis of this guide so far has largely been upon the clinician in isolation—on the importance of their mentalizing stance, the need to maintain that stance, and the onus on them to recognize their own mentalizing lapses and difficulties. In this chapter, we set out how the network within which the clinician works has a role to play in supporting MBT practice. One of the points we have returned to throughout the book is the fact that we all experience fluctuations in our mentalizing capacities, and we may all need support in maintaining or restoring mentalizing in the face of interpersonally challenging situations. A mentalizing team around the clinician is crucial, we argue, if the clinician is to be expected to maintain a mentalizing stance across their clinical work—which entails, by necessity, constant exposure to the nonmentalizing modes of psychic equivalence, pretend mode, and teleological mode. In principle—at least in the individual MBT session—the patient and clinician are isolated in a room, albeit with bidirectional social influence—the clinician is in a position to enhance the patient's capacity to reflect, to question, and to focus simultaneously on both other and self, inside and outside. However, the reality is that the clinician becomes part of the patient's (dysfunctional) social system, and therefore mentalizing alone will not be sufficient; systemic intervention may be required to address the situational constraints. This problem can be even further exaggerated in the context of group therapy. Clinicians require their own system of support relationships, primarily from other clinicians, in order to scaffold their capacity to mentalize and facilitate epistemic trust.

One of the defining characteristics of personality disorder is that patients' patterns of social dysfunction are enduring. Indeed, borderline personality disorder (BPD) was traditionally regarded as being almost untreatable; this is one of the factors that have contributed to the stigma experienced by those receiving a BPD diagnosis. We now have effective therapies for BPD: at least nine forms of treatment have been tested in at least 20 randomized controlled trials (Stoffers et al., 2012), and patients with BPD should no longer be regarded as being beyond help. We would argue that the reason for the apparent contradiction of a condition that appeared to be untreatable also appearing to be more responsive to therapy than most mental disorders is to be found in the way the nonmentalizing actions of BPD patients can create nonmentalizing social systems that sustain their condition.

The impact of nonmentalizing on the social system, not the unchangeability of nonmentalizing per se, makes both BPD and antisocial personality disorder (ASPD) the challenging conditions they are, and causes the clinician to experience sustained demands on their mentalizing capacities. We suggest that it is unrealistic to expect a clinician to maintain an effective mentalizing stance in the medium to long term if they are not supported adequately by their surrounding team. Indeed, there is considerable evidence that clinicians can find it very difficult to maintain their mental equilibrium while working with patients with BPD. Clinicians have been found to struggle with negative responses toward their patients, and to experience patients with BPD as being less responsive and more withdrawn (Bourke & Grenyer, 2010). Further pressures are generated by either hostility or increased dependency (and fluctuations between the two, as different prementalizing modes emerge), and a context of heightened risk of suicide or self-harm. Given the demands involved in this work, we argue that the task of supporting the clinician and maintaining a mentalizing team (see Box 15.1) is a critical element of MBT.

Supervision

MBT integrates supervision within its structure. All clinicians and teams are expected to be well supported and supervised: good supervision systems are regarded as an integral element of the implementation of MBT. The supervisor

---

Box 15.1 The system around the clinician

Different layers of supervision and support together form an essential component of MBT practice:

1 Individual supervision: supervisor works with supervisee to help maintain a mentalizing stance in the course of their work

2 Supervision of the team:

- Group discussion of cases: focuses on techniques, practice, and knowledge, often in relation to particular patients

- Intervision: aims to improve individual team members' mentalizing of themselves and each other.

---

is expected to be a senior member of the MBT team or, alternatively, a member of a different MBT program. For example, if an MBT team runs two groups, the lead clinician from one group supervises the other group and vice versa, bringing with it the advantage of cross-fertilization of ideas.

The main aim of supervision within an MBT context is to help the clinician maintain his/her mentalizing stance in the face of the potential disruptions and obstructions thrown up in the course of his/her work. Mentalizing supervision seeks to support the clinician's mentalizing capacity in relation to a particular patient. In other words, like MBT itself, supervision is carefully focused on mentalizing the relationship rather than seeking to make broader judgments or directions about practice. If corrections need to be made, these are rooted in the supervisee's loss of mentalizing in the specific moment(s) of the treatment. The supervisee requires assistance to recover mentalizing and, once this is achieved, the process can be assumed to continue spontaneously. Thus, it is not for the supervisor to tell the supervisee what it was in the patient's discourse that "they had missed": that would entail the supervisor taking a nonmentalizing stance.

The task of the supervisor is to take the perspective of the supervisee as his/her starting point, to validate that perspective before offering an alternative, in just the same way as the clinician starts the recovery of mentalizing by validating the patient's understanding. The clinician gives an account of his/her experience as close to verbatim as possible (ideally, taped sessions are used). The supervisor listens for loss of mentalizing on the part of the clinician, stops the account at that point, and "rewinds" to the moments before mentalizing was lost. The supervisor asks for details about the interactions *before* the loss of mentalizing in the patient–clinician pair, and supervisor and supervisee both reflect on the context, identify the problem, and create an alternative course of action that might not have led the conversation down a nonmentalizing path. Little effort is made in speculating about the "causes" of the loss of mentalizing or divining the putative motivations of the patient in generating a nonmentalizing discourse, or wondering about the reasons for the clinician's "failure" to address the gap in mentalizing. None of these strategies are considered helpful in dealing with the next occasion when this might happen. They are also parallel strategies to trying to address nonmentalizing discourse in the patient by implicitly demanding mentalizing from him/her through asking the patient to reflect on his/her thoughts or feelings. It is far better and more productive to think about how the clinician could have avoided being drawn into nonmentalizing discourse. For example, if a clinician found him/herself disputing the patient's version of events (even if the clinician was justified in terms of historical accuracy), the supervisor can start by being sympathetic about the difficulty in being forced to accept an inaccurate account, and the extent to which it can generate anger and lead to a gap in sympathy with the patient. Then he/she can gently wonder if there would have been a major problem in partly implicitly agreeing with the patient's version of events, at least in terms of sympathizing with the patient's reactions to the events as he/she had perceived them. The inquisitive stance is as relevant to supervision as it is to therapy. The aim of supervision is the reinstatement of mentalizing; it is not offered to obtain insight into either the patient's or the clinician's psyche. There is a role for the general enhancement of mentalizing capacity, but this is best offered in the context of the team, and we consider it as part of the intervision process (discussed later in the "Supervision of the team" section).

The structure of supervision for MBT involves supervising individual and group clinicians together to encourage understanding of different perspectives. The most commonly expected number of clinicians in a supervisory group would be four—two individual clinicians and the two group clinicians who work with the same patients. Role-play figures heavily in MBT supervision. It is a useful way of obtaining feedback on one's practice of mentalizing. In the role-play, a clinician will bring to the group an example of a recent experience with a patient to which the clinician was unsure how best to respond. The clinician concerned takes on the role of the patient and a colleague will role-play the clinician's role. The process can help to indicate how mentalizing might be reinstated, or may indeed be blocked, by different kinds of intervention.

Supervision of the team

As well as regular supervisions in relation to individual cases, a fundamental aspect of MBT practice involves the supervision of the team. There are two different forms of team supervision that need to be implemented.

The first form of team supervision involves a focus on MBT techniques, knowledge, and case discussion. The team might discuss patients who are presenting particular challenges at that time, and role-play might be used to consider the kinds of interventions that might be helpful in the face of such challenges. In these supervisions, aspects of MBT theory or practice might also be discussed, with the aim of maintaining and improving clinicians' understanding of and engagement with the model, and help them develop their skills in the practice of MBT.

The second form of team supervision is known as *intervision*. The aim of intervision is to improve individual team members' mentalizing of themselves and each other. The issues raised in this type of supervision may be more personal than the theory and practice-oriented discussions of the first form of team supervision. Intervision seeks to improve the cohesion and mentalizing levels of the team; it may well involve discussion of disagreements that might be occurring within the team. The purpose of intervision is to encourage consideration of the meaning behind these disagreements—that is, what the factors behind them are, whether poor communication, the effects of a patient's internal processes, or a team member's unresolved transferences, or a mixture of various factors (as is often the case). Intervision attempts to shed light on some of these processes and restore mentalizing in relation to them.

A team around the worker

Here we borrow heavily from the ideas advanced by the developers of adolescent mentalization-based integrative treatment (AMBIT) (Bevington, Fuggle, Fonagy, Target, & Asen, 2013). AMBIT is a practice developed to provide help for adolescents with severe, complex, and multiple needs. The AMBIT model places a strong emphasis on the role of the keyworker, that is, an individual who is the primary clinician delivering and overseeing the patient's treatment, and the mentalizing-based relationship he/she forms with the patient. However, according to this model, this central keyworker relationship must be sustained by a responsive and supportive team; for all its emphasis on the keyworker, the model can be applied only within the context of an AMBIT team. Supervision is one way in which the clinician's work can be supported by the team; the team process is discussed in Chapter 5. But mentalizing treatment can effectively be sustained in practice only if it is backed up by a more broadly mentalizing system. In understanding how a system can mentalize, we draw on the ideas of the systems scientist Peter Senge, a seminal thinker in the area of how organizations work, how they learn, and how their cultures can develop, change, and progress (Senge, 1990). We suggest that this systems thinking is highly congruent with a mentalizing approach. The systems approach describes how organizations are underpinned by their interactive, interconnected relationships and the consequences of these relationships. An example for the clinician working with a patient with BPD or ASPD might be the involvement of another service—for instance, psychiatric, social, or medical—and the impact of an intervention instigated by one service on the work of another. An individual whose capacity to mentalize is regularly challenged can undermine the capacity of the system to function effectively. Adopting a psychic equivalence or pretend mode of thinking in relation to interpreting the actions of other clinicians or professionals working with a patient will quickly lead to a disintegration of network working and to nonproductive attributions being made. An absence of doubt or curiosity about actions can displace trust; being "certain" why fellow professionals acted in particular ways or, equally, mentally throwing one's hands up in a gesture of total incomprehension will generate conflict and, without doubt, hinder progress. Of course, even a clinician working within the most supportive of MBT teams cannot hope to mentalize the whole network of agencies that their patient may come into contact with. But, by creating a mentalizing environment, a team approach to MBT practice can create a structure in which the anxieties and pressures that arise from working within a challenging wider system can be partially mitigated.

A mentalizing team culture can support and maintain effective practice. Mentalizing is all about relationships and our intrinsically interactive and communicative state of being; the way we mentalize, or stop mentalizing, constitutes a form of social learning, in that it is something we change and adapt to according to the social climate around us. The collaboration essential for the clinical and social management of people with complex mental health problems is facilitated by understanding the actions of colleagues as well as patients in terms of the mental states that motivated their actions.

Mentalizing the system around the patient

In Chapter 1, we built on our thinking about how therapeutic processes may work and suggested that effective therapeutic interventions can be broken down into three types of communication system change. To recap, the first communication system involves providing the patient with a model for thinking about the mind and understanding their disorder, including fostering skills and competencies to improve their adaptation. This process of providing valued explanation and support requires the clinician to communicate in a way that makes the patient feel that their difficulties have been understood, which in turn generates a sense that their sense of self and "agentiveness" have been recognized. Being made to feel agentive is a cue for enhanced social communication, which encourages the acceptance and acquisition of information that can be generalized beyond the current situation (in other words, it may have a long-term impact on behavior). The first phase is an implicitly mentalizing process that is rich in ostensive cues. It brings forth the second communication system, in which the patient's epistemic trust gradually increases to the point that their capacity to mentalize is recovered and they can start to engage in open social exchanges, initially with the clinician— allowing their mind to be changed by another mind. The patient is now open to change, and their ability to learn from social information (rather than discarding all knowledge inconsistent with their expectations) is regenerated and supported within the intervention. We suggested that the real benefits of the relearning of mentalizing in this way are fully reaped only via the third communication system, when the patient is able to experience and apply their social learning beyond their relationship with the clinician, to create a virtuous circle of improved interpersonal relations in their wider social interactions. The increase in epistemic trust allows the patient to build on and respond to social situations in a more constructive manner and to mentalize themselves and others around them, serving to build stronger and more supportive relationships. However, this final communication system, outside the clinical setting, is dependent upon the patient's social environment being sufficiently benign for balanced mentalizing to be applied constructively: that is, it has to be an environment in which reduced epistemic hypervigilance and the maintenance of epistemic trust are justified.

The implication of this thinking about the third system of communication is that what happens within any therapeutic intervention cannot, on its own, be expected to be enough for any lasting significant improvement in the patient's state to occur. The conceptualization of the three communication systems therefore involves an acknowledgment of the inherent limitations of clinical interventions in cases where the patient is faced with a social environment that does not support mentalizing. Indeed, certain circumstances make it maladaptive for the individual to continue to mentalize in a fully balanced way—for example, in social environments characterized by high levels of aggression or violence, which require the individual to prioritize an external, nonreflective, rapidly responding focus on the control of others, as opposed to interest in the affective states of self or others, as a survival strategy.

This emphasis on the role of the social environment points to the value of thinking about ways in which social climates can be encouraged to become more mentalizing. Clearly, families are one social system to which the mentalizing approach can be applied, as discussed in Chapter 14. Beyond the family, one obvious example of where mentalizing can practically be applied more systemically is in schools. Creating a mentalizing institutional climate in a school may be a way of triggering the three communication systems that we suggest are involved in bringing about therapeutic change (see Box 15.2).

Box 15.2 Dealing with the school climate: assumptions, aims, and adjuncts

- To reduce violence in schools, we need to systemically increase awareness of the mental states that underpin behavior
- The whole school community contributes to unthinking, bullying-related dysfunction
- Peaceful collaboration with others requires prioritizing their subjective states, thus placing limits upon the urge to violently control the behavior of less powerful members of the group.

Making a social system more mentalizing: a schools program

A mentalizing individual will reflect, empathize with the self and others, modulate affect storms, set boundaries, and have a strong sense of agency. This same principle can be applied to social groups. Dysfunctional social systems cause the collapse of mentalizing and result in the highly reactive, tense, and defensive interactions that can lead to violence. A school in which violence, aggression, and bullying are the norm is by definition a social environment that works to close down mentalizing in staff members and pupils.

The mentalizing approach to schools we shall discuss here is Creating a Peaceful School Learning Environment (CAPSLE), a program designed to address bullying and violence in schools. The emphasis of CAPSLE, which differentiates it from the many other anti-bullying programs that have been devised and applied in schools, is that it focuses on the whole school community, and seeks to create a mentalizing climate and a group dynamic that can resist and limit the potency and currency carried by individual acts of violence or aggression (Twemlow, Fonagy, & Sacco, 2005a, 2005b) (see Box 15.3). CAPSLE is a teacher-implemented, school-wide program made up of four components:

1   A "positive climate" campaign, which uses reflective classroom discussions of immediate past experiences, in lessons led by counselors, to create a shift in the language and thinking of students and personnel.

2   A classroom management plan, which assists the teachers' discipline skills by focusing on understanding and correcting problems at the root rather than punishing and criticizing only the behavior that is apparent. For example, a behavior problem in a single child is conceptualized as a problem for all the pupils in the class, who, often unwittingly, participate in bully, victim, or

---

Box 15.3 Creating A Peaceful School Learning Environment (CAPSLE)

- A manualized psychodynamic social systems approach to bullying in schools
- Assumes that all members of the school community, including teachers, play a role in interpersonal violence
- Aims to improve the capacity of all community members to mentalize
- Assumes that greater awareness of other people's feelings will counteract the temptation to bully others.

---

bystander roles. This approach reduces scapegoating, and insight into the meaning of the behavior becomes paramount.

3 A physical education program, derived from a combination of role-playing, relaxation, and self-defense techniques, which teaches children skills to deal with victimization and bystanding behavior. This component of the program helps children to protect themselves and others by using nonaggressive physical and cognitive strategies. For example, enacting bully–victim–bystander roles provides pupils with the opportunity to role-play and work out alternative actions to fighting. Learning ways to physically defend oneself (e.g., when grabbed, pushed, or punched), coupled with classroom discussion, teaches personal self-control as well as respect and helpfulness toward others.

4 Schools may put in place one or two support programs: peer mentorship or adult mentorship. These relationships provide additional containment and modeling to assist children in mastering the skills and language to deal with power struggles. For example, mentors instruct children in refereeing games, resolving playground disputes, and the importance of helping others.

In a cluster-randomized control trial involving 1345 children across nine elementary schools in a city in the United States (Fonagy et al., 2009), the CAPSLE program was found to substantially reduce aggression and improve classroom behavior. There was a reduction in children's experience of aggression and victimization. The program's effectiveness was indicated by a reduction in the number of children nominated by their peers as being aggressive, victimized, or engaging in aggressive bystanding. This was confirmed by the observation of reduced disruptive and off-task classroom behavior in schools implementing CAPSLE. The program develops a school-wide awareness of the omnipresence of power struggles and their effects on individuals' capacity to think about others' points of view. The study's findings suggested that empathic mentalizing increased in schools using the CAPSLE program. This is consistent with the view that the emotional and cognitive skills learned in handling interpersonal power struggles enhance both the emotional and the cognitive empathic aspects of mentalizing and self-agency (Baron-Cohen, 2005) and thus may reduce the likelihood of an individual resorting to physical aggression (Fonagy, 2003).

CAPSLE focuses on the power dynamics in the relationship between bullies, victims, and bystanders, and emphasizes the role of bystanders in restoring mentalizing within this dynamic. Through the components of the program outlined earlier, bystanders are trained to act to encourage bullies, victims, and other bystanders to be aware of and move away from "pathological" roles. In a nonmentalizing environment, the witness to a power struggle—that is, the bystander—may experience sadistic feelings of pleasure in seeing another's difficulty or suffering. This is possible only when the witness feels distanced from the internal world of the other person, and is then able to use the victim to contain the unwanted (usually frightened) part of him/herself. The enjoyment and excitement that bystanding groups often show when witnessing fights or aggression in violent schools—for example, the crowding around fights and stirring up of grudges that often take place—does not involve *complete* mentalizing failure: some level of empathy is necessary for this projective identification with the victim's pain to take place. However, the mentalizing that does take place is highly limited by the social setting, such that the victim's pain is not fully represented as a mental state in the witness's own consciousness; that is, the victim's pain is *recognized* but not *felt* by the witness. It should not surprise us that such a dynamic unfolds in schools: mentalizing is a fragile capacity until early adulthood (or even later in life), and it requires a social environment to scaffold it and make sure that the mental states of both the self and other can be reflected upon. The CAPSLE intervention constitutes a deliberate attempt to scaffold the unbalanced, fluctuating, and incompletely emerging mentalizing capacities of children and young people (and the teachers reacting to them), creating a social environment in which more balanced mentalizing can be practiced and reinforced, and its benefits experienced.

We will illustrate our thinking with a case study (which we have previously published; Twemlow et al., 2005b).

The child concerned in this example, "Billy," is a large, round-faced 11-year-old, well known by his teacher, "Ms. Jones," to be disruptive in class. He has a long history of behavioral problems. When interacting with his peers, he seeks to dominate, and he disrupts games with constant complaints and power struggles. His bullying manner has made him unpopular with his peers, so he seeks to build social status by acting as "bodyguard" to the leader of the "most popular" clique, something not always appreciated by the child concerned. Billy attends a large middle school (2000 students aged between 11 and 14 years) in a low-income, medium-sized city in the United States. The school environment is tense: there are high levels of physical aggression, including acts of outright violence, and both teachers and pupils report feeling frightened for their safety. The teachers feel underqualified and unsupported in dealing with high numbers of children who appear seriously disturbed.

Billy arrives late to class one Monday morning, stomps to his desk, and sits down, shouting "I hate Mondays, school is such a waste of time!" The class is supposed to be catching up on their English Language project work, one of the subjects Billy dislikes most. Ms. Jones perceives, partly on the basis of previous experience, that Billy is planning to misbehave, cause conflict, and avoid doing any work. She tries to ignore him, but his disruptive behavior continues and Ms. Jones's irritation with him is rapidly rising, as this is the latest of many similar recent experiences with Billy. When Ms. Jones says that she will call Billy's mother, he becomes rude and indignant, adding that he couldn't care less because his mother thinks the school is "stupid" anyway. Ms. Jones's frustration is made worse by the fact that Billy's mother has also made her life difficult: she feels that, along with other parents, Billy's mother has made an inordinate number of aggressive, unreasonable complaints and made no attempt to engage in conversations about improving Billy's behavior. Billy's mother has been so hostile to the school, and to Ms. Jones in particular, that all her communications are now made directly to the school principal. Ms. Jones has felt unsupported and frustrated by the way the school management has handled both Billy and his mother, both of whom she sees as being allowed to get away with undermining and destructive behavior.

Every time Ms. Jones intervenes in an attempt to deter Billy's outbursts, his behavior worsens. She asks him to sit down and keep quiet so that the other students can do their work without distraction. With increasing emphasis, she tells him to "Stop making that noise!" but to no avail. She shouts: "Billy, JUST SIT DOWN! NOW! AND I MEAN IT!" But again, this has no impact. The continued bad behavior that results from these failed interventions causes constant upheaval in the classroom, leaving the remainder of the pupils unattended for considerable amounts of time. Eventually, Ms. Jones has no choice but to send Billy to the principal. Unhelpfully, he is then essentially "baby-sat" in the principal's office for the remainder of that lesson, and then sent on to his next class.

From Ms. Jones's point of view, Billy is bullying and manipulative, capable of "playing the system" by getting his mother and even the principal to protect him from discipline and, as a result, he is allowed to continue to disrupt the whole classroom and undermine Ms. Jones as a professional. She understands that

Billy has social problems, and at one level she does not blame him: she feels the fault lies with his mother, who communicates a destructive and truculent attitude to authority to her son. Ms. Jones also recognizes that Billy's behavior is partly fueled by his difficulties with his peers and his misjudged desire to achieve esteem through aggression and domination.

The difficulty with Ms. Jones's interpretation of Billy's behavior is that it is based on the assumption that Billy is an averagely competent mentalizer, as she herself is. As such, she is making assumptions about the thoughts and feelings that drive Billy's actions: that he is acting at a rational level in his pursuit of avoiding getting any work done. While some of Ms. Jones's conclusions are not unreasonable—she certainly seems to be able to predict what Billy is going to do (i.e., cause further mayhem)—she is not able to fully mentalize him, for the understandable reason that she is highly stressed in her encounters with him, particularly when she is having to respond to him while also being responsible for an entire classroom of pupils. As a result, she has become inflexible in her thinking. Although she feels certain that Billy's exclamation "I hate Mondays!" is born of his desire to create turmoil, motivated by his wish to avoid unpleasurable work, she cannot know this for certain. Indeed, Ms. Jones cannot and does not know that before he left home that morning Billy's mother had screamed at him to get out of the house, to go to school, to leave her alone, adding for good measure that she wished Billy "had never been born." Billy's provocative and aggressive behavior, driven by his emotional arousal, and the anxiety this gave rise to in Ms. Jones in relation to her responsibilities to the other students in the class, prevented her from exploring possible alternative intentions behind Billy's behavior. It never occurred to her to ask him what the matter was. Her reaction was to inhibit mentalizing, to simplify matters and assume immediately that the past was repeating itself. "Here we go again," she said to herself, without thinking of the specific instance. Billy gives only the faintest of indications of the nature of the turmoil he feels. When threatened with his mother's involvement, he outwardly expresses little apparent concern.

But Ms. Jones's anxieties, which undermine her capacity to envision mental states, go beyond the interaction with Billy. Her failure to consider alternative accounts for Billy's behavior may be linked to the threat that she experiences in relation to Billy's mother and all the other parents who aggressively manipulate teachers, making thinking about beliefs and desires, thoughts, and feelings well-nigh impossible. In such acrimonious situations, thinking about the intentions of someone who harbors malevolent intent toward one would be unbearable. As a result, Ms. Jones protects herself by refusing to have contact with Billy's mother, but at the same time she deprives herself of the opportunity to think about the mother and about what it might be like for an 11-year-old to be subject to the mother's raging temper. Unlike Ms. Jones, Billy does not have the opportunity to route all communications with his mother via the principal. Perhaps at the beginning of the class when he made the commotion he was still feeling the impact of his mother's vitriolic onslaught and was not fully aware of the impact his behavior was having on others but was simply trying to make himself feel better—and not, as Ms. Jones assumed, to create an upheaval to conceal his inadequacy at school work. Contrary to Ms. Jones's belief, far from being able to manipulate the behavior of his peers through creating distraction, Billy, with his limited capacity to mentalize, is actually not able to see their minds clearly; nor is he able to anticipate their behavior on the basis of their mental states, but, instead, only on the basis of their concrete behaviors.

Little wonder, then, that Ms. Jones' interaction with Billy was unsuccessful. The kind of self-regulation she was demanding of him was quite simply beyond his capability at this point. He experiences the rebuke as an assault from yet another hostile mind, which simply confirms his need to shut off, to make a noise, to disrupt, to protect himself from what is unbearably painful. Unable to tolerate hostile cognitions about him, he closes himself off to the entire person whose mind he experiences as malevolent. Ms. Jones, in feeling unheeded, naturally increases her wish to control, and becomes increasingly physical or teleological in her attempts to control Billy's behavior. She finds herself caring less and less about what Billy thinks or how he feels, and just wishes his body to cease to be an obstacle to her overarching goal of education and communication. Were she able to reflect at this stage, she would recognize that her attitude simply pushes Billy further in a nonmentalizing direction. Thus, the classroom drama continues along its predictable path of emphasizing physical control as opposed to influence through modifying feelings and ideas. Each party feels deprived of the capacity to think, and they react by depriving the other of their ability to do so, until little remains beyond the controlling power relationship that is usually called bullying.

Looking at Billy as an agent whose rationality is limited by his impoverished ability to mentalize, particularly at times when he feels upset or anxious, helps us to have a somewhat different appreciation of not only his current behavior but also his history. Billy's father is absent, and thus not there to protect him from his mother, but also not there to help Billy see his situation from an alternative standpoint. The presence of another adult, or even a more mature individual (such as an older sibling) can help a child to think about his/her relationship with a parent if he/she finds this relationship overwhelming. Billy has neither older siblings nor a father present to play this role. In fact, none of the adult figures around him assist him with the terror he sometimes feels in relation to his mother. Even the principal appears to be frightened of Billy's mother, and so does Ms. Jones, although neither of these well-intentioned people recognizes that their acquiescence to Billy's mother further exaggerates Billy's fear of her. They do not think about it—not because they are unthinking people, but because they apparently have specific difficulty in thinking about thoughts and feelings in relation to Billy.

Billy lacks the capacity to be attuned to his peers, often reacting to them in ways that they find disturbing. Occasionally, he appears overanxious to please. He might then repeatedly do the wrong thing, making him an object of ridicule. He inadequately defends against this state by creating a position for himself through coercion and sometimes cruelty. No one notices that these instances of cruelty are almost invariably linked to moments where he feels profoundly humiliated by those around him. They fail to notice because the kind of teleological physical strategies that he uses to control the minds of those around him are precisely those that exclude the possibility of mentalizing. Billy has created a system around him that increasingly responds solely to physical threats rather than reason. Unlike most other boys, Billy is not able to set aside social criticism, which he experiences as a direct attempt to destroy him. Although Ms. Jones links her own difficulties with Billy with his earlier experiences of shame and humiliation, she has lost sight of just how devastating humiliation is for this 11-year-old with severely unbalanced mentalizing skills.

In seeking to help Billy—and Ms. Jones in dealing with him—it would be impractical to try to explain the intricate communication patterns we have outlined above. Ms. Jones is far too busy having to cope with an entire class. Would Billy benefit from individual therapy? Experience shows that boys like Billy respond poorly to such efforts, however skilled, if they do not take place in the context of concurrent family and social interventions. We feel that disrupting the vicious cycle that a child such as Billy finds himself in should be undertaken in school. Furthermore, it may be best, given Billy's sensitivity to humiliation, if the intervention does not directly concern Billy at all but, rather, the whole class.

It may seem like using a sledgehammer to crack a nut to modify the behavior of the class rather than imposing consequences on Billy alone. Yet, if we take a broader view, we can see that it is not just Billy, but all those interacting with him, who have difficulty in considering thoughts and feelings. The problems may originate in Billy, but Ms. Jones, normally a sensitive and caring person, finds herself reacting to Billy by shouting and bullying him. Her reactions in turn paralyze the other children to a point where there is little expectation on anyone's part that thinking about what is going on could achieve anything more than imposing physical consequences.

The procedure in the context of our program would have been for Ms. Jones to stop the class immediately after Billy started creating a commotion, and mark some space for reflection on what was happening. In other words, she would recognize the assault on her own mentalizing that she was experiencing, and she would attempt to restore her own capacity for controlled, cognitive mentalizing, and in the process seek to draw upon the collective mentalizing capacity of her classroom to create an environment in which Billy's arousal could reduce.

We would argue it would be far more realistic to expect Ms. Jones to make such an intervention if she felt that such an approach was supported and understood by her colleagues and senior management. The chaotic relationship between Billy's mother and the school authorities is symptomatic of a social system that is not functional. In effect, the principal is veering between being in effect a victim of Billy and his mother and their overwhelming affect; acting as a bystander in relation to Billy's behavior toward Ms. Jones, which allows Billy to continue to dominate her and the class; and then, when the situation is no longer tenable, turning on Billy in a punitive, bullying manner for his behavior, possibly ultimately culminating in school exclusion. The mentalizing approach to the school system requires the staff involved to be able to recognize the distorted power dynamics that arise as a result of the mentalizing challenges presented by individuals like Billy and his mother.

Understanding social environments in terms of mentalizing

In a social system, we are all attuned to whom we can trust and whom we cannot. In contrast to the widespread assumption that young children are prone to uncritical credulity, recent evidence shows that they extend trust with appropriate selectivity. Even preschoolers monitor the reliability of a particular individual who is providing them with information, differentiate between informants on the basis of validity of their past claims, and are guided by their interpretation of informants' minds when evaluating new information from these people (Koenig & Harris, 2005). There are sound biological reasons for prioritizing this ability to be selective in social attention. As humans we are part of a wider ecosystem. At all levels the system is characterized by levels of flexibility, which in turn reflect the system's capacity to respond to challenges to the system in an appropriate way. For social systems to be effective socializing structures—that is, supportive, flexible, and responsive to the needs of the individual people within them—they have to be characterized by high levels of epistemic trust. It is the good understanding of the self by the other (i.e., mentalizing) that generates epistemic trust in relation to that person.

There is a potential virtuous cycle in relation to this process that empowers the individual by empowering the social context of that person, which ultimately feeds back at the level of the individual. As we described in Chapter 1, social communications that create epistemic trust tend to be ostensive cues marked by recognition of the listener as an intentional agent; the use of such ostensive cues will in turn increase the likelihood of subsequent communications from the speaker being coded as relevant, generalizable, and to be retained in the procedural or semantic memory of the listener as influential—that is, relevant to them (Csibra & Gergely, 2009). Enhancement of such responsiveness naturally promotes the general flexibility of the system and increases the likelihood that individuals in the system can be responded to as individual intentional agents. To put this simply, if communications directed at me make me feel that my preferences are being taken into account and that my state of mind is a source of concern to the person who is speaking to me, then I will take those communications to be relevant to organizing my future social behavior (i.e., I will "learn the rules"), which will thus increase my chances of being appropriately aware of the preferences of others in my social group. Their reactions to my communications will in turn be more *deferential*—that is, they will take seriously and internalize what I have to say, and accurately perceive and recognize my position, and in future communications will address me with greater accuracy, making me feel agentive and thereby responsive to social influence.

So, what are the characteristics of a social system that is able to mentalize and generate a high level of epistemic trust (see Box 15.4)? The system is relaxed and flexible, not "stuck" in one point of view. It permits modifications of convention, at least on a temporary basis. Thus, interactions can be playful, with humor that engages rather than being hurting or distancing. The group can solve problems through "give and take" between one's own and others' perspectives. The

Box 15.4 Some features of a successfully mentalizing system

- Relaxed and flexible, not "stuck" in one point of view
- Can be playful, with humor that engages rather than being hurtful or distracting
- Can solve problems by "give and take" between own and others' perspectives
- Advocates describing one's own experience, rather than defining other people's experience or intentions
- Conveys individual "ownership" of behavior rather than a sense that it "happens" to them
- Is curious about other people's perspectives, and expects to have one's own views extended by others' views.

system values describing every member's experience, rather than defining other people's experience or intentions. By the same token, it conveys individual "ownership" of behavior, rather than a sense of highlighting events or forces beyond the individual that just "happen" to them and explain individual actions. Perhaps as a consequence of this, the system is endlessly curious about other people's perspectives, and people expect to have their own views extended by those of others. The relational strengths of a mentalizing social system include curiosity, safe uncertainty, contemplation and reflection, perspective-taking, forgiveness, impact awareness, and non-paranoid attitudes. General values and attitudes required to promote epistemic trust are tentativeness, humility (moderation), playfulness and humor, flexibility, and "give and take," coupled with individual responsibility and accountability.

At the heart of our social model is the interchangeable character of the individual and the group. The different levels of the human ecological system* (Bronfenbrenner, 1979) (see Figure 15.1) are similar in relation to the property of epistemic trust. Mentalizing develops and is sustained by the social system

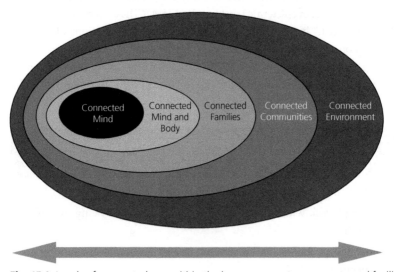

Fig. 15.1 Levels of connectedness within the human ecosystem promote and facilitate each other.

---

* The levels of the system can be considered as: (a) microsystem: interactions between the child and other people in the immediate setting; (b) mesosystem: interactions between the various microsystems (e.g., between the child's family and the school, or between the child's peers and his/her family); (c) exosystem: involves the institutions in which the child does not directly participate, but which have an indirect influence on the child; and (d) macrosystem: involves the interaction of children with the beliefs, values, expectations, and lifestyles of their cultural setting.

> **Box 15.5 Mentalizing and nonmentalizing social systems**
>
> ◆ Mentalizing develops and is sustained by the social system we live in
>
> ◆ Social systems that are compassionate (care about us) have physical (oxytocin) and psychological (feel "held in mind") effects, which enhance accurate self-awareness and awareness of the mental state of others
>
> ◆ Social systems that disrespect human subjectivity (how a person is likely to feel) recreate the evolutionary environment that encodes for self-sufficiency (dismissing of subjectivity) and create an environment for bullying.

we live in (see Box 15.5). Social systems that are compassionate (i.e., that care about us) have both physical (e.g., at the level of neuropeptides such as oxytocin) and phenomenological (e.g., feeling "held in mind") effects that enhance accurate self-awareness and awareness of the mental state of others. Social systems that do not respect human subjectivity and agency (e.g., those that pay no attention to how a person is likely to feel in response to an action) recreate the evolutionary environment that encodes the need for self-sufficiency (dismissing of subjectivity) and closes down social attention to the communication of others. This makes for a rigid, unresponsive system in which individuals are primed to consider communications as not generalizable or relevant to them beyond the context of the particular situation.

We have considered the characteristics of social systems that are imbued with mentalizing and capable of generating an environment of trust. So, what can we expect from social environments that are not saturated with mentalizing and the sense of general epistemic trust that follows from it?

Some social environments are inchoate, vague, confused, and disorganized (see Box 15.6). Individuals circulate within them in a kind of Brownian motion (the random motion of particles suspended in a liquid or a gas resulting from their collision with the quickly moving atoms or molecules in the liquid or gas). People experience their thoughts and feelings as having no consequence for others, leading ultimately to the experience of an empty and meaninglessness social existence: this is a social system that is operating in the pretend mode (Box 15.7).

Selfishness and extreme egocentrism then emerge out of the unreality of anything other than one's own thoughts and feelings. Lack of reality of internal experience permits interpersonal aggression and deliberate harm because other minds are not felt to exist and the mind is no longer felt to be contingent on the continued existence of the physical self. Frequently there is endless "communication" and searching but it is destined to yield no change. Christopher

---

Box 15.6 Nonmentalizing disorganized social systems

- Social systems that create fear and hyperactivate attachment can destroy the capacity for higher-order cognition and force the system back to pre-mentalizing modes of social thinking
- Such social systems can be self-reinforcing and therefore highly stable in their instability
- They undermine the very social mechanism that could alter their character: human collaboration (negotiation and creativity).

Lasch (1965, 1978) has described such societies in his acclaimed analyses of late twentieth-century North American culture:

> When government was centralized and politics became national in scope, as they had to be to cope with the energies let loose by industrialism, and when public life became faceless and anonymous and society an amorphous democratic mass, the old system of paternalism (in the home and out of it) collapsed, even when its semblance survived intact. The patriarch, though he might still preside in splendor at the head of his board, had come to resemble an emissary from a government which had been silently overthrown. The mere theoretical recognition of his authority by his family could not alter the fact that the government which was the source of all his ambassadorial powers had ceased to exist. (Lasch, 1965, p. 111)

Box 15.7 Nonmentalizing disorganized social systems: pretend mode systems

- Ideas fail to form a bridge between inner and outer reality; the mental world is decoupled from external reality
- People think and feel, but this can have no consequence, leading to an empty and meaningless social existence
- There is selfishness and extreme egocentrism emerging out of the unreality of anything other than one's own thoughts and feelings
- Lack of reality of internal experience permits interpersonal aggression and deliberate harm because other minds are not felt to exist and the mind is no longer felt to be contingent on the continued existence of the physical self
- Frequently, there is endless "communication" and searching but it is destined to yield no change.

> ## Box 15.8 Nonmentalizing disorganized social systems: psychic equivalence systems
>
> Mental reality and outer reality become blurred, such that internal thoughts have the power of external reality:
>
> + Thoughts are real and therefore they have to be controlled
> + There are singular solutions to social reality, there are no alternative ways of seeing things, there is intolerance of perspectives
> + Models of minds are simple (black and white), schematic, and rigidly held—leads to acts of prejudice
> + Negative ideas (threats) become terrifying.

By contrast, social systems that create fear and hyperactivate attachment can destroy higher-order cognition (thinking capacity) and force the system back to prementalizing modes of social thinking. Such social systems can be self-reinforcing and therefore highly persistent in their instability. They undermine the very social mechanism that could alter their character: human collaboration (negotiation and creativity). Sometimes a mind–world isomorphism is created and psychic equivalence becomes institutional (see Box 15.8). George Orwell's dystopian novel *Nineteen Eighty-Four* comes close to this formulation, in which thoughts and feelings acquire the significance and power of the external. If thoughts are real, it makes sense that they have to be controlled. There are singular solutions to all social realities, there are no alternative ways of seeing things, and there can be dramatic intolerance of other perspectives. But models of minds that are simple (black-and-white thinking), schematic, and rigidly held readily generate dramatic social acts of individual prejudice. Because thoughts are close to the realm of the physical, negative ideas (any threats or images of danger) become terrifying and have to be physically defended against.

Expectations concerning the agency of the other are present but these are largely formulated in terms restricted to the physical world, so protection against hostility is primarily physical: this is operating in the teleological mode of prementalizing (see Box 15.9). Because thoughts and feelings are so close to the material world, only what is material comes to be considered socially meaningful: only what I physically obtain counts. The gestures of others matter to the extent they are observable, but in that context only the actions, rather than potential motives behind them, are meaningful; they are taken to be the only true index of the intentions of the other. Since only action that has a physical

---

Box 15.9 Nonmentalizing disorganized social systems: teleological systems

Only behavior that has a physical impact is considered meaningful:

♦ Physical acts of harm: aggression is seen as legitimate

♦ Demand for physical demonstrations of intent by others: payment, acts of subservience, retributive justice.

---

impact is felt potentially capable of altering the mental state of others, threats of physical acts of harm or actual acts of aggression are seen as legitimate. Social demand is for physical acts to demonstrate intent. Punishment is by payment, acts of subservience, and retributive (as opposed to restorative) justice.

Making peace in communities

It follows from the previous section that communities contribute to aggression-related dysfunction. Peaceful collaboration with others requires prioritizing others' subjective states, thus placing limits upon the urge to physically control the behavior of less powerful members of the group. Secure social environments aim to focus on the mental states of all those involved in power dynamics of interpersonal violence.

Is there a recipe for creating a peaceful community? Following our model, the process should start with activating the systems of attachment by creating an attitude of caring and compassion—a social prerequisite for sensitive responsiveness to individual needs, particularly in the context of stress. In general, we should aim to enhance the curiosity that members of the community have about each other's social experience, and their thoughts and feelings about those around them. This curiosity must be coupled with respectful not-knowing, avoiding assumptions, as reflected in social prejudice, generalizations about groups, the absence of doubt, and black-and-white, all-or-nothing thinking.

A good example of overcoming nonmentalizing social processes is the radical approach to criminal accountability of restorative justice (Sherman & Strang, 2007). The simple expedient of confronting the offender with the victim, in the form of face-to-face conferences, victim–offender mediation, restitution, or reparation payment, forces the offender to create an image of the person he/she harmed. In many tests, offenders who receive restorative justice commit fewer repeat crimes than offenders who do not, which is consistent with our earlier-mentioned suggestions. In one study of young adult offenders in Canada, the reoffending rates after 2 years were 11% for those who had gone through restorative justice versus 37% for those who served their sentence in prison (Sherman & Strang, 2007). Restorative justice reduces repeat offending more consistently for violent crimes than for less serious crimes, suggesting—in accordance with our thesis in relation to ASPD—that the loss of mentalizing is particularly marked in relation to acts of violence. Diversion of offenders from the traditional route of prosecution to restorative justice is a pragmatic solution because evidence suggests that it also substantially increases the odds of an offender being brought to justice.

There are few things that turn out to be more practical than mentalizing solutions to social problems. The reason for this is that mentalizing underpins the way we have evolved to function as a society.

References

Baron-Cohen, S. (2005). Autism. In B. Hopkins (Ed.), *Cambridge encyclopedia of child development* (pp. 398–401). Cambridge, UK: Cambridge University Press.

Bevington, D., Fuggle, P., Fonagy, P., Target, M., & Asen, E. (2013). Innovations in Practice: Adolescent Mentalization-Based Integrative Therapy (AMBIT)—a new integrated approach to working with the most hard to reach adolescents with severe complex mental health needs. *Child and Adolescent Mental Health*, **18**, 46–51.

Bourke, M., & Grenyer, B. F. S. (2010). Psychotherapists' response to borderline personality disorder: A core conflictual relationship theme analysis. *Psychotherapy Research*, **20**, 680–691.

Bronfenbrenner, U. (1979). *The ecology of human development: Experiments by nature and design*. Cambridge, MA: Harvard University Press.

Csibra, G., & Gergely, G. (2009). Natural pedagogy. *Trends in Cognitive Sciences*, **13**, 148–153.

Fonagy, P. (2003). Towards a developmental understanding of violence. *British Journal of Psychiatry*, **183**, 190–192.

Fonagy, P., Twemlow, S. W., Vernberg, E. M., Nelson, J. M., Dill, E. J., Little, T. D., & Sargent, J. A. (2009). A cluster randomized controlled trial of child-focused psychiatric consultation and a school systems-focused intervention to reduce aggression. *Journal of Child Psychology and Psychiatry*, **50**, 607–616.

Koenig, M. A., & Harris, P. L. (2005). The role of social cognition in early trust. *Trends in Cognitive Sciences*, **9**, 457–459.

Lasch, C. (1965). *The new radicalism in America, 1889–1963. The intellectual as a social type*. New York, NY: W. W. Norton.

Lasch, C. (1978). *The culture of narcissism: American life in an age of diminishing expectations*. New York, NY: W. W. Norton.

Senge, P. (1990). *The fifth discipline: The art and practice of the learning organization*. New York, NY: Doubleday.

Sherman, L., & Strang, H. (2007). *Restorative justice: The evidence*. London, UK: Smith Institute.

Stoffers, J. M., Vollm, B. A., Rucker, G., Timmer, A., Huband, N., & Lieb, K. (2012). Psychological therapies for people with borderline personality disorder. *Cochrane Database of Systematic Reviews*, **8**, CD005652.

Twemlow, S. W., Fonagy, P., & Sacco, F. C. (2005a). A developmental approach to mentalizing communities: I. A model for social change. *Bulletin of the Menninger Clinic*, **69**, 265–281.

Twemlow, S. W., Fonagy, P., & Sacco, F. C. (2005b). A developmental approach to mentalizing communities: II. The Peaceful Schools experiment. *Bulletin of the Menninger Clinic*, **69**, 282–304.

Recommended further reading

Allen, J. G. (2013). *Mentalizing in the development and treatment of attachment trauma.* London, UK: Karnac Books.

Allen, J. G., & Fonagy, P. (2014). Mentalizing in psychotherapy. In R. E. Hales, S. C. Yudofsky, & L. Roberts (Eds.), *Textbook of psychiatry* (6th edn., pp. 1095–1118). Washington, DC: American Psychiatric Publishing.

Allen, J. G., Fonagy, P., & Bateman, A. W. (2008). *Mentalizing in clinical practice.* Washington, DC: American Psychiatric Publishing.

Asen, E., & Fonagy, P. (2012). Mentalization-based therapeutic interventions for families. *Journal of Family Therapy,* **34,** 347–370.

Bateman, A., Bolton, R., & Fonagy, P. (2013). Antisocial personality disorder: A mentalizing framework. *Focus: The Journal of Lifelong Learning in Psychiatry,* **11,** 178–186.

Bateman, A., & Fonagy, P. (2008). 8-year follow-up of patients treated for borderline personality disorder: Mentalization-based treatment versus treatment as usual. *American Journal of Psychiatry,* **165,** 631–638.

Bateman, A., & Fonagy, P. (2008). Comorbid antisocial and borderline personality disorders: Mentalization-based treatment. *Journal of Clinical Psychology,* **64,** 181–194.

Bateman, A., & Fonagy, P. (2009). Randomized controlled trial of outpatient mentalization-based treatment versus structured clinical management for borderline personality disorder. *American Journal of Psychiatry,* **166,** 1355–1364.

Bateman, A., & Fonagy, P. (2010). Mentalization based treatment for borderline personality disorder. *World Psychiatry,* **9,** 11–15.

Bateman, A., & Krawitz, R. (2013). *Borderline personality disorder: An evidence-based guide for generalist mental health professionals.* Oxford, UK: Oxford University Press.

Bateman, A. W. (2012). Treating borderline personality disorder in clinical practice. *American Journal of Psychiatry,* **169,** 560–563.

Bateman, A. W. & Fonagy, P. (Eds.). (2012). *Handbook of mentalizing in mental health practice.* Washington, DC: American Psychiatric Publishing.

Bateman, A. W., Gunderson, J., & Mulder, R. (2015). Treatment of personality disorder. *Lancet,* **385,** 735–743.

Bevington, D., Fuggle, P., & Fonagy, P. (2015). Applying attachment theory to effective practice with hard-to-reach youth: The AMBIT approach. *Attachment and Human Development,* **17,** 157–174.

Fonagy, P. & Allison, E. (2014). The role of mentalizing and epistemic trust in the therapeutic relationship. *Psychotherapy,* **51,** 372–380.

Fonagy, P., Gergely, G., Jurist, E., & Target, M. (2002). *Affect regulation, mentalization, and the development of the self.* New York, NY: Other Press.

Fonagy, P., & Luyten, P. (2016). A multilevel perspective on the development of borderline personality disorder. In D. Cicchetti (Ed.), *Development and psychopathology* (3rd ed.). New York, NY: John Wiley & Sons.

Fonagy, P., Luyten, P., & Allison, E. (2015). Epistemic petrification and the restoration of epistemic trust: A new conceptualization of borderline personality disorder and its psychosocial treatment. *Journal of Personality Disorders, 29,* 575–609.

Fonagy, P., Rossouw, T., Sharp, C., Bateman, A., Allison, L., & Farrar, C. (2014). Mentalization-based treatment for adolescents with borderline traits. In C. Sharp & J. L. Tackett (Eds.), *Handbook of borderline personality disorder in children and adolescents* (pp. 313–332). New York, NY: Springer.

Gergely, G. (2013). Ostensive communication and cultural learning: The natural pedagogy hypothesis. In J. Metcalfe & H. S. Terrace (Eds.), *Agency and joint attention* (pp. 139–151). Oxford, UK: Oxford University Press.

Ha, C., Sharp, C., Ensink, K., Fonagy, P., & Cirino, P. (2013). The measurement of reflective function in adolescents with and without borderline traits. *Journal of Adolescence, 36,* 1215–1223.

Rossouw, T. I., & Fonagy, P. (2012). Mentalization-based treatment for self-harm in adolescents: A randomized controlled trial. *Journal of the American Academy of Child and Adolescent Psychiatry, 51,* 1304–1313.e3.

Sharp, C., Ha, C., Carbone, C., Kim, S., Perry, K., Williams, L., & Fonagy, P. (2013). Hypermentalizing in adolescent inpatients: Treatment effects and association with borderline traits. *Journal of Personality Disorders, 27,* 3–18.

Sharp, C., & Venta, A. (2012). Mentalizing problems in children and adolescents. In N. Midgley & I. Vrouva (Eds.), *Minding the child: Mentalization-based interventions with children, young people and their families* (pp. 35–53). London, UK: Routledge.

Index